A Histological Approach to Human Body Barriers

nova
Medicine & Health
New York

Cell Biology Research Progress

More information about this series can be found at
https://novapublishers.com/product-category/series/cell-biology-research-progress/

Pathology and Laboratory Medicine

More information about this series can be found at
https://novapublishers.com/product-category/series/pathology-and-laboratory-medicine/

İlknur Keskin
Editor

A Histological Approach to Human Body Barriers

nova
Medicine & Health
New York

DOI: https://doi.org/10.52305/EZIY1518

Library of Congress Cataloging-in-Publication Data

ISBN: 979-8-89530-738-0 (Hardcover)
ISBN: 979-8-89530-810-3 (eBook)

Published by Nova Science Publishers, Inc. † New York

Contents

Preface

A Histological Approach to Human Body Barriers aims to investigate the histological features of barriers in the human body with the most up-to-date information. In the book, cellular diversity of barriers, cell properties, protein expression profiles of cells, cellular changes in barriers in pathological conditions, current immunohistochemical markers and imaging methods for imaging barriers is discussed. In this book, in addition to revealing the histological characteristics of body barriers, the changes that molecular parameters in the barriers undergo in pathological conditions is emphasized. In addition, the relationships between different barriers is examined. Information is given on how digital histology can be used to visualize barriers and which types of microscopes are used. Important points regarding histopathological, immunohistochemical and molecular biomarkers that can be used in the diagnosis of damaged barriers will be explained. As a result, the histological features of barrier structures seen in almost all systems are collected in a single book, presenting the most up-to-date protocols to researchers who plan to work in the relevant field.

Chapter 1

The Barrier Systems

İlknur Keskin*, **MD, PhD**
Department of Histology and Embryology, The School of Medicine,
Istanbul Medipol University, İstanbul, Türkiye

Abstract

Blood-tissue barriers are vital physiological structures that regulate the transport of substances between the circulatory system and tissues and ensure the maintenance of a tissue-specific environment. These barriers allow the controlled transport of gases, water, nutrients, molecules and metabolites critical for cellular functions while preventing the entry of potentially harmful substances such as toxins, pathogens and various immune cells through their selective permeability. The selective permeability of these barriers is critical for maintaining tissue homeostasis and preventing systemic or local inflammatory responses.

The structure of blood-tissue barriers is highly specialised depending on the function and location of the organ. For example, the blood-brain barrier has a specialised structure to protect the central nervous system while the blood-air barrier in the lungs is specialised to protect the tissue against harmful particles and pathogens while allowing effective gas exchange. Despite the specific adaptations to these organs, the basic structure of these barriers consists mainly of tightly connected epithelial and endothelial cells. These cells form a selective barrier that regulates the bidirectional transport of substances and maintains the structural and functional integrity of the tissue.

An important aspect of the functionality of the blood-tissue barrier is the formation of tight junctions between cells, which prevent unwanted leakage and enable selective permeability. There are two important

* Corresponding Author's Email: ilknurkeskin@medipol.edu.tr

In: A Histological Approach to Human Body Barriers
Editor: İlknur Keskin
ISBN: 979-8-89530-738-0

groups of components that provide these intercellular connections. The first group consists of cell junctions such as tight junctions, adherens junctions, desmosomes, and hemidesmosomes. These junctions physically connect cells and regulate the passage of substances. These junctions are important in that the barrier can adjust its permeability according to physiological needs. The second group includes plasma membrane proteins such as connexin, E-cadherin, occludin, claudin, and junctional adhesion molecules (JAMs) (Figure 2). These proteins further strengthen cell junctions and regulate communication between neighbouring cells. These proteins not only contribute to the physical stability of the barrier but also play a critical role in the dynamic regulation of permeability and signalling in response to environmental stimuli.

These two groups of components form a complex and highly coordinated network that ensures the proper functioning of the blood-tissue barrier. This complex mechanism plays a vital role in maintaining tissue homeostasis, preventing the uncontrolled passage of substances, and protecting the tissue from damage caused by external factors. Furthermore, any disruption or interruption in the integrity of these barriers can result in increased permeability, tissue inflammation, and the development of diseases such as multiple sclerosis, acute lung injury, or infertility.

This chapter examines the common features of all blood-tissue barriers and discusses their structural components, functional mechanisms, and critical roles in protecting tissues in different organ systems. A comprehensive understanding of these barriers will allow us to better understand their importance in health and disease processes and to explore their potential as therapeutic targets in clinical medicine.

Keywords: barrier systems, blood-tissue barriers, cellular junctions, selective permeability

Introduction

Proper control of the composition of the internal environment is essential for the survival and maintenance of health of the organism. Parenchymal cells of many organs in the body face a wide variety of environments on their luminal side, while on their basal side they face a constant internal environment created by the bloodstream and interstitial spaces. The exchange of waste products and nutrients between the bloodstream and organs is regulated by highly selective organ-blood barriers that are specifically adapted to support homeostasis and organ function. Therefore, the structure of these barriers and the forces regulating transport across the barrier vary considerably.

Blood-tissue barriers are specialized structural and functional units that play a crucial role in protecting various tissues and organs in the body and regulating their functions. Blood-tissue barriers control the entry and exit of certain substances into the tissue by providing selective permeability through cells, intercellular connections and various molecules. Each barrier has its own unique structure and is specialized according to the needs of the tissue or organ to be protected (Figure 1).

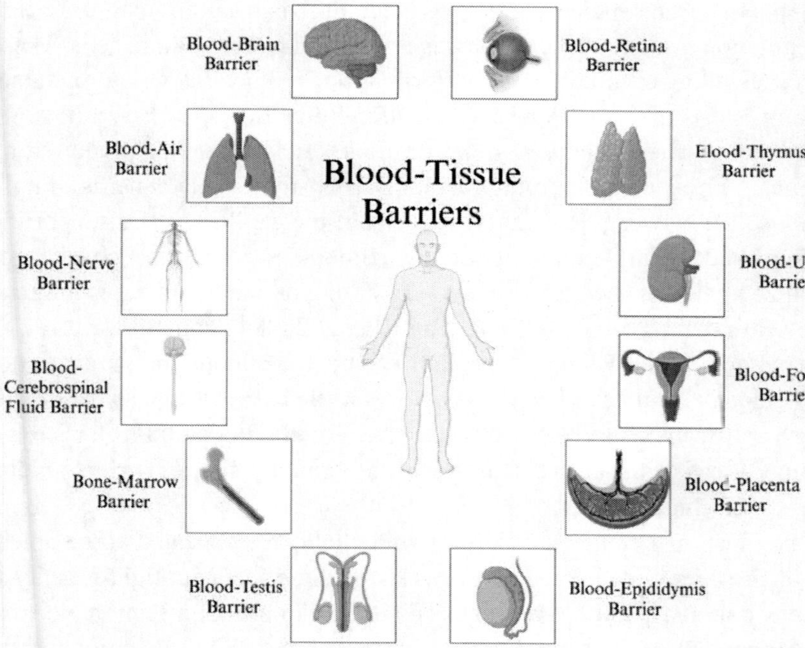

Figure 1. Blood-tissue barriers (Created with BioRender.com).

The existence of a blood-tissue barrier is a concept that was put forward in the early 20th century when it was observed that the brain and testicles were not completely stained with vital dyes. Paul Ehrlich, who first administered the vital dye trypan blue to animals intravenously in 1880, observed that all organs except the brain were stained and suggested that there was a selectively permeable structure between the blood and the brain. Edwin Goldmann, a student of Ehrlich, injected the same dye into the cerebrospinal fluid (CSF) in 1913 and observed that the brain was stained but the other organs were not

(Chin & Goh, 2018; Dobbing, 1961). Over the years, it has been shown that there are different blood-tissue barriers in different parts of the body. Common examples of blood barriers are; Blood Testis Barrier, Blood Epididymis Barrier, Blood Urine Barrier, Blood Follicle Barrier, Blood Placenta Barrier, Blood Nerve Barrier, Blood Brain Barrier, Blood Cerebrospinal Fluid Barrier, Blood Retina Barrier, Bone Marrow Barrier, Blood Air Barrier, Blood Thymus Barrier, Blood Tumor Barrier (Caceres et al., 2017; Watson et al., 2024) (Figure 1).

Each barrier consists of cells and junctional complexes specific to the tissue in which it is located. Barriers exhibit specialized functions according to the specific needs of the tissue they protect. Each barrier provides protection and regulation by controlling the passage of certain molecules and cells. These differences allow each barrier to perform specific functions and to maintain the homeostasis of the relevant tissue. Different epithelial cells significantly change their barrier structures to perform the specific functions required by the organ. For example, the Blood-Brain Barrier in the body consists of tight junctions (TJ) between the endothelial cells of the capillaries and supporting pericytes and basal lamina, while the Blood-Testis Barrier consists of specialized junctions between Sertoli cells sitting on the basement membrane in the seminiferous tubules (Siu & Yan Cheng, 2008; Thomas et al., 2022). Barriers such as the Blood-Testis Barrier and the Blood-Brain Barrier are highly selective and have low permeability, while barriers such as the blood-tumor barrier can be more permeable. Therefore, the Blood-Brain Barrier and the Blood-Testis Barrier are considered the strongest tissue barriers among barriers (Mescher, 2021).

The junctional complex of simple epithelial cells is located at the apical edge of the lateral membrane and consists of three sections: tight junctions, adherens junctions, and desmosomes (Figure 2). In ultrathin section electron micrographs, which are the initial electron microscopic descriptions, tight junctions are observed as a series of apparent fusions where the outer leaflets of the plasma membranes of adjacent cells merge (Farquhar & Palade, 1963; Tsukita et al., 2001). TJs, also known as zonulae occludentes, are crucial structures in epithelial and endothelial cells, forming a continuous, belt-like barrier at the interface between the basolateral and apical membrane domains. These junctions regulate the paracellular pathway, creating distinct compartments in multicellular organisms and facilitating controlled exchange between the internal and external environments through tissue-specific transport proteins and channels. The transmembrane proteins of TJs are connected to the cytoskeleton, linking cell-substratum and cell-cell adhesion sites (Förster, 2008). Apical tight junctions connect adjacent cells to create the blood-CSF barrier, blocking the unrestricted passage of molecules from the systemic circulation into the cerebrospinal fluid. The basolateral region forms interlocking folds, with the cell resting on a basal lamina (Kierszenbaum & Tres, 2020).

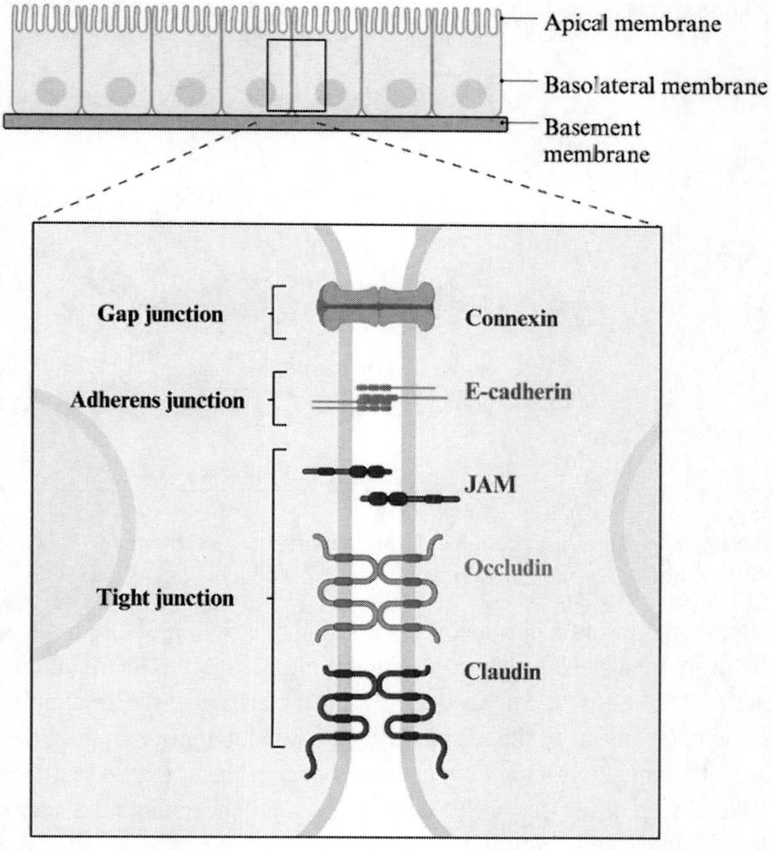

Figure 2. Schematic representation of the junctional complex at the lateral surface of two epithelial cells. (Created with BioRender.com).

Barriers emerge during the embryonic stage through a complex process, as seen in the blood brain barrier (BBB). The development of the BBB occurs in multiple stages, beginning with pre-existing vessels sprouting into the embryonic neuroectoderm to form new vessels. These initial vessels have already shown several BBB characteristics, such as the presence of tight junction (TJ) proteins and nutrient transporters. They also have high levels of leukocyte adhesion molecules and numerous transcytotic vesicles. As these new vessels mature through interactions with pericytes and astroglia, the barrier properties of the BBB are refined. This maturation process involves the development of tight junctions, a reduction in transcytosis, a decrease in leukocyte adhesion molecules, and an increase in efflux transporter levels. The final sealing of interendothelial tight junctions occurs during this maturation phase and must be preserved throughout life (Obermeier et al., 2013).

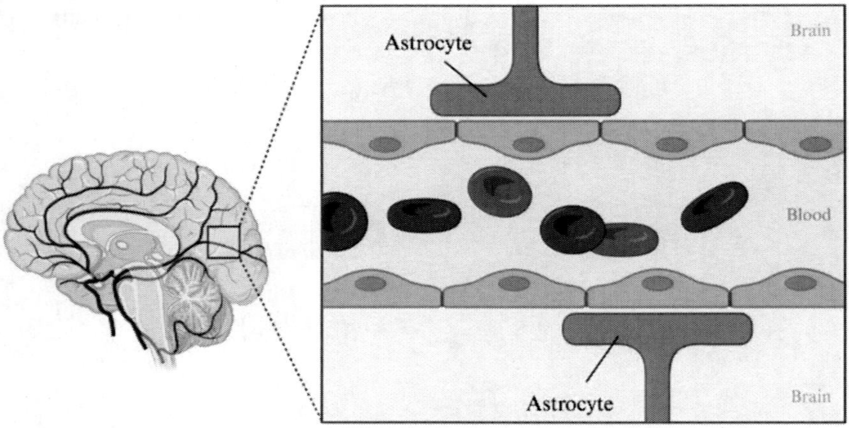

Figure 3. A schematic view of the blood-brain barrier. (Created with BioRender.com).

Three types of brain permeability barriers have been identified: the blood-CSF barrier, in which the choroid epithelium is involved in regulating the proteins and solutes that can access the ventricular space; the arachnoid-CSF barrier, which consists of the arachnoid membrane that prevents the CSF from coming into contact with the extracellular space of the arachnoid villi and the dura mater that allow the CSF to pass through the endothelial cells and arachnoid barrier cells; and the BBB, which seals the interendothelial space with tight junctions. Additionally, the end-feet of astrocytes in contact with the capillary wall contribute to BBB (Kierszenbaum & Tres, 2020).

The blood-retinal barrier (BRB) is crucial for preserving the integrity of the retina. Similar to the BBB, the BRB protects the retina from harmful chemicals and large molecules in the capillary blood by tightly regulating the transport of molecules into the tissue. It is composed of outer and inner components and serves an important role in the homeostatic regulation of the retinal microenvironment (Kaur et al., 2008; Nagymihály et al., 2021).

The retinal pigment epithelium (RPE) cells have extensions surrounding the processes of cones and rods in the eye. These adjacent RPE cells form the blood-retinal barrier, a junctional complex consisting of gap junctions and elaborate zonulae occludentes and adherentes. Molecules exceeding 20–30 kDa cannot penetrate the retinal vessels due to the BRB (Pawlina, 2024). The BRB is a restrictive and tight barrier that regulates protein, ion, and water dynamics within and outside the retina. The complex interaction of vascular endothelial cells and RPEs and their TJs are crucial for maintaining the unique environment of the eye, unlike other barrier systems. Especially in functional studies, it is essential to specify the role RPEs play in physiology and disease, maintenance of oxidative balance and phagocytosis (Nagymihály et al., 2021).

In the thymus, lymphocytes that reach the thymic cortex are protected from interacting with antigens by a physical barrier known as the blood-thymus barrier (BTB). This barrier is composed of cortical thymic epithelial cells (cTECs), basal laminae, and endothelial cells. Macrophages located near the capillaries prevent antigens from leaking out of the blood vessels into the thymus and interacting with developing thymocytes in the cortex, thereby reducing the risk of autoimmune reactions (Kierszenbaum & Tres, 2020; Pawlina, 2024).

The blood-air barrier consists of the cells and cellular components that gasses must pass through to diffuse between the alveoli and the capillaries. The thinnest blood-air barrier is composed of a thin layer of surfactant, a type I epithelial cell with its basal lamina, and a capillary endothelial cell along with its basal lamina. In acute interstitial pneumonia, the blood-air barrier is disrupted by injury to type I pneumocytes or the endothelial epithelium, resulting in the exudation of plasma proteins into the alveolar space (Pawlina, 2024).

The human placenta changes constantly throughout pregnancy to ensure the normal evolution and maturation of the fetus. The effective functioning of the placenta is maintained by a balance between differentiation, proliferation and cell death. The placental tissue barrier is formed by the capillary endothelium of the villi, the loose connective tissue surrounding the endothelium, the cytotrophoblast, and the syncytiotrophoblast (Gorbunov, 2021; Smith et al., 1997). This barrier is analogous to the blood-air barrier in the lungs, serving a similar role in facilitating the exchange of carbon dioxide and oxygen between fetal and maternal blood (Pawlina, 2024).

The BBB is important in neuronal function and protection by tightly controlling the movement of molecules, cells and ions between the blood and brain parenchyma. The complex properties that define the BBB may alter in disease states and BBB dysfunction is recognized as a key factor in various neurological disorders. Disruption of the BBB causes swelling, ion imbalance, and neuroinflammation, potentially resulting in neuronal impairment, neuronal degeneration, and elevated intracranial pressure (Profaci et al., 2020).

The BBB is basically categorized into four distinct barriers: the vascular BBB (BBB), whose main unit is the brain endothelial cell (BEC), located in vertebrate capillary beds and nearby venules and arterioles; the blood-cerebrospinal fluid (CSF) barrier, whose main unit is the ependymal cell, located in the choroid plexus; the tanycytic barrier, whose main unit is the tanycyte, it separates the circumventricular organs (small brain regions without a BBB) from the surrounding barrier-protected brain regions; and the meningeal barrier, whose main unit is the epithelial cell, located in primarily in the arachnoid mater. In addition, there are specialized extensions or regions of the BBB, including the otic barrier and the blood–retinal barrier. It is put forward that all of these barriers change with aging (Banks et al., 2021).

The perineurium acts as a diffusion barrier that is metabolically active, contributing to the formation of the blood-nerve barrier, which protects the ionic environment of the nerve fibers. Perineurial cells contain receptors, transporters, and enzymes that enable the active transport of substances, similar to the endothelial cells of the brain capillaries giving rise to blood brain barrier. Tight junctions between cells within the same layer of the perineurium provide the structural basis for the blood-nerve barrier (BNB) (Pawlina, 2024).

Disruption of the blood-tissue barrier can seriously affect the functions of the tissues and organs they protect. Disruption of the barriers can lead to various diseases, infections, inflammation and tissue damage (Figure 4). For example, diseases such as multiple sclerosis, Alzheimer's disease and Parkinson's disease are associated with disruption of the Blood-Brain Barrier. The decrease in the permeability of the blood-tumor barrier can make it difficult for chemotherapy drugs to reach the tumor tissue and reduce the effectiveness of the treatment, while at the same time facilitating the passage of cancer cells into the bloodstream and leading to metastasis. Disruption of the blood-testis barrier can affect the spermatogenesis process and lead to male infertility. Therefore, preserving the integrity of these barriers and preventing their disruption is of critical importance for health. Studying their anatomical structures and understanding their physiological functions are important for the protection of these barriers and the treatment of their disruption (Rönnbäck & Hansson, 2019).

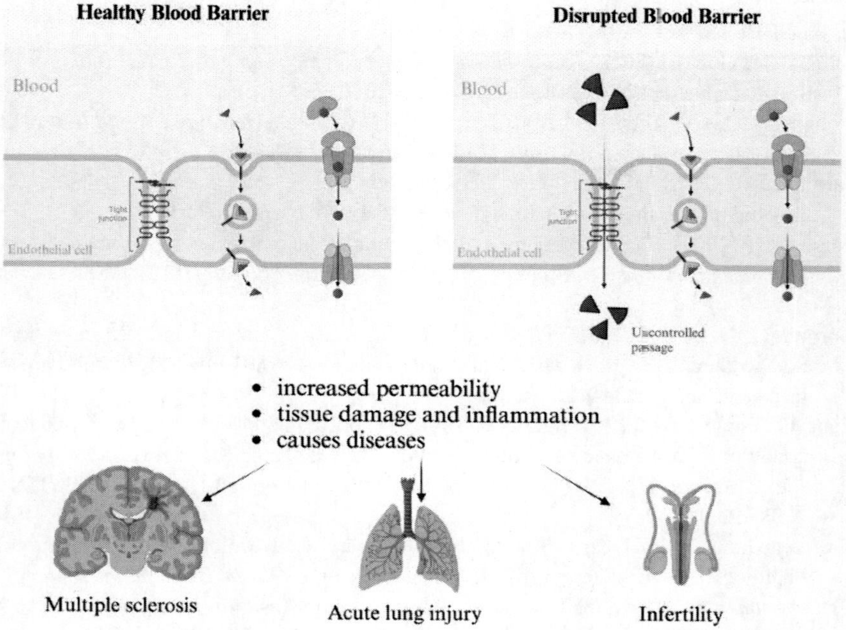

Figure 4. Disruption of the blood-tissue barriers can cause various tissue damage, inflammation and diseases.

Conclusion

This book will cover the types of blood-tissue barriers, their structures, the molecules they contain, their functions, and the potential consequences of their disruption. Understanding the factors that affect these barriers and implementing strategies to preserve their integrity is essential for understanding human health and disease.

References

Banks, W. A., Reed, M. J., Logsdon, A. F., Rhea, E. M., & Erickson, M. A. (2021). Healthy aging and the blood-brain barrier. *Nature Aging,* 1(3), 243–254. https://doi.org/10.1038/S43587-021-00043-5.

Caceres, P. S., Benedicto, I., Lehmann, G. L., & Rodriguez-Boulan, E. J. (2017). Directional Fluid Transport across Organ–Blood Barriers: Physiology and Cell

Biology. *Cold Spring Harbor Perspectives in Biology,* 9(3). https://doi.org/10.1101/CSHPERSPECT.A027847.

Chin, E., & Goh, E. (2018). Blood-brain barrier on a chip. *Methods in Cell Biology,* 146, 159–182. https://doi.org/10.1016/BS.MCB.2018.06.003.

Dobbing, J. (1961). The Blood-Brain Barrier. *Developmental Medicine & Child Neurology,* 3(4), 311–314. https://doi.org/10.1111/J.1469-8749.1961.TB15323.X.

Farquhar, M. G., & Palade, G. E. (1963). Junctional complexes in various epithelia. *The Journal of Cell Biology,* 17(2), 375–412. https://doi.org/10.1083/JCB.17.2.375.

Förster, C. (2008). Tight junctions and the modulation of barrier function in disease. *Histochemistry and Cell Biology,* 130(1), 55–70. https://doi.org/10.1007/S00418-008-0424-9.

Gorbunov, N. V. (2021). Tissue Barriers in Disease, Injury and Regeneration | ScienceDirect. https://www.sciencedirect.com/book/9780128185612/tissue-barriers-in-disease-injury-and-regeneration.

Kaur, C., Foulds, W. S., & Ling, E. A. (2008). Blood-retinal barrier in hypoxic ischaemic conditions: basic concepts, clinical features and management. *Progress in Retinal and Eye Research,* 27(6), 622–647. https://doi.org/10.1016/J.PRETEYERES.2008.09.003.

Kierszenbaum, A., & Tres, L. (2020). Hisyology and Cell Biology: An Introduction to Phatology. In Elsevier (Ed.), *Paper Knowledge. Toward a Media History of Documents.* https://www.nobelkitabevi.com.tr/histoloji-ve-embriyoloji/23618-histology-and-cell-biology-an-introduction-to-pathology-5th-edition.html.

Mescher, A. L. (2021). Junqueira's Basic Histology: Text and Atlas (16th ed.). McGraw-Hill. https://www.nobelkitabevi.com.tr/histoloji-ve-embriyoloji/7903-junqueira-s-basic-histology-text-and-atlas16th-edition-9781264269280.html.

Nagymihály, R., Nemesh, Y., Ardan, T., Motlik, J., Eidet, J. R., Moe, M. C., Bergersen, L. H., Lytvynchuk, L., & Petrovski, G. (2021). The retinal pigment epithelium: at the forefront of the blood-retinal barrier in physiology and disease. *Tissue Barriers in Disease, Injury and Regeneration,* 115–146. https://doi.org/10.1016/B978-0-12-818561-2.00003-5.

Obermeier, B., Daneman, R., & Ransohoff, R. M. (2013). Development, maintenance and disruption of the blood-brain barrier. *Nature Medicine,* 19(12), 1584–1596. https://doi.org/10.1038/NM.3407.

Pawlina, Wojciech. (2024). Histology: a text and atlas : with correlated cell and molecular biology. *Wolters Kluwer.* https://www.nobelkitabevi.com.tr/histoloji-ve-embriyoloji/24398-histology-a-text-and-atlas-with-correlated-cell-and-molecular-biology-9-edition.html.

Profaci, C. P., Munji, R. N., Pulido, R. S., & Daneman, R. (2020). The blood-brain barrier in health and disease: Important unanswered questions. *The Journal of Experimental Medicine,* 217(4). https://doi.org/10.1084/JEM.20190062.

Rönnbäck, C., & Hansson, E. (2019). The Importance and Control of Low-Grade Inflammation Due to Damage of Cellular Barrier Systems That May Lead to Systemic Inflammation. *Frontiers in Neurology,* 10(MAY), 533. https://doi.org/10.3389/FNEUR.2019.00533.

Siu, M. K. Y., & Yan Cheng, C. (2008). Extracellular Matrix and Its Role in Spermatogenesis. *Advances in Experimental Medicine and Biology*, 636, 74. https://doi.org/10.1007/978-0-387-09597-4_5.

Smith, S. C., Baker, P. N., & Symonds, E. M. (1997). Placental apoptosis in normal human pregnancy. *American Journal of Obstetrics and Gynecology,* 177(1), 57–65. https://doi.org/10.1016/S0002-9378(97)70438-1.

Thomas, S., Sadanandan, J., Blackburn, S. L., McBride, D. W., Dienel, A., Hong, S., Zeineddine, H. A., & Thankamani, P. K. (2022). Glyoxal Fixation Is Optimal for Immunostaining of Brain Vessels, Pericytes and Blood-Brain Barrier Proteins. *International Journal of Molecular Sciences,* 23(14). https://doi.org/10.3390/IJMS23147776/S1.

Tsukita, S., Furuse, M., & Itoh, M. (2001). Multifunctional strands in tight junctions. Nature Reviews. *Molecular Cell Biology,* 2(4), 285–293. https://doi.org/10.1038/35067088.

Watson, B. E., Miles, J. A., & Moss, M. A. (2024). Human in vitro blood barrier models: architectures and applications. *Tissue Barriers,* 12(2). https://doi.org/10.1080/21688370.2023.2222628.

Chapter 2

The Blood-Testis Barrier

Bircan Kolbaşı Erkan*, PhD
Department of Histology and Embryology, Istanbul Medipol University, Istanbul, Turkey

Abstract

The blood-testis barrier (BTB) is an important element of the male reproductive system and is responsible for creating the microenvironment necessary for spermatogenesis. BTB consists of specialized junctional complexes between adjacent Sertoli cells in the seminiferous tubule epithelium and separates the seminiferous tubule epithelium into adluminal and basal compartments. BTB acts as a barrier that regulates the exchange of substances between the blood vessels in the interstitial space and the seminiferous epithelium (adluminal compartment). This barrier protects the developing germ cells from potential toxins and immune system attacks during the process of spermatogenesis, ensuring proper sperm development. BTB is an active structure and allows preleptotene spermatocytes to pass into the adluminal compartment while performing its protective function. BTB integrity disruptions are associated with male infertility and various testicular pathologies. This section aims to provide information about the structure and function of BTB and its effects in both physiological and pathological conditions. It provides an overview for researchers and clinicians interested in male reproductive biology.

Keywords: blood-testis barrier, male reproductive system, Sertoli cell, testis

---

* Corresponding Author's Email: bkolbasi@medipol.edu.tr

In: A Histological Approach to Human Body Barriers
Editor: İlknur Keskin
ISBN: 979-8-89530-738-0

Introduction

The male reproductive system consists of a pair of testes, intra- and extra-testicular ducts, accessory glands and the penis. Testes are oval-shaped organs located outside the body in the scrotum, a sac like structure covered with skin (Durairajanayagam et al., 2015). The reason they are located outside the body is that the testes are responsible for sperm production through the spermatogenesis process. The temperature of the testes is maintained at 34.4°C, slightly below body temperature, because temperatures above 36.7°C inhibit spermatogenesis. Intra- and extra-testicular ducts are responsible for transmitting the sperm produced in the testes to the penis, allowing them to be expelled from the body by ejaculation. In addition, sperm produced in the testes do not have the ability to fertilize the oocyte, and they undergo some changes within the male ducts before entering the female reproductive tract. Accessory glands contribute to the formation of semen.

Testes, which are organs of the male reproductive system, have two basic functions: exocrine and endocrine. Exocrine function is the production of sperm cells from spermatogonia at the end of the spermatogenesis process. The endocrine function is that Leydig cells in the interstitial area produce the testosterone hormone (Ge et al., 2021).

Spermatogenesis occurs in the seminiferous tubules located in the testes. The epithelium lining the seminiferous tubules has a unique organization to enable the production of sperm cells. This section aims to explain the cells lining the seminiferous tubule epithelium, the structure of the blood-testis (BTB) barrier formed by Sertoli cells, the function of the BTB, and its clinical significance.

Testis

The testes are a pair of organs in the male reproductive system where spermatogenesis and steroidogenesis (testosterone production) occur. The testes are surrounded by a thick tunica albuginea made up of dense connective tissue. Fibrous extensions from this capsule structure divide the testis into approximately 250 lobules. Each lobule contains 1-4 seminiferous tubules. The seminiferous tubule structures are surrounded by a connective tissue called interstitial tissue. The interstitial tissue contains Leydig cells (interstitial cells) responsible for testosterone production, as well as blood and lymph vessels, and nerve endings. Leydig cells are large, polygonal, eosinophilic cells that contain abundant lipid droplets. Testosterone secretion is under the control of luteinizing Hormone (LH) released from the anterior lobe of the pituitary gland. Leydig cells differentiate in the early fetal period and are important in the development of male reproductive organs in the embryonic period. During puberty, they are responsible for the start of sperm production, the secretion of accessory sex glands, and the development of secondary sex characteristics (Pawlina et al., 2016). In adults, testosterone secretion is necessary for the continuity of spermatogenesis and the maintenance of secondary sex characteristics. The number of seminiferous tubules in each testis is approximately 250-1000 and each 150-250 µm in diameter. The seminiferous tubules are convoluted structures, and their straight, narrow ends are called tubuli recti. The tubuli recti connect the seminiferous tubules to the labyrinth called the rete testis. Through these structures, the sperm produced in the testes is transferred to the canal system for ejaculation (Marieb & Hoehn, 2007) (Figure 1).

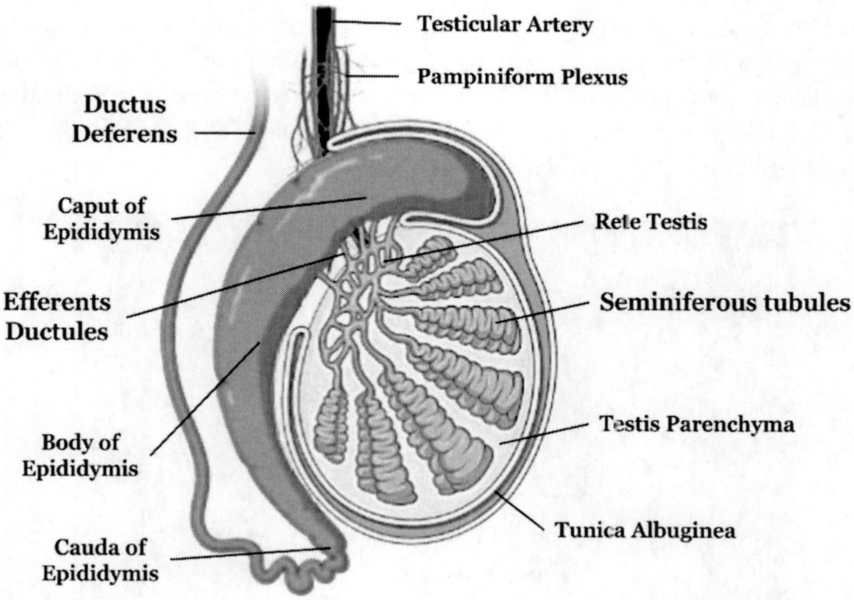

Figure 1. Structure and organization of the testis (Horvath-Pereira et al., 2023).

Seminiferous Epithelium

There are two types of cells in the seminiferous epithelium lining the seminiferous tubule wall: somatic Sertoli cells (support cells), and spermatogenic series cells (Wong & Khan, 2020) (Figure 2). Sertoli cells sit on the basement membrane of the seminiferous tubules, with their apical surface extending into the tubule lumen (Mruk & Cheng, 2004). They have an extensive surface area because they support the developing sperm cells (Wong & Russell, 1983). Because of their cytoplasmic projections and complex three-dimensional structure, cell boundaries cannot be distinguished at the light microscopic level (Mruk & Cheng, 2004). They are distinguished by their darkly stained euchromatic nuclei and prominent nucleoli in routine histological staining (Hess & França, 2005) (Figure 3). Sertoli cells have many important functions, one of the most important of which is to form the BTB. The functions of Sertoli cells include supporting, nourishing, creating a suitable microenvironment for developing spermatozoa (via the BTB), phagocytosis of residual bodies formed during spermiogenesis, production of androgen-binding protein, which helps concentrate testosterone in the seminiferous tubules, ensuring its availability for spermatogenesis, production of anti- Müllerian hormone, inhibin and aromatase binding protein and formation of the BTB (França et al., 2016).

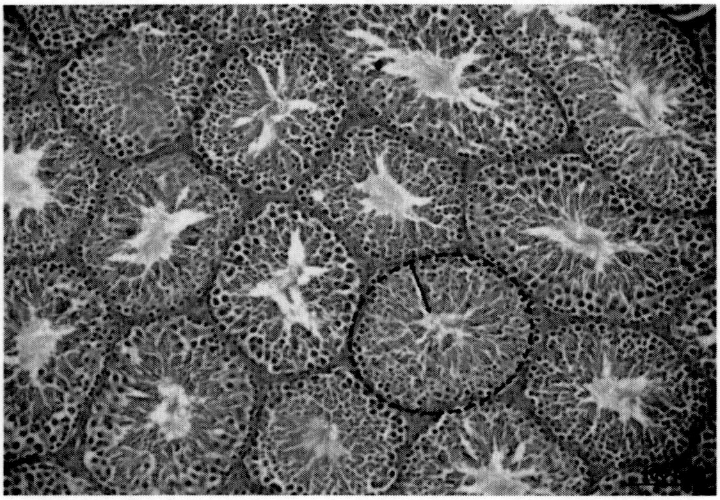

Figure 2. Cross section of testis stained with hematoxylin-eosin. Dashed circle: Seminiferous tubule, Double sided arrow: Seminiferous epithelium. Captured with: 20x.

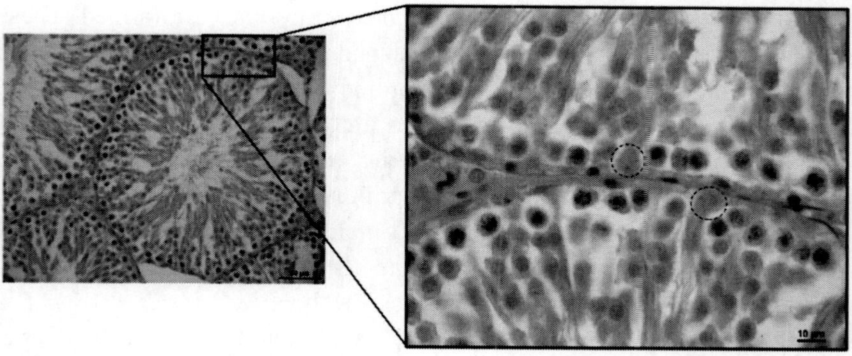

Figure 3. Cross-section of seminiferous epithelium stained with hematoxylin-eosin. The image on the right is an enlargement of the area marked with a rectangle in the image on the left. Dashed circle: Sertoli cell nucleus. Left: 40x. Right:100x.

Spermatogenesis

Spermatogenesis is a complex and well-organized process that takes place in the seminiferous tubules of the testes. In humans, spermatogenesis takes about 72-74 days, while in mice it takes about 35 days (Hogarth & Griswold, 2010). It is divided into three important stages; 1) self-renewal of spermatogonial stem cells, 2) reduction of diploid chromosome number to haploid by meiosis (spermatogenesis) and 3) spermiogenesis (differentiation of round spermatids into sperm). In mice, undifferentiated stem cells are called type A, and in humans, type A_{dark} spermatogonia. Spermatogonia that enter the differentiation phase are called A_{pale} in humans and A_1 in mice. In mice, differentiated spermatogonia undergo 5 mitotic divisions before differentiating into preleptotene spermatocytes. Following these divisions, spermatocytes enter meiosis. From this stage on, divisions and the spermiogenesis phase continue in the same way in both mice and humans (Hogarth & Griswold, 2010). Prophase of the first meiotic division lasts about 10 days. The prophase stage consists of leptotene (chromosomes consisting of two sister chromatids), zygotene (pairing of chromosomes), pachytene (thickening of chromosomes), diplotene (separation of paired chromosomes), and diakinesis (chromosomes moving away from each other) stages (Bergmann, 2006). During this division, cells migrate along the BTB structure as they pass from the preleptotene stage to the leptotene stage. During this transition, the proteins that form the barrier are disassembled and reassembled at the base of the newly formed cell (Mruk & Cheng, 2015). As a result of meiosis I, secondary spermatocytes with n chromosomes are formed. These secondary spermatocytes then enter the second meiosis II and produce round spermatids, each containing n haploid chromosomes (Schlegel & Katzovitz, 2020). During spermatogonial divisions, the incomplete completion of cytokinesis results in spermatogenic series remaining connected through cytoplasmic bridges of approximately 1 μm diameter, forming a syncytium. This syncytium structure allows ions and molecules to pass easily between cells, enabling synchronous maturation. In other words, there is a synchronized cell cycle in spermatogenesis (Kubota & Brinster, 2018). The head regions of mature sperm cells, formed as a result of the spermatogenesis, interact with the Sertoli cell membrane and are oriented toward the seminiferous tubule basement membrane, while their tails extend into the seminiferous tubule lumen.

Blood-Testis Barrier Structure

BTB forms in the human testicle between the ages of 12 and 14 (Cheng & Mruk, 2010). In murines, this process begins approximately on days 15-16 *postpartum*, and its complete formation at around day 18 to 21 (Bergmann & Dierichs, 1983; Russell et al., 1989; Toyama et al., 2001). The BTB is an essential structure for functional adult sperm production and the creation of an isolated microenvironment, which represents its most critical role. This is because soluble molecules and pathogens from the blood vessels in the interstitial area can pass through the basement membrane and damage the developing sperm cells. In order to prevent this, the junctional complexes between the Sertoli cells form the BTB, creating the tightest barrier structure in the body (Cheng & Mruk, 2012). Another important function of the BTB is to prevent the formation of anti-sperm antibodies (ASA) by inhibiting the interaction between membrane proteins of developing germ cells and the body's immune cells (AS et al., 2019). ASAs may interfere with early embryonic development and cause infertility by inducing agglutination, reducing sperm motility, preventing sperm passage through cervical mucus, and inhibiting fertilization (Chen et al., 2023; Kremer & Jager, 1992; Rümke et al., 1984; Taneichi et al., 2002; Verón et al., 2016; Yoshitake et al., 2016). ASAs may also activate the immune system, leading to the lysis and destruction of sperm cells (Chiu & Chamley, 2004; D'Cruz et al., 1991). During spermatogenesis, the creation of an isolated microenvironment by the

BTB is of crucial to prevent the developing sperm cells from being recognized by the immune system.

The BTB consist of four types of junctions: tight junctions, ectoplasmic specializations, desmosomes, and gap junctions (Cheng et al., 2011) (Figure 4).

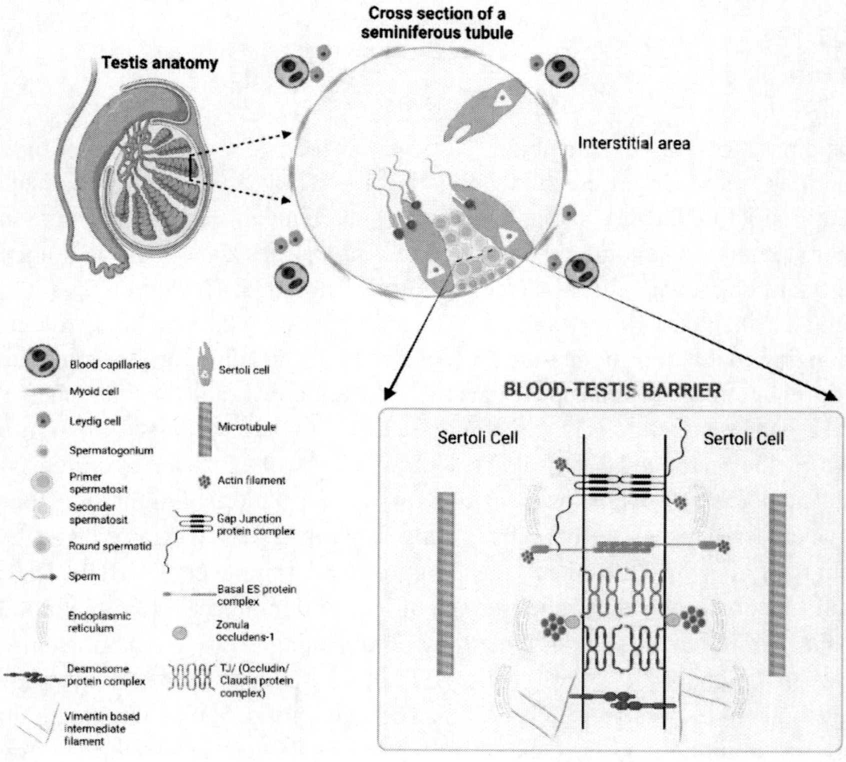

Figure 4. The organization of BTB. This figure shows the general male reproductive system anatomy and BTB organization in detailed. (TJ: Tight junctions; Es: Ectoplasmic specializations) Created with BioRender.com.

Tight Junctions

Ultrastructurally, tight junctions are areas of contact between neighboring Sertoli cells. They function both as a barrier and as a means of establishing polarity in the Sertoli cell membrane by dividing it into two regions, the apical (adluminal) and the basolateral. They perform their barrier function by providing controlled passage of water, ions, and solutes (Balda & Matter, 2008) (Furuse, 2010; Tsukita et al., 1999). BTB tight junction proteins include occludin, claudin, and junctional adhesion molecules (Mruk & Cheng, 2010). Occludin is a 65 kDa integral membrane protein (Furuse et al., 1993). Occludin is expressed in mouse and rat testes, but not in Guinea pig and human testes (Moroi et al., 1998).

Claudins

Claudins are integral membrane proteins responsible for forming tight junctions and charge-selective pores in the BTB. Studies to date have identified 23 different claudins in humans and chimpanzees, and 23 more in other mammals. Claudins are expressed in many tissues and organs, including the brain, epithelial cells, and testes (Florin et al., 2005; Hellani et al., 2000; Meng et al., 2005; Van Itallie & Anderson, 2006). Claudins are proteins belonging to the transmembrane protein family, responsible for the formation of tight junctions between epithelial and endothelial cells and the maintenance of the barrier structure (Günzel & Yu, 2013). They are expressed by Sertoli cells in the testis and are proteins with a weight of 22 kDa, containing 4 transmembrane domains, responsible for the formation of tight junctions between neighboring Sertoli cells (Cheng & Mruk, 2002). Claudins originate from the Latin word 'claudere', meaning 'to stand' (Gupta et al., 2019). Their main function is to control the passage of ions and molecules from the blood to the seminiferous tubule lumen by establishing tight junction strands between neighboring Sertoli cells (Lui et al., 2003). In this way, they contribute to the establishment of an immune-privileged environment to prevent immune system elements from attacking cells formed by spermatogenesis (Kaur et al., 2018). Claudins, one of the important proteins of the tight junction complexes in the BTB structure, interact with cytoskeletal components (Morrow et al., 2010). Expressed by Sertoli cells, Claudin-11 first begins to be expressed in the testes from the 3rd postnatal day and reaches a constant level between the 6th and 16th days of development (Hellani et al., 2000). Parallel to the expression of Claudin-11 seen in mouse and rat testes, the expression of Claudin-11 has also been observed in human testicular BTB structure. It has been reported that Claudin-11 knockout mice are infertile (Morita et al., 1999). In the absence of claudin-11, the integrity of tight junctions between Sertoli cells is lost, leading to loss of the epithelial phenotype (Hellani et al., 2000). In another study, it was observed that Sertoli cell polarity and tight junction function were impaired and the distance between Sertoli cells increased in Claudin-11-null mice. And also, this study showed that germ cell apoptosis increased in Claudin-11-/- testes (Mazaud-Guittot et al., 2010). When the levels of Claudin-11 were examined in biopsy samples of patients with intraepithelial neoplasia areas in the testicular tissue, it was seen that there was an increase in mRNA and protein levels and when examined with the immunogold staining method, it was seen that the expression of Claudin-11 was concentrated in the cytoplasm of Sertoli cells. The reason for the deterioration in the BTB structure was attributed to the change in the level of Claudin-11 and the change in the protein location (Fink et al., 2009). In another study, the expression level of Claudin-11 was compared in healthy male patients who had children and in patients with prostate cancer, orchiectomy and obstructive azoospermia. It was observed that there was an increase in the level of Claudin-11 in the patient group and that there was only arrest in the Sertoli cells and spermatogenic series in many seminiferous tubules (Nah et al., 2011). In a study using the varicocele model, an increase in the level of Claudin-11 mRNA and protein was observed in the testicle with varicocele (Oh et al., 2016). In a study investigating the effects of bilateral varicocele on the BTB in rats, it was reported that Claudin-11 was significantly downregulated in the varicocele group compared to the control group, the integrity of the BTB was impaired, and the degree of destruction increased over time (Pan et al., 2018). A study in cryptorchid rats reported that dysregulation of Claudin-11 may limit BTB function, leading to spermatogenic impairment (Kato et al., 2020). Considering the above-mentioned information and the studies provided, it is shown that Claudin-11, one of the BTB tight junction proteins, is an indispensable element for maintaining the integrity of the BTB.

Zonula Ocludens-1 and Zonula Ocludens-2

Zonula occludens-1 (ZO-1, TJP1) (220 kDa) and Zonula occludens-2 (ZO-2) (160 kDa) are adaptor proteins that link integral membrane proteins such as Occludin and Claudin to the cytoskeletal element actin (Segretain et al., 2004). ZO-1 and ZO-2 are associated with the cytoplasmic faces of tight junction proteins (Mruk & Cheng, 2015). It colocalizes with connexin-43 and regulates communication between gap junctions (Umeda et al., 2006). They also regulate claudin polymerization, which is necessary for the establishment of tight junctions. Cell adhesion in BTB is mediated by the presence of various integral membrane proteins, such as tight junction protein complexes (Ocludin-ZO-1, Claudin-ZO-1, JAM-ZO-1) and their adaptors (Cheng & Mruk, 2012). In the absence of Claudin polymerization resulting from complete/partial loss of ZO-1 and ZO-2, epithelial cells become polarized but tight junction complexes cannot be formed (Umeda et al., 2006). In the testis, ZO-1 is localized to the BTB and the apical ectoplasmic specializations surrounding elongated spermatids. Disruption of the BTB has been reported to be associated with a decrease in ZO-1 in diabetic mice (Zhou et al., 2020). In a study conducted to investigate BTB permeability in rats with autoimmune orchitis, germ cell shedding and decreased occludin expression in the testes, as well as delocalization of Claudin-11 and ZO-1 were detected. It was shown that BTB permeability was increased in these rats (Pérez et al., 2012). The ZO-1 protein plays a crucial role in the integrity of the BTB by binding the Occludin and Claudin-11 proteins to actin filaments within Sertoli cells, making ZO-1 extremely important for spermatogenesis.

Ectoplasmic Specializations

Ectoplasmic specializations are testis-specific adhesion junctions composed of hexagonally arranged filamentous actin microfilaments between the cisternae of the endoplasmic reticulum and the plasma membrane. Sertoli-Sertoli specializations are called basal ectoplasmic specializations, and those between Sertoli-elongating spermatids are called apical ectoplasmic specializations (Mruk & Cheng, 2011b). They consist of cadherin-catenin complexes. They are usually found in association with ZO-1 proteins. They take part in the process of breaking down and rebuilding the barrier during the passage of preleptotene spermatocytes to the adluminal compartment during spermatogenesis (Yan & Cheng, 2005; Yan et al., 2008). E-Cadherin expression has been shown to increase before the development of adhesion junctions, desmosomes, and gap junctions, thus suggesting that E-Cadherin expression is important for the development of BTB (Ha et al., 2011). α, β and ɣ catenins are proteins that are important in maintaining cell-cell adhesion by connecting E-Cadherin to the actin cytoskeleton. Hirano et al. showed that cells lacking α-catenin were unable to form stable adherens junctions despite normal E-Cadherin and β-catenin expression; however, when α-catenin expression was restored by cDNA transfection, adherens junctions became stable (Hirano et al., 1992).

Desmosomes

Desmosomes are the type of junction that connects cell-cell intermediate filaments like Vimentin in Sertoli cells. Desmosomes are cell-cell junctions that provide strong adhesion between neighboring Sertoli cells in the BTB structure (Mruk & Cheng, 2004, 2011a; Vogl et al., 2008). They include the integral membrane proteins desmoglein-2 (122.2 kDa) and desmocollin-2 (110 kDa). Recent studies have shown that desmosomes in the BTB structure not only connect cell-cell intermediate filaments but also regulate the functions of other junction proteins such as N-cadherin and occludin in regions where tight junctions and basal ectoplasmic specializations are seen (Lie et al., 2011; Mruk & Cheng, 2011a).

Gap Junctions

The GJ is a cell-cell actin-based communication junction composed of two opposing connexons between neighboring Sertoli cells in the BTB and responsible for cell communication with each other (Vinken et al., 2011).These channels allow the diffusion of solutes with a molecular mass of less than 1–1.5 kDa. However, large molecules, including siRNA duplexes, cyclic nucleotides, and polypeptides, can pass through these channels with selective and specific permeability (Harris, 2007; Maeda & Tsukihara, 2011). The most important gap junction protein is connexin 43 (Cx43) (39 kDa), which forms the connexin structure (Qi et al., 2023). Connexin-43 and connexin-46 are the most studied types of gap junctions in testis (Mruk & Cheng, 2011b; Mruk et al., 2011). A study in rats suggested that Cx43 is structurally associated with the desmosome proteins plakophilin-2, the basal ectoplasmic specializations N-cadherin and β-catenin, but has no structural relationship with tight junction proteins. According to the results of the study, knockdown of Cx43 did not affect the function of tight junctions, basal ectoplasmic specializations or desmosome-like junctions. However, the knockdown of both Cx43 and plakophilin-2 simultaneously resulted in transient disruption of tight junctions in Sertoli cells. They stated that this disruption was due to the mislocalization of occludin and ZO-1. In summary, Cx43 and plakophilin-2 form a protein complex to regulate cell adhesion in the BTB, in part through their effects on the occludin/ZO-1 complex. This facilitates the passage of preleptotene spermatocytes (Li et al., 2009). Loss of Cx43 during embryonic development results in a decrease in germ cell numbers, whereas loss of Cx43 expression in Sertoli cells in adults can result in complete inhibition of spermatogenesis (Kidder & Cyr, 2016; Rode et al., 2018).

Implications in Physiological and Pathological Conditions

As mentioned in the above sections, BTB is an indispensable element for the spermatogenesis process and mature sperm production. In this section, we will focus on the parameters that some conditions/agents that cause damage to the testicle and especially the BTB structure are effective on. Damage that may occur in BTB affects testicular histopathology and sperm parameters (concentration, motility, progressive motility, chromosome integrity, etc.). Examples of the most common conditions affecting the male reproductive system include varicocele, torsion/detorsion, increased oxidative stress in the testis as a result of some environmental toxicants, metabolic diseases like high-fat diet (obesity) and chronic stress (Carrageta et al., 2024; Huang et al., 2024; Kaltsas, 2023; Kang et al., 2022; Minas et al., 2023). Although studies investigating the effects of these damages are currently carried out on experimental animals, it is also thought that the effects of some promising therapeutics can be tested on humans through phase studies. Varicocele is defined as dilatation of the internal spermatic vein that drains the testicle (Soares et al., 2013). Varicocele, which is detected in less than 1% of children, is seen in ~14% of adolescent males and 20% of adults (Jensen et al., 2017). 89.4% of varicoceles are seen in the left testicle (Gat et al., 2004). Increased venous pressure due to the expansion of testicular veins in the scrotum disrupts the venous valves and causes venous reflux. As a result, varicocele develops. While the right internal spermatic vein ends at a more horizontal angle with the low-pressure inferior vena cava, the left internal spermatic vein opens at a right angle to the higher-pressure left renal vein. The reason why clinical varicoceles are seen more frequently on the left side is explained by this anatomical difference (Leslie et al., 2017). Increased hydrostatic pressure, increased scrotal temperature, hypoxia and accumulated toxic metabolites resulting from varicocele cause increased oxidative stress, leading to deterioration in testicular structure and function (Fretz & Sandlow, 2002; Jensen et al., 2017; Marmar, 2001; Turner, 2001). In studies investigating the effects of varicocele on the testis, a decrease in seminiferous tubule diameter, thinning of the seminiferous epithelium, increase in Fas/FasL, Caspase-3 levels (Zhang et al., 2018) and decrease in androgen receptor (AR) expression levels (down-regulation) were observed (Soares et al., 2013). In a study evaluating the effects of varicocele on inflammatory cytokines, apoptosis and BTB tight junction proteins, an increase in TNFα, IL-1α and IL-6 levels was observed. In addition, an increase in the mRNA levels of proapoptotic genes Bad and Bax and a decrease in the mRNA levels of prosurvival apoptotic genes Bcl-2 and Bcl-xl were detected. While an increase in the amount and mRNA expression of BTB proteins, Claudin-11, was observed, they reported that the production of this protein may have increased in order to rearrange BTB that was damaged by the destructive effects of cytokines. This is because, while Klaudin-11 expression was organized in the periphery of the seminiferous tubule epithelium in the control group, Claudin-11 expression was seen in the cytoplasm of Sertoli cells in the varicocele group. Similarly, an increase in the levels of Zonula Occludens-1 (ZO-1), Occludin and N-cadherin has also been reported (Oh et al., 2016). In another study conducted by Koo Ha et al., E-cadherin and α-catenin expressions were evaluated. It was observed that the expression levels of these proteins decreased as a result of the increase in the level of reactive oxygen species (ROS). The results obtained show that varicocele increases the level of ROS and that BTB damage occurs due to the changing intracellular ion concentration. It was determined that the impaired BTB and/or increased ROS levels negatively affect sperm and that these changes may play a role in the infertility problem in varicocele patients. However, the effect of ROS on transmembrane proteins and especially on the cadherin/catenin complex has not been fully elucidated (Ha et al., 2011).

Testicular torsion is a medical term that describes a significant urological condition in which the testicle rotates around its longitudinal axis and the spermatic cord twists, resulting in a significant reduction in blood flow to the testicle and perfusion of testicular tissue (Laher et al., 2020). If immediate intervention is not sought, irreversible ischemic damage to the testicle occurs. The incidence is estimated to be 1 in 4000 in individuals under the age of 25 (Ekşi et al., 2020). During testicular torsion, testicular tissue is affected by ischemia, heat stress, hypoxia, oxidative and nitrosative stress (Minas et al., 2023). There are studies reporting disruption and damage to the BTB as a result of testicular torsion (Hadžiselimović et al., 1986; Reda et al., 2017; Visser & Heyns, 2003). In one study, it was reported that testicular torsion resulted in the deterioration of the BTB structure and the formation of ASA in the semen. It was reported that ASA levels increased significantly after torsion, and this ASA targeted the developing sperm cells, causing infertility and remained high for at least 26 weeks (Fu et al., 2006).

Obesity is a pathological condition that causes hormonal changes that can affect the reproductive system. Obesity is a pathological condition that causes hormonal changes that can affect the reproductive system (Hammoud et al., 2008). Some studies have shown that the accumulation of fat tissue in men causes a decrease in total and free testosterone levels in the serum and an increase in estradiol levels (SCHNEIDER et al., 1979). Some studies in humans have indicated that this change in hormone levels can cause a decrease in sperm count (Jensen et al., 2004; Magnusdottir et al., 2005). Other animal studies have shown that animals fed a high-fat diet exhibited morphological deterioration in sperm, decreased sperm motility, progressive motility, acrosome reaction and significantly decreased testosterone levels (Erdemir et al., 2012; Fan et al., 2015). In addition to the findings mentioned in the previous sentence, Fan et al.'s study revealed atrophic seminiferous tubules in the histopathological analysis of the testis. Ultrastructural analyses showed that the connections between Sertoli cells and spermatogenic series cells were loosely arranged. They showed that the BTB tight junction proteins occludin and ZO-1 expression level, were quantitatively decreased (Fan et al., 2015). In a study investigating the effect of exercise on a high-fat diet, it was shown that high-fat diet increased body weight, apoptotic cell count and DNA fragmentation, while decreasing FSH, LH, testosterone levels, and immunoreactivity of BTB proteins ZO-1, occludin and Cx43. It was suggested that exercise reduced testicular cytotoxicity by regulating hormone and oxidant/antioxidant levels, improved impaired testicular function, reduced apoptotic cell count and preserved barrier integrity (Elmas et al., 2022).

Stress is defined as the body's response to various stressors coming from the environment. Stress is divided into two categories: acute and chronic stress. Although some studies have shown that the effects of acute stress can be eliminated, long-term exposure to stressors (chronic) causes irreversible damage. In studies showing the effects of the chronic stress model on the male reproductive system, there are studies showing that stress causes a decrease in sperm count and affects reproductive functions (Gollenberg et al., 2010; Lampiao, 2009). Hou et al.'s morphological examinations have shown that chronic stress causes deterioration in seminiferous tubule dimensions, vacuolization, and difficulty in distinguishing spermatogenic series cells from each other (Hou et al., 2014). Another study has shown that stress causes a decrease in superoxide dismutase (SOD), catalase, glutathione, testosterone, serotonin, steroidogenic acute-regulatory (StAR) gene protein expression levels and sperm motility, and an increase in malondialdehyde (MDA) and corticosterone levels. In the same study, it has been shown that resveratrol increases antioxidant levels, serotonin, StAR gene expression levels, sperm motility and number, and decreases MDA and corticosterone levels (Sakr et al., 2015). In another study investigating the effects of chronic stress on the male reproductive system, it was shown that chronic stress significantly decreased the levels of ZO-1 and Claudin-11 quantitatively, which are BTB tight junction proteins (Kolbasi et al., 2021). Antisperm antibodies (ASA) play a role as immunological infertility factors (AS et al., 2019). The basic finding of the presence of antisperm antibodies in semen is the observation of agglutination of sperm cells (Gupta et al., 2022). In this study, it was also shown that in the group subjected to chronic stress, intense agglutination was observed during the microscopic examination of sperm obtained from the epididymis for concentration analysis, and due to the destruction of BTB, immune cells passed into the seminiferous tubule lumen and from there into the male conduction channels, and antisperm antibodies were formed (Kolbasi et al., 2021).

Conclusion

The BTB structure is an indispensable element of the male reproductive system. One of its most important roles is to create an immune-privileged, isolated microenvironment for spermatogenesis to occur within the seminiferous tubules. The tight junctions in the BTB structure, on the one hand, prevent harmful substances and immune cells from reaching the developing germ cells, while on the other hand, they are responsible for regulating the selective passage of ions, water, nutrients, solutes and regulatory molecules into the adluminal compartment of the seminiferous tubules. One of the most important features of the BTB structure is that it is an active structure that adapts to the spermatogenic cycle. While preleptotene spermatocytes migrate from the basal compartment to the adluminal compartment, the BTB structure is temporarily destroyed and immediately closed after the transition to the adluminal part. This destruction/construction is also regulated by many signaling pathways and structural proteins. This active process is an important event required for spermatogenesis to continue and sperm cells to mature. In some studies, the effects of metabolic diseases such as varicocele, torsion/detorsion, environmental toxicants, obesity, and environmental factors such as stress on BTB permeability have been investigated. In addition, these studies have shown that the disrupted BTB structure affects sperm parameters and can lead to infertility. Therefore, more detailed studies are needed on how these factors affect BTB integrity. Developments in molecular biology and microscopy allow the investigation of the complex protein network that forms the BTB structure and the signaling pathways that play a role in maintaining BTB integrity. Claudin, occludin, and zonula occludens play key roles in maintaining barrier integrity and the active construction/destruction of the barrier. Future studies should focus on investigating the mechanisms regulating BTB dynamics and male fertility. Targeted treatments can be developed to restore BTB integrity by elucidating these pathways. The dramatic decrease in the number of sperm considered normal with each passing year necessitates more detailed investigation of the conditions affecting male fertility. In conclusion, the BTB structure is a unique structure that creates an isolated and regulated environment required for sperm production. Elucidation of the BTB structure and its regulatory pathways will greatly contribute to the understanding of the biology of the male reproductive system and the development of treatments for infertility and other related diseases.

References

AS, V., Dhama, K., Chakraborty, S., Abdul Samad, H., K. Latheef, S., Sharun, K.,…Bhatt, P. (2019). Role of antisperm antibodies in infertility, pregnancy, and potential for contraceptive and antifertility vaccine designs: Research progress and pioneering vision. *Vaccines*, *7*(3), 116.

Balda, M. S., & Matter, K. (2008). Tight junctions at a glance. *Journal of cell science*, *121*(22), 3677-3682.

Bergmann, M. (2006). Physiology of spermatogenesis. In *Andrology for the Clinician* (pp. 272-281). Springer.

Bergmann, M., & Dierichs, R. (1983). Postnatal formation of the blood-testis barrier in the rat with special reference to the initiation of meiosis. *Anatomy and embryology*, *168*, 269-275.

Carrageta, D. F., Pereira, S. C., Ferreira, R., Monteiro, M. P., Oliveira, P. F., & Alves, M. G. (2024). Signatures of metabolic diseases on spermatogenesis and testicular metabolism. *Nature Reviews Urology*, 1-18.

Chen, Y., Hasegawa, A., Honda, H., Wakimoto, Y., & Shibahara, H. (2023). Characterization of a spontaneously occurring self-reactive antibody against sperm in mice. *Journal of Reproductive Immunology*, *157*, 103930.

Cheng, C. Y., & Mruk, D. D. (2002). Cell junction dynamics in the testis: Sertoli-germ cell interactions and male contraceptive development. *Physiological reviews*, *82*(4), 825-874.

Cheng, C. Y., & Mruk, D. D. (2010). A local autocrine axis in the testes that regulates spermatogenesis. *Nature Reviews Endocrinology*, *6*(7), 380-395.

Cheng, C. Y., & Mruk, D. D. (2012). The blood-testis barrier and its implications for male contraception. *Pharmacological reviews*, *64*(1), 16-64.

Cheng, C. Y., Wong, E. W., Lie, P. P., Li, M. W., Mruk, D. D., Yan, H. H.,…Lui, W.-y. (2011). Regulation of blood-testis barrier dynamics by desmosome, gap junction, hemidesmosome and polarity proteins: An unexpected turn of events. *Spermatogenesis*, *1*(2), 105-115.

Chiu, W. W.-C., & Chamley, L. W. (2004). Clinical associations and mechanisms of action of antisperm antibodies. *Fertility and sterility*, *82*(3), 529-535.

D'Cruz, O., Haas Jr, G., Wang, B., & DeBault, L. (1991). Activation of human complement by IgG antisperm antibody and the demonstration of C3 and C5b-9-mediated immune injury to human sperm. *Journal of immunology (Baltimore, Md.: 1950)*, *146*(2), 611-620.

Durairajanayagam, D., Rengan, A. K., Sharma, R. K., & Agarwal, A. (2015). Introduction to the Male Reproductive System. *Unexplained Infertility: Pathophysiology, Evaluation and Treatment*, 29.

Ekşi, E., Yalçın Cömert, H. S., Imamoğlu, M., Alver, A., Aydin Mungan, S., & Sarıhan, H. (2020). Effects of myricetin on testicular torsion-detorsion injury in rats. *Andrologia*, *52*(10), e13775.

Elmas, M. A., Ozakpinar, O. B., Kolgazi, M., Sener, G., Arbak, S., & Ercan, F. (2022). Exercise improves testicular morphology and oxidative stress parameters in rats with testicular damage induced by a high-fat diet. *Andrologia*, *54*(11), e14600.

Erdemir, F., Atilgan, D., Markoc, F., Boztepe, O., Suha-Parlaktas, B., & Sahin, S. (2012). The effect of diet induced obesity on testicular tissue and serum oxidative stress parameters. *Actas Urológicas Españolas (English Edition)*, *36*(3), 153-159.

Fan, Y., Liu, Y., Xue, K., Gu, G., Fan, W., Xu, Y., & Ding, Z. (2015). Diet-induced obesity in male C57BL/6 mice decreases fertility as a consequence of disrupted blood-testis barrier. *PloS one*, *10*(4), e0120775.

Fink, C., Weigel, R., Fink, L., Wilhelm, J., Kliesch, S., Zeiler, M.,…Brehm, R. (2009). Claudin-11 is over-expressed and dislocated from the blood–testis barrier in Sertoli cells associated with testicular intraepithelial neoplasia in men. *Histochemistry and cell biology*, *131*, 755-764.

Florin, A., Maire, M., Bozec, A., Hellani, A., Chater, S., Bars, R.,… Benahmed, M. (2005). Androgens and postmeiotic germ cells regulate claudin-11 expression in rat Sertoli cells. *Endocrinology*, *146*(3), 1532-1540.

França, L. R., Hess, R. A., Dufour, J. M., Hofmann, M., & Griswold, M. (2016). The Sertoli cell: one hundred fifty years of beauty and plasticity. *Andrology*, *4*(2), 189-212.

Fretz, P. C., & Sandlow, J. I. (2002). Varicocele: current concepts in pathophysiology, diagnosis, and treatment. *Urologic Clinics*, *29*(4), 921-937.

Fu, G., Qian, L., Cui, Y., Xu, Z., Xuan, H., Zhu, J., & Zhang, W. (2006). Antisperm-antibodies induced by testicular torsion and its influence on testicular function. *Zhonghua nan ke xue= National Journal of Andrology*, *12*(11), 988-991.

Furuse, M. (2010). Molecular basis of the core structure of tight junctions. *Cold Spring Harbor perspectives in biology*, *2*(1), a002907.

Furuse, M., Hirase, T., Itoh, M., Nagafuchi, A., Yonemura, S., Tsukita, S., & Tsukita, S. (1993). Occludin: a novel integral membrane protein localizing at tight junctions. *The Journal of cell biology*, *123*(6), 1777-1788.

Gat, Y., Bachar, G. N., Zukerman, Z., Belenky, A., & Gornish, M. (2004). Varicocele: a bilateral disease. *Fertility and sterility*, *81*(2), 424-429.

Ge, R.-S., Li, X., & Wang, Y. (2021). Leydig cell and spermatogenesis. *Molecular Mechanisms in Spermatogenesis*, 111-129.

Gollenberg, A. L., Liu, F., Brazil, C., Drobnis, E. Z., Guzick, D., Overstreet, J. W.,…Swan, S. H. (2010). Semen quality in fertile men in relation to psychosocial stress. *Fertility and sterility*, *93*(4), 1104-1111.

Günzel, D., & Yu, A. S. (2013). Claudins and the modulation of tight junction permeability. *Physiological reviews*, *93*(2), 525-569.

Gupta, S., Dhanda, S., & Sandhir, R. (2019). Anatomy and physiology of blood-brain barrier. In *Brain targeted drug delivery system* (pp. 7-31). Elsevier.

Gupta, S., Sharma, R., Agarwal, A., Boitrelle, F., Finelli, R., Farkouh, A. a.,…Zilaitiene, B. (2022). Antisperm antibody testing: a comprehensive review of its role in the management of immunological male infertility and results of a global survey of clinical practices. *The world journal of men's health*, *40*(3), 380.

Ha, H. K., Park, H. J., & Park, N. C. (2011). Expression of E-cadherin and α-catenin in a varicocele-induced infertility rat model. *Asian journal of andrology*, *13*(3), 470.

Hadžiselimović, F., Snyder, H., Duckett, J., & Howards, S. (1986). Testicular histology in children with unilateral testicular torsion. *The Journal of Urology*, *136*(1), 208-210.

Hammoud, A. O., Wilde, N., Gibson, M., Parks, A., Carrell, D. T., & Meikle, A. W. (2008). Male obesity and alteration in sperm parameters. *Fertility and sterility*, *90*(6), 2222-2225.

Harris, A. L. (2007). Connexin channel permeability to cytoplasmic molecules. *Progress in biophysics and molecular biology*, *94*(1-2), 120-143.

Hellani, A., Ji, J., Mauduit, C., Deschildre, C., Tabone, E., & Benahmed, M. (2000). Developmental and hormonal regulation of the expression of oligodendrocyte-specific protein/claudin 11 in mouse testis. *Endocrinology*, *141*(8), 3012-3019.

Hess, R. A., & França, L. R. (2005). Structure of the Sertoli cell. *Sertoli cell biology*, *40*.

Hirano, S., Kimoto, N., Shimoyama, Y., Hirohashi, S., & Takeichi, M. (1992). Identification of a neural α-catenin as a key regulator of cadherin function and multicellular organization. *Cell*, *70*(2), 293-301.

Hogarth, C. A., & Griswold, M. D. (2010). The key role of vitamin A in spermatogenesis. *The Journal of clinical investigation*, *120*(4), 956-962.

Horvath-Pereira, B. d. O., Almeida, G. H. D. R., Silva Júnior, L. N. d., do Nascimento, P. G., Horvath Pereira, B. d. O., Fireman, J. V. B. T.,…Miglino, M. A. (2023). Biomaterials for Testicular Bioengineering: How far have we come and where do we have to go? *Frontiers in Endocrinology*, *14*, 1085872.

Hou, G., Xiong, W., Wang, M., Chen, X., & Yuan, T. F. (2014). Chronic stress influences sexual motivation and causes damage to testicular cells in male rats. *The journal of sexual medicine*, *11*(3), 653-663.

Huang, J., Li, X., Zhang, D., Wang, L., Li, Z., & Song, Z. (2024). Depression-related Testosterone Deficiency is Linked to Reduced Cholesterol Levels in Leydig Cells of CUMS Mice. *Reproduction*, *1*(aop).

Jensen, C. F. S., Østergren, P., Dupree, J. M., Ohl, D. A., Sønksen, J., & Fode, M. (2017). Varicocele and male infertility. *Nature Reviews Urology*, *14*(9), 523-533.

Jensen, T. K., Andersson, A.-M., Jørgensen, N., Andersen, A.-G., Carlsen, E., & Skakkebæk, N. E. (2004). Body mass index in relation to semen quality and reproductive hormonesamong 1,558 Danish men. *Fertility and sterility*, *82*(4), 863-870.

Kaltsas, A. (2023). Oxidative stress and male infertility: the protective role of antioxidants. *Medicina*, *59*(10), 1769.

Kang, C., Punjani, N., Lee, R. K., Li, P. S., & Goldstein, M. (2022). Effect of varicoceles on spermatogenesis. Seminars in Cell & Developmental Biology.

Kato, T., Mizuno, K., Nishio, H., Moritoki, Y., Kamisawa, H., Kurokawa, S.,…Hayashi, Y. (2020). Disorganization of claudin-11 and dysfunction of the blood-testis barrier during puberty in a cryptorchid rat model. *Andrology*, *8*(5), 1398-1408.

Kaur, G., Wright, K., Greer, R. H., Mueller, K., Haynes, A., & Dufour, J. M. (2018). Sertoli cell immune regulation within the testis. In *Spermatogenesis* (pp. 81-93). CRC Press.

Kidder, G. M., & Cyr, D. G. (2016). Roles of connexins in testis development and spermatogenesis. *Seminars in cell & developmental biology*.

Kolbasi, B., Bulbul, M. V., Karabulut, S., Altun, C. E., Cakici, C., Ulfer, G.,…Keskin, I. (2021). Chronic unpredictable stress disturbs the blood–testis barrier affecting sperm parameters in mice. *Reproductive BioMedicine Online*, *42*(5), 983-995.

Kremer, J., & Jager, S. (1992). OPINION: The significance of antisperm antibodies for sperm-cervical mucus interaction. *Human reproduction*, *7*(6), 781-784.

Kubota, H., & Brinster, R. L. (2018). Spermatogonial stem cells. *Biology of reproduction*, *99*(1), 52-74.

Laher, A., Ragavan, S., Mehta, P., & Adam, A. (2020). Testicular torsion in the emergency room: a review of detection and management strategies. *Open Access Emergency Medicine*, 237-246.

Lampiao, F. (2009). Variation of semen parameters in healthy medical students due to exam stress. *Malawi Medical Journal*, *21*(4).

Leslie, S. W., Sajjad, H., & Siref, L. E. (2017). *Varicocele.*

Li, M. W., Mruk, D. D., Lee, W. M., & Cheng, C. Y. (2009). Connexin 43 and plakophilin-2 as a protein complex that regulates blood–testis barrier dynamics. *Proceedings of the National Academy of Sciences*, *106*(25), 10213-10218.

Lie, P. P., Cheng, C. Y., & Mruk, D. D. (2011). The biology of the desmosome-like junction: a versatile anchoring junction and signal transducer in the seminiferous epithelium. *International review of cell and molecular biology*, *286*, 223-269.

Lui, W.-Y., Mruk, D., Lee, W. M., & Cheng, C. Y. (2003). Sertoli cell tight junction dynamics: their regulation during spermatogenesis. *Biology of reproduction*, *68*(4), 1087-1097.

Maeda, S., & Tsukihara, T. (2011). Structure of the gap junction channel and its implications for its biological functions. *Cellular and Molecular Life Sciences*, *68*, 1115-1129.

Magnusdottir, E. V., Thorsteinsson, T., Thorsteinsdottir, S., Heimisdottir, M., & Olafsdottir, K. (2005). Persistent organochlorines, sedentary occupation, obesity and human male subfertility. *Human reproduction*, *20*(1), 208-215.

Marieb, E. N., & Hoehn, K. (2007). *Human anatomy & physiology*. Pearson education.

Marmar, J. L. (2001). Varicocele and male infertility: part II: the pathophysiology of varicoceles in the light of current molecular and genetic information. *Human Reproduction Update*, *7*(5), 461-472.

Mazaud-Guittot, S., Meugnier, E., Pesenti, S., Wu, X., Vidal, H., Gow, A., & Le Magueresse-Battistoni, B. (2010). Claudin 11 deficiency in mice results in loss of the Sertoli cell epithelial phenotype in the testis. *Biology of reproduction*, *82*(1), 202-213.

Meng, J., Holdcraft, R. W., Shima, J. E., Griswold, M. D., & Braun, R. E. (2005). Androgens regulate the permeability of the blood–testis barrier. *Proceedings of the National Academy of Sciences*, *102*(46), 16696-16700.

Minas, A., Mahmoudabadi, S., Gamchi, N. S., Antoniassi, M. P., Alizadeh, A., & Bertolla, R. P. (2023). Testicular torsion in vivo models: Mechanisms and treatments. *Andrology*, *11*(7), 1267-1285.

Morita, K., Sasaki, H., Fujimoto, K., Furuse, M., & Tsukita, S. (1999). Claudin-11/OSP-based tight junctions of myelin sheaths in brain and Sertoli cells in testis. *The Journal of cell biology*, *145*(3), 579-588.

Moroi, S., Saitou, M., Fujimoto, K., Sakakibara, A., Furuse, M., Yoshida, O., & Tsukita, S. (1998). Occludin is concentrated at tight junctions of mouse/rat but not human/guinea pig Sertoli cells in testes. *American Journal of Physiology-Cell Physiology*, *274*(6), C1708-C1717.

Morrow, C. M., Mruk, D., Cheng, C. Y., & Hess, R. A. (2010). Claudin and occludin expression and function in the seminiferous epithelium. *Philosophical Transactions of the Royal Society B: Biological Sciences*, *365*(1546), 1679-1696.

Mruk, D. D., & Cheng, C. (2010). Tight junctions in the testis: new perspectives. *Philosophical Transactions of the Royal Society B: Biological Sciences*, *365*(1546), 1621-1635.

Mruk, D. D., & Cheng, C. Y. (2004). Sertoli-Sertoli and Sertoli-germ cell interactions and their significance in germ cell movement in the seminiferous epithelium during spermatogenesis. *Endocrine reviews*, *25*(5), 747-806.

Mruk, D. D., & Cheng, C. Y. (2011a). Desmosomes in the testis: Moving into an unchartered territory. *Spermatogenesis*, *1*(1), 47-51.

Mruk, D. D., & Cheng, C. Y. (2011b). The myotubularin family of lipid phosphatases in disease and in spermatogenesis. *Biochemical Journal*, *433*(2), 253-262.

Mruk, D. D., & Cheng, C. Y. (2015). The mammalian blood-testis barrier: its biology and regulation. *Endocrine reviews*, *36*(5), 564-591.

Mruk, D. D., Su, L., & Cheng, C. Y. (2011). Emerging role for drug transporters at the blood–testis barrier. *Trends in pharmacological sciences*, *32*(2), 99-106.

Nah, W. H., Lee, J. E., Park, H. J., Park, N. C., & Gye, M. C. (2011). Claudin-11 expression increased in spermatogenic defect in human testes. *Fertility and sterility*, *95*(1), 385-388.

Oh, Y. S., Jo, N. H., Park, J. K., & Gye, M. C. (2016). Changes in inflammatory cytokines accompany deregulation of claudin-11, resulting in inter-sertoli tight junctions in varicocele rat testes. *The Journal of Urology*, *196*(4), 1303-1312.

Pan, J., Zhu, Z., Xu, G., Niu, L., Yu, L., Luo, Z., & Yan, J. (2018). Expression of claudin-11 in a rat model of varicocele and its effects on the blood-testis barrier. *Molecular Medicine Reports*, *18*(6), 5647-5651.

Pawlina, W., Ross, M., & Kaye, G. (2016). Histology: a text and atlas. *With Correlated Cell and Molecular Biology*, *7*.

Pérez, C. V., Sobarzo, C. M., Jacobo, P. V., Pellizzari, E. H., Cigorraga, S. B., Denduchis, B., & Lustig, L. (2012). Loss of occludin expression and impairment of blood-testis barrier permeability in rats with autoimmune orchitis: effect of interleukin 6 on Sertoli cell tight junctions. *Biology of reproduction*, *87*(5), 122, 121-112.

Qi, C., Gutierrez, S. A., Lavriha, P., Othman, A., Lopez-Pigozzi, D., Bayraktar, E.,…Bortolozzi, M. (2023). Structure of the connexin-43 gap junction channel in a putative closed state. *Elife*, *12*, RP87616.

Reda, S., Hashem, H., Elnegris, H., & Elshal, L. (2017). Role of bone marrow derived mesenchymal stem cells in protection of spermatogenic and Sertoli cells against histological alterations induced by torsion/detorsion in rats. *Journal of medical histology*, *1*(2), 154-169.

Rode, K., Weider, K., Damm, O. S., Wistuba, J., Langeheine, M., & Brehm, R. (2018). Loss of connexin 43 in Sertoli cells provokes postnatal spermatogonial arrest, reduced germ cell numbers and impaired spermatogenesis. *Reproductive Biology*, *18*(4), 456-466.

Rümke, P., Renckens, C. N., Bezemer, P. D., & van Amstel, N. (1984). Prognosis of fertility in women with unexplained infertility and sperm agglutinins in the serum. *Fertility and sterility*, *42*(4), 561-567.

Russell, L., Bartke, A., & Goh, J. (1989). Postnatal development of the Sertoli cell barrier, tubular lumen, and cytoskeleton of Sertoli and myoid cells in the rat, and their relationship to tubular fluid secretion and flow. *American Journal of Anatomy*, *184*(3), 179-189.

Sakr, H. F., Abbas, A., Elsamanoudy, A., & Ghoneim, F. (2015). Effect of fluoxetine and resveratrol on testicular functions and oxidative stress in a rat model of chronic mild stress-induced depression. *J Physiol Pharmacol*, *66*(4), 515-527.

Schlegel, P. N., & Katzovitz, M. A. (2020). Male reproductive physiology. *Urologic Principles and Practice*, 41-62.

Schneider, G., Kirschner, M. A., Berkowitz, R., & Ertel, N. H. (1979). Increased estrogen production in obese men. *The Journal of Clinical Endocrinology & Metabolism*, *48*(4), 633-638.

Segretain, D., Fiorini, C., Decrouy, X., Defamie, N., Prat, J., & Pointis, G. (2004). A proposed role for ZO-1 in targeting connexin 43 gap junctions to the endocytic pathway. *Biochimie*, *86*(4-5), 241-244.

Soares, T., Fernandes, S., Lima, M., Stumpp, T., Schoorlemmer, G., Lazari, M., & Porto, C. (2013). Experimental varicocoele in rats affects mechanisms that control expression and function of the androgen receptor. *Andrology*, *1*(5), 670-681.

Taneichi, A., Shibahara, H., Hirano, Y., Suzuki, T., Obara, H., Fujiwara, H.,…Sato, I. (2002). Sperm immobilizing antibodies in the sera of infertile women cause low fertilization rates and poor embryo quality in vitro. *American Journal of Reproductive Immunology*, *47*(1), 46-51.

Toyama, Y., Ohkawa, M., Oku, R., Maekawa, M., & Yuasa, S. (2001). Neonatally administered diethylstilbestrol retards the development of the blood-testis barrier in the rat. *Journal of andrology*, *22*(3), 413-423.

Tsukita, S., Furuse, M., & Itoh, M. (1999). Structural and signalling molecules come together at tight junctions. *Current opinion in cell biology*, *11*(5), 628-633.

Turner, T. (2001). The study of varicocele through the use of animal models. *Human Reproduction Update*, *7*(1), 78-84.

Umeda, K., Ikenouchi, J., Katahira-Tayama, S., Furuse, K., Sasaki, H., Nakayama, M.,…Tsukita, S. (2006). ZO-1 and ZO-2 independently determine where claudins are polymerized in tight-junction strand formation. *Cell*, *126*(4), 741-754.

Van Itallie, C. M., & Anderson, J. M. (2006). Claudins and epithelial paracellular transport. *Annu. Rev. Physiol.*, *68*, 403-429.

Verón, G. L., Molina, R. I., Tissera, A. D., Estofan, G. M., Marín-Briggiler, C. I., & Vazquez-Levin, M. H. (2016). Incidence of sperm surface autoantibodies and relationship with routine semen parameters and sperm kinematics. *American Journal of Reproductive Immunology*, *76*(1), 59-69.

Vinken, M., Decrock, E., De Vuyst, E., Ponsaerts, R., D'hondt, C., Bultynck, G.,… Rogiers, V. (2011). Connexins: sensors and regulators of cell cycling. *Biochimica et Biophysica Acta (BBA)-Reviews on Cancer*, *1815*(1), 13-25.

Visser, A., & Heyns, C. (2003). Testicular function after torsion of the spermatic cord. *BJU international*, *92*(3).

Vogl, A., Vaid, K., Guttman, J., & Cheng, C. (2008). Molecular mechanisms in spermatogenesis. Springer.

Wong, V., & Russell, L. D. (1983). Three-dimensional reconstruction of a rat stage V Sertoli cell: I. Methods, basic configuration, and dimensions. *American Journal of Anatomy*, *167*(2), 143-161.

Wong, W. J., & Khan, Y. S. (2020). *Histology, sertoli cell.*

Yan, H. H., & Cheng, C. Y. (2005). Blood–testis barrier dynamics are regulated by an engagement/disengagement mechanism between tight and adherens junctions via peripheral adaptors. *Proceedings of the National Academy of Sciences*, *102*(33), 11722-11727.

Yan, H. H., Mruk, D. D., Lee, W. M., & Cheng, C. Y. (2008). Cross-talk between tight and anchoring junctions—lesson from the testis. *Molecular Mechanisms in Spermatogenesis*, 234-254.

Yoshitake, H., Oda, R., Yanagida, M., Kawasaki, Y., Sakuraba, M., Takamori, K.,…Araki, Y. (2016). Identification of an anti-sperm auto-monoclonal antibody (Ts4)-recognized molecule in the mouse sperm acrosomal region and its inhibitory effect on fertilization in vitro. *Journal of Reproductive Immunology*, *115*, 6-13.

Zhang, J., Jin, P., Gong, M., Guo, J., Fang, K., Yi, Q., & Zhu, R. (2018). Roles of Fas/FasL-mediated apoptosis and inhibin B in the testicular dysfunction of rats with left-side varicocele. *Andrologia*, *50*(2), e12850.

Zhou, J., Xi, Y., Zhang, J., Tang, J., Zhou, X., Chen, J.,… Ma, B. (2020). Protective effect of Dioscorea zingiberensis ethanol extract on the disruption of blood–testes barrier in high-fat diet/streptozotocin-induced diabetic mice by upregulating ZO-1 and Nrf2. *Andrologia*, *52*(3), e13508.

Chapter 3

The Blood-Epididymal Barrier

Arife Ahsen Kaplan[1,*], PhD
and Suat Utku Keskin[2]
[1]Department of Histology and Embryology, Faculty Medicine,
Bolu Abant İzzet Baysal University, Bolu, Türkiye
[2]The School of Medicine, Koç University, İstanbul, Türkiye

Abstract

The male reproductive system, especially the testis and epididymis, plays a critical role in sperm production and maturation. Spermatozoa produced in the testis are initially immobile and dysfunctional. They gain their fertilization potential and mobility during their passage through the epididymis. The epididymis, a highly segmented and convoluted canal adjacent to the testis, is surrounded by an epithelium composed of various cell types, including principal cells, clear cells, narrow cells, apical cells, basal cells, halo, and mononuclear phagocytes. The epithelial cells and the blood-epididymal barrier provide a special microenvironment for sperm maturation by selectively transporting and protecting them from harmful agents. The blood-epididymis barrier is conducted by tight junctions (TJs) between epithelial cells, regulates the paracellular transport of ions, molecules, and water, and provides polarity to the cells. In addition, epididymosomes, exosomes secreted by epididymal epithelial cells, play an essential role in sperm development by delivering critical proteins. In this chapter, the structure of the blood-epididymal barrier is presented in detail.

* Corresponding Author's Email: ahsenkaplan@gmail.com

In: A Histological Approach to Human Body Barriers
Editor: İlknur Keskin
ISBN: 979-8-89530-738-0

Keywords: blood-epididymal barrier, principal cell, clear cell, apical cell, epididymis

Introduction

The male reproductive system consists of external and internal reproductive organs; the testis and epididymis are functional units for sperm production (Ramírez-González & Sansone, 2022; Rehfeld et al., 2017). Spermatogonia and spermatocyte male gonads are produced in the seminiferous epithelium of the testis, then it is followed by maturing sperm in the epididymis (Suede et al., 2023). Sertoli cells are located within the seminiferous epithelium to conduct the blood testis barrier and monitor the production and development of germ cells (Plant et al., 2016).

In vertebrates that perform internal fertilization, sperm produced in the testis are dysfunctional, and they gain fertilization and motility abilities by passing through the epididymis (Esteves & Miyaoska, 2015) The epididymis consists of a single long, convoluted tubule with a central lumen lined with convoluted pseudostratified epithelium that protects sperm cells and is located next to the testis (Carvelli et al., 2023; Esteves & Miyaoska, 2015; Sullivan & Belleannée, 2018). Sperm passing through the epididymis takes approximately 3-12 days. It takes approximately 3-12 days for sperm to pass through the epididymis (Sullivan & Belleannée, 2018).

The epididymis is connected to the rete testis via efferent ducts and is surrounded by the tunica vaginalis and connective tissue (Esteves & Miyaoska, 2015). The epididymis consists of four main anatomical segments with structural and regional differences in cell types: initial segment (proximal region), head (caput), body (corpus) and tail (cauda) (Elbashir et al., 2021) (Figure 1). The epididymal epithelium is composed of different cell types and their distribution varies according to the segment. The cells in the epididymal epithelium have been named as apical cells, principal cells, clear cells, basal cells, halo cells and narrow cells (Carvelli et al., 2023; Esteves & Miyaoska, 2015). In recent studies, new cells have been identified at the base of the epithelium; these are epididymal mononuclear phagocytes (eMPS), monocytes/macrophages (M/M) and dendritic cells (Carvelli et al., 2023).

1. The Function of the Epididymis

The epididymis, which includes the rete testis and vas deferens, transports sperm through the male reproductive system by peristaltic movements of the epididymal tubules and contraction of smooth muscle layers. Spermatozoa in the testis and epididymis are nonmotile. In the caudal segment and around the vas deferens, epididymal smooth muscle layers have developed around the epididymal tubule to help propel sperm during ejaculation.(Sullivan & Belleannée, 2018).

The epididymis is very important for the male reproductive health. Although spermatozoa entering the caput region of the epididymis are fully differentiated, they are immobile and cannot induce fertilization (Liu et al., 2020; Orgebin-Crist, 1967). In vitro fertilization, studies with epididymal spermatozoa show sperm functionality increases during the epididymal passage (Sullivan & Belleannée, 2018). Spermatozoa gain fertilizing capacity as they pass through the epididymis, and this is called sperm maturation (Kohane et al., 1979). With sperm maturation, structural changes occur in the size and appearance of the nucleus and acrosome, the plasma membrane, chromatin condensation, migration of the cytoplasmic droplet along the tail, and intracellular organelles (Esteves & Miyaoska, 2015). The microenvironment of the epididymis affects the maturation progress. The corpus segment contains the first fertilization-capable sperm. Due to the tight packaging of DNA and the absence of some organelles such as the ribosomes, Golgi and endoplasmic reticulum, spermatozoa emerging from the testes are transcriptionally and translationally inactive cells and cannot perform protein synthesis (Sullivan & Belleannée, 2018). The blood-epididymal barrier (BEB) functions to regulate the transport of nutrients, hormones and other essential molecules to support sperm maturation and to prevent the entry of harmful substances and pathogens (Gregory & Cyr, 2014; Kim et al., 2022; Manfrevola et al., 2021). Extracellular factors secreted by epithelial cells and proteins secreted into the intraluminal environment provide a suitable environment for sperm maturation (Sullivan & Belleannée, 2018). Recent studies showed that the maturation process is androgen-dependent and mediated by factors produced by the epididymis (Kohane et al., 1979; Roberts & Chauvin, 2018). Autocrine, paracrine, and endocrine factors are important for sperm maturation (Esteves & Miyaoska, 2015). Secretory products identified in the luminal fluid include cystatin-related epididymal spermatogenic protein (CRES), WAP four disulfide core domain 2 (Wfdc2 or HE4), associated antigen 11 (Spag 11 or HE2), protein B/C and glutathione peroxidase 5

(GPX5), and cysteine-rich secretory protein 1 (Roberts & Chauvin, 2018). In addition, most of these proteins are produced in specific regions in the epididymis (Roberts & Chauvin, 2018). On the other hand, biochemical changes critical for sperm maturation and survival.

For example, high levels of compounds such as L-carnitine, glycerophosphorylcholine, sialic acid, lactate, inositol, glutamate, and taurine have been identified in the composition of epididymal fluid (Esteves & Miyaoska, 2015; Kohane et al., 1979).

The BEB protects maturing spermatozoa from the immune system by sequestering sperm antigens and restricting the entry of immunoglobulins and immune cells into the epididymal lumen. This immunological barrier is essential to prevent autoimmune reactions against sperm. It is also affected by cytokines released during inflammation (Gregory & Cyr, 2014).

The epididymis has many vital functions, such as sperm transportation, sperm concentration, motility gain, fertilization abilities, and sperm protection (James et al., 2020). The length of cell modifications in each region, region-specific modifications, and sperm survival time are critical for epididymal functions related to sperm maturation (Carvelli et al., 2023). Water is reabsorbed by the epithelium surrounding the intraluminal compartment of the epididymis; the diameter of this region increases distally, and the sperm concentration (hematocrit) increases significantly throughout the epididymis (Sullivan & Belleannée, 2018). This channel carries, concentrates, stores and protects sperm; it also ensures sperm motility and fertility (Carvelli et al., 2023). The membrane phospholipid composition and cholesterol/phospholipid ratio of spermatozoa changes during maturing in the epididymis, with increases in disulfide bonds and net surface negative charge, repositioning of surface antigens, and modification, removal, and addition of surface proteins (Sullivan et al., 2007).

The epididymal mucosa is a highly dynamic environment where sperm, epithelial fragility, and immune capabilities are broadly regulated. This order ensures the maintenance of homeostasis and the separation of stress from its structure. One of the most exciting aspects of male reproductive biology is that the long and segmented epididymis can inhibit the development of autoimmune responses against antigenic sperm while initiating highly effective metabolism against pathogenic microorganisms and cancer. Epididymal epithelial lumen (CCs) rapidly develop proinflammatory mediators such as Cxcl10, Cxcl1, Cxcl2, Ccl5, and Il6 against genetics; this indicates that they are located near macrophages (MPs) to maintain their native stability. Furthermore, lipopolysaccharide (LPS) from Escherichia coli screening into the vas deferens and distal epididymis increased proinflammatory factors such as Il6, Tnfa, and Il1b in the rat and mouse epididymal tail region. These molecules are critical for expanding pores in the epididymis during heat exposure.

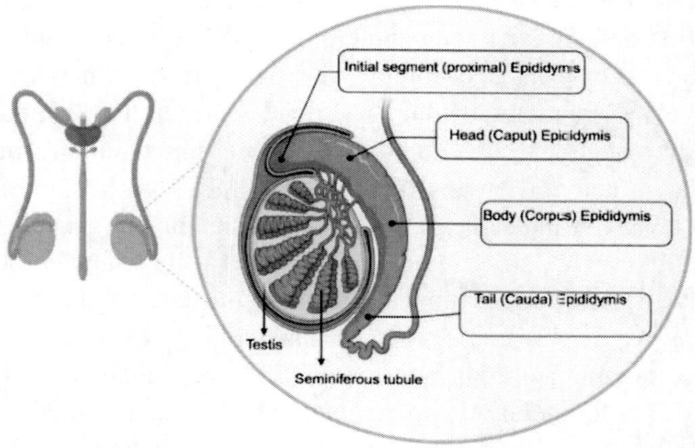

Figure 1. The schematic view of the epididymis, which is divided into the initial segment, head, body, and tail. (Created in BioRender. Kaplan, A. (2023) BioRender.com/m74h770).

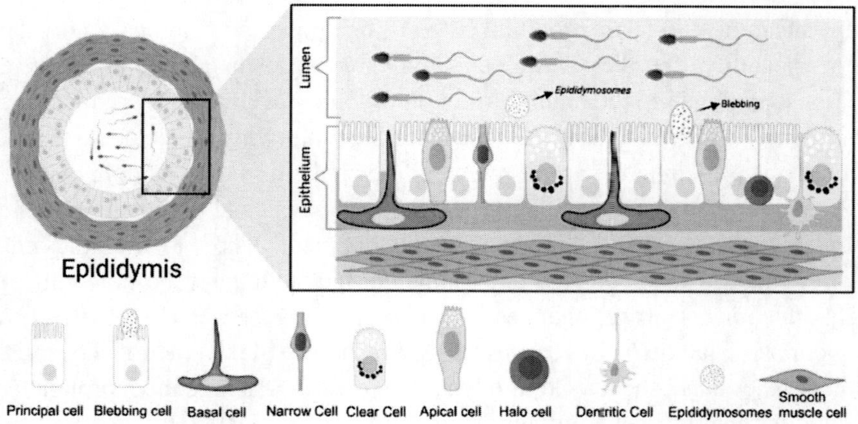

Figure 2. The structure of the epididymal epithelium. The epithelium consists of principal cell (columnar shape), basal cell (shorter, pyramid-shaped), narrow cell (elongated and narrow, champagne glass shaped), clear cell (numerous vesicles (white color) and lysosomes (black color)), apical cell (spherical nucleus at apical pole), halo cell (round cell at basal zone), dentritic cell (with dense dendritic network). (Created in BioRender. Kaplan, A. (2024) BioRender.com/t28u72).

2. The Epididymal Epithelium and the Blood-Epididymal Barrier

The blood-epididymal barrier (BEB) is in the epididymis, which controls the passage of molecules and cells through the blood vessels. It is a morphological structure first defined by Friend and Gilula (1972) (Friend & Gilula, 1972). BEB is formed by zonula occludens and tight junctions between adjacent epithelial cells surrounding the lumen (Friend & Gilula, 1972; Hinton, 1985). These tight junctions are composed of transmembrane proteins and intracellular proteins. Claudins (Cldns), MARVEL proteins, occludin, and junctional adhesion molecules (JAM) are transmembrane proteins for tight junction (Breton et al., 2019; Gregory & Cyr, 2014). Junctional proteins carry out selective transport to the lumen and control the level of organic molecules (Gregory & Cyr, 2014). This barrier maintaining the microenvironment required for sperm maturation and storage (Sullivan et al., 2007).

The BEB is formed by tight junctions (TJs) between epithelial cells. The BEB establishes and maintains the luminal environment necessary for spermatozoa. Tight junctions separate the apical and basolateral regions of cells, regulate the paracellular transport of ions, molecules, and water, and maintain the polarity of cells (Breton et al., 2019). There are differences in the ultrastructure of tight junctions throughout the epididymis. In rats, the impermeability in the proximal region on postnatal day 14 and the impermeability in the entire epididymis on postnatal day 21 were demonstrated using lanthanum during embryonic development. In mice, the epididymal lumen is shown to form during embryonic development and occludin is present in the apical region of the epithelium. It is thought that the BEB structure begins to form during fetal development and that changes in the ultrastructure occur during postnatal development. The blood-epididymis barrier changes with age, and environmental factors disrupt the functions of tight junctions, causing changes in the barrier (Breton et al., 2019). The depletion of Claudin (Cldn) causes the disappearance of the junctional strands. On the other hand, the knockout of occludin does not change the morphology of the junction but causes inflammation (Breton et al., 2019).

A two-layered pseudostratified epithelium surrounds the lumen of the epididymis. The base of the epithelium is separated from the connective tissue (smooth muscle and blood vessels). The apical pole of the epithelium is in direct contact with the lumen, which contains sperm and luminal fluid. The BEB, constituted by the tight junctions between adjacent cells in the epididymal epithelium, controls the composition of the luminal microenvironment crucial for sperm maturation and plays a crucial role in male fertility (Meng et al., 2023). There is also a gap junction between cells along the entire length of the epididymal tubule, which ensures the communication and coordination of cells (Sullivan & Belleannée, 2018). The ultrastructure of cells in the epithelium varies depending on the epididymis segment; the epithelium's function is different through the epididymis. Water absorption is at a high level in the proximal segment, and there are many cells with long stereocilia and many mitochondria in their basal sides. On the other hand, in the distal region, cells are small, and their function is to clear cellular debris (Esteves & Miyaoska, 2015).

2.1. Principal Cell

The cell constituting 80% of the epididymal epithelium are principal cells (Esteves & Miyaoska, 2015). They take part in the blood barrier with the tight junction between cells. These cells are the most studied cells; they secrete proteins into the lumen of the epididymis (Esteves & Miyaoska, 2015). The ultrastructure of principal cells has been identified as having an abundant rough endoplasmic reticulum in the intranuclear compartments. In contrast, the supranuclear compartments have many highly developed Golgi complexes and mitochondria (Esteves & Miyaoska, 2015). They produce glyceryl phosphorylcholine, sialic acid, carnitine, and various glycoproteins (Esteves & Miyaoska, 2015).

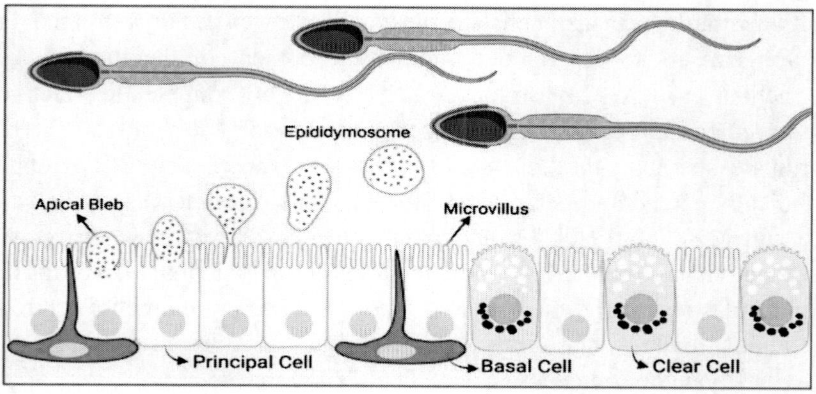

Figure 3. Principal cells secrete a complex recipe of molecules in epididymosome for sperm maturation. (Created in BioRender. Kaplan, A. (2024) BioRender.com/a88y754).

2.2. Epididymal Epithelial Clear Cells

Clear cells (CCs) are endocytotic cells involved in the clearance of proteins from the epididymal lumen (Esteves & Miyaoska, 2015). They also play a role in the acidification process in the lumen, with narrow and apical cells, to maintain spermatozoa in a quiescent state (Esteves & Miyaoska, 2015). When the ultrastructure of clear cells is examined, it is characterized by a specialized apical pole with many mitochondria. In addition, coated pits, numerous vesicles, multivesicular bodies, endosomes, and lysosomes have been identified, and the structure of the cell membrane consists of special microvillus (Sullivan & Belleannée, 2018). Apical microvillar projections elongate to secrete protons into the lumen (Roy et al., 2013; Sullivan & Belleannée, 2018). Their function could be affected by hormonal (angiotensin II (ANG II)) and nonhormonal (ATP, adenosine, bicarbonate, and H+) luminal factors (Belleannée et al., 2010; Roy et al., 2013). The effect of circulating aldosterone on the cauda and caput regions of the epididymis is different; it has been shown to affect the elongation of CC microvilli in the caput region but not in the caudal CCs (Roy et al., 2013).

2.3. Basal Cell

Basal cells (BC), pyramidal-shaped cells, line the base of the epididymal epithelium and connect with principal and clear cells by gap junction(Sullivan & Belleannée, 2018). These cells, which extend into the lumen with axiopodia, function with the principal cells and clear cells. However, they cross the tight junction barriers to control and sample the content of the luminal fluid (Barrachina et al., 2022; Breton et al., 2019). For example, it effectively controls the appropriate chloride concentration of the luminal fluid to coordinate sperm maturation events. It is well known that BC axiopodia periodically extend and retract over time, that this movement is regulated by cSrc and MEK1/2-ERK1/2, and that the axiopodia retract when tyrosine kinase activity is inhibited. Periodic axial motility (PAM) is a novel form of cellular plasticity in which BCs in pseudostratified epithelia send out "antennae" to survey the luminal environment and subsequently affect the behavior of neighboring cells (Breton et al., 2019).

2.4. Apical Cells

Apical cells are stained goblet-shaped, and thin-structured cells extending from the basement membrane to the lumen, with nuclei close to the apical compartment (Adamali & Hermo, 1996; Akbarsha et al., 2015; Picut & Remick, 2016). They are specialized with numerous mitochondria, called 'mitochondria rich cells'. The connection of these cells to the basement membrane is not definite (Picut & Remick, 2016), and the primary function is unknown (Lin & Troyer, 2014). When examined histologically, these cells appear at an apical location and are defined as apical cells They are located in the caput region of the epididymis (Adamali & Hermo, 1996) and participate in endocytosis with narrow and clear cells (Akbarsha et al., 2015).

2.5. Narrow Cells

Narrow (or pencil) cells are characterized by long nuclei and are found in the initial segment of the epididymis (Picut & Remick, 2016; Sullivan & Belleannée, 2018). Ultrastructures of these cells have been described and shown to contain numerous vesicles and mitochondria. Like clear cells, they are involved in endocytosis, acidification of epididymal luminal fluid, and proton pumping (Akbarsha et al., 2015; Sullivan & Belleannée, 2018).

2.6. Halo Cells and Mononuclear Phagocytes

The epididymal epithelium consists of many different cell types; two are lymphocytes and macrophages, also called halo cells (Lin & Troyer, 2014). Halo cells are the primary immune cell type (Esteves & Miyaoska, 2015), present at all levels of the epididymal epithelium (Akbarsha et al., 2015) and located at the basal compartment of the epithelium (Picut & Remick, 2016). Mononuclear phagocytes (dendritic cells, monocytes, macrophages) are involved in maintaining homeostasis of the epididymal mucosa and also play an essential role in protecting sperm cells from environmental factors (Barrachina et al., 2023).

2.7. Epididymosomes

Epithelial cells in the epididymis produce specific exosomes. These are called epididymosomes or apical blebs. Exosomes play an essential role in sperm maturation, promoting forward progressive motility and capacitation sperm–oocyte interaction (James et al., 2020; Luo et al., 2022). Epididymosomes are primarily secreted by principal cells (Luo et al., 2022). Epididymosomes can move to neighboring epithelial cells and do specific functions together. Epididymosomes can be exterminated by lysosomal degradation (Carvelli et al., 2023). It is secreted into the intraluminal region by small membrane vesicles of 50-500 nm diameter containing epididymal proteins secreted by epithelial cells in a merocrine manner. Vesicles interacting with the sperm surface were shown by electron microscopy in 1985 (Yanagimachi et al., 1985), and the proteins interacting with the sperm head and tail are schematically illustrated (Figure 4). For example, proteins such as P25b and P26h can reach the sperm head via the epididymosomes, and the accumulation of these proteins in the acrosome increases the ability of the sperm to bind to the zona pellucida and increases the fertilization rate (Sullivan et al., 2007).

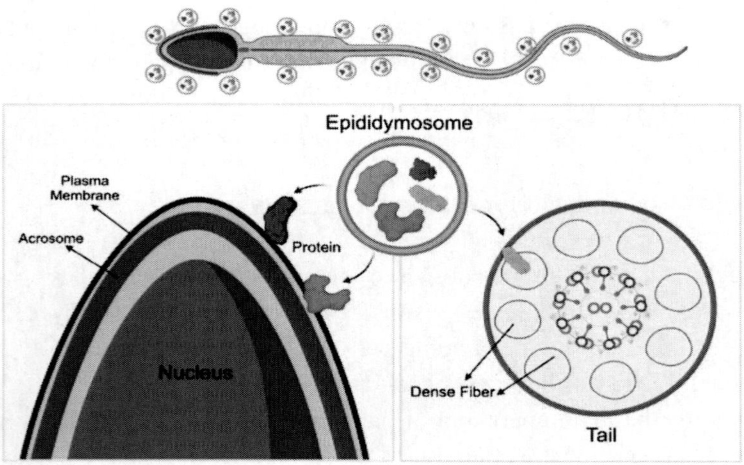

Figure 4. Epididymosome transport and release proteins interacting with the sperm head and tail. (Created in BioRender. Kaplan, A. (2024) BioRender.com/d07g320).

There are a variety of proteins associated with the epididymosome that play different roles. Some of these identified include Murine sperm adhesion molecule 1 (SPAM1), which is involved in cumulus-oocyte complex interactions, polyol pathway enzymes and macrophage migration inhibitory factor (MIF), which are involved in modulating sperm motility within the epididymis, HE5/CD52, which is involved in modulating immunological fertility, Type 5 glutathione peroxidase (GPX5), which is involved in protection against oxidative stress, and ubiquitin, which is involved in the elimination of defective spermatozoa (Sullivan et al., 2007).

3. Epididymal Microenvironment

The epididymal tube is a highly organized structure consisting of different segments, each acting as a separate "organ" with its microenvironment. These segments communicate with each other through paracrine systems to allow the sperm to mature. This process changes sperm morphology, motility, biochemistry, permeability, concentration and metabolism (Elbashir et al., 2021). Many factors ensure microenvironmental homeostasis.

3.1. Zinc

Zinc is essential for the continuation of life, reproduction, and the maintenance of immune system activities. Systemic and cellular zinc balance control is vital for all biological systems (Yazğan et al., n.d.). Zinc homeostasis is maintained by the free movement of zinc ions across the cytoplasm or organelle membranes through zinc transporters. In mammals, the transport of zinc across cell membranes is facilitated by ZnT proteins. The levels of zinc and ZnT expression vary in different regions of the epididymis. There is a high expression of ZnT1 in almost all pseudostratified ciliated columnar epithelium of the epididymis, especially in the principal and basal cells. ZnT2 expression is high in the lumen of the epididymal duct, mainly in principal and myoid cells. It has been shown that in the caput and cauda regions of the epididymis of diabetic mice, zinc levels and ZnT2 mRNA and protein levels decrease. It was identified that zinc homeostasis was disrupted in the epididymis of diabetic mice (Zhang et al., 2024).

3.2. Heparan Sulfate

The glycoprotein and glycolipid layer that covers the cell surface and consists of polysaccharides linked to lipids or proteins is defined as the glycocalyx.

Heparan sulfate (HS), a glycosaminoglycan (GAG) family member, forms heparan sulfate proteoglycans (HSPGs) by binding covalently to core proteins. GAG molecules are long, unbranched polysaccharides containing repeating disaccharide units, containing glucuronic or L-iduronic acid which are linked to N-acetyl glucosamine via a β1,4 glycosidic bond. Structural diversity is achieved by sulfation of disaccharides at various positions (Carvelli et al., 2023). Heparan sulfate (HS) enzyme structure deteriorations are associated with lysosomal storage diseases and neurodegenerative mucopolysaccharidosis.

Heparan sulfate proteoglycans (HSPG) are now known to function as cell surface receptors for a variety of macromolecular cargoes. In many cell types, small membrane vesicles, called exosomes or extracellular vesicles, derived from the cell surface and/or multivesicular bodies, provide cells with a wide variety of biologically active molecules, proteins, lipids, and mRNAs and microRNA (Dilsiz, 2022). These vesicles can enter cells via HSPG-mediated endocytosis. In this context, various possibilities can be put forward that endocytosed heparan sulfate originates from epididymal epithelial cells (Carvelli et al., 2023).

4. Factors Affecting the Blood-Epididymal Barrier

Many different conditions affect the BEB. Hormonal changes, inflammatory conditions (Gregory & Cyr, 2014; Lotti et al., 2018), oxidative stress, anti-cancer drugs (Fang et al., 2017), environmental factors (Breton et al., 2019), genetic factors could disrupt the BEB (Dubé et al., 2008). Testosterone and estrogen control the permeability of the blood-epididymal barrier. Imbalances in hormone levels can disrupt barrier function, affecting nutrient transport, sperm maturation, and motility (Gregory & Cyr, 2014; Marty et al., 2003).

Disruption of the BEB, such as through inflammation, can lead to the formation of sperm granulomas and decreased sperm function, contributing to male infertility (Gregory & Cyr, 2014). Altered immune privilege may lead to autoimmune reactions against sperm, causing infertility (Zhao et al., 2020). The BEB is more permeable than the blood-testis barrier but still provides an effective barrier to regulate the epididymal microenvironment and protect sperm (Lotti et al., 2018).

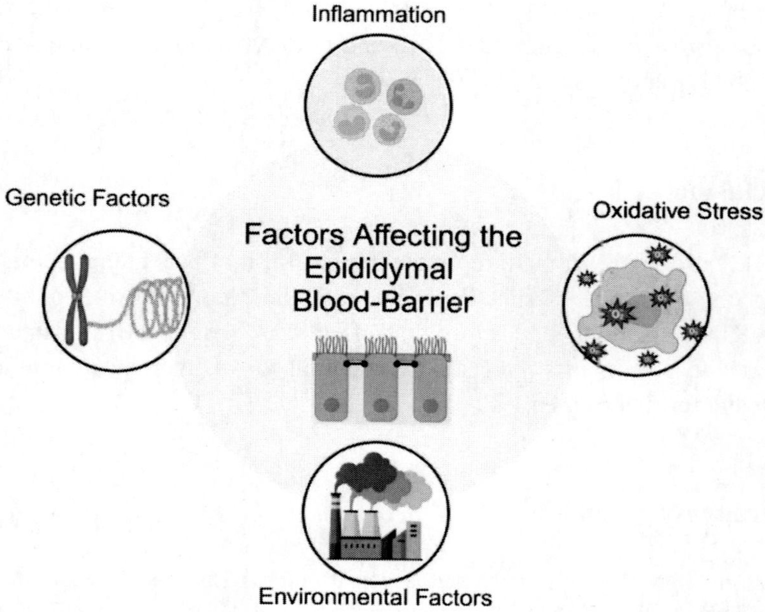

Figure 5. Factors Affecting the Blood-Epididymal Barrier. (Created in BioRender. Kaplan, A. (2024) BioRender.com/e87h806).

In normal cellular processes, reactive oxygen species (ROS) are produced by mitochondria, taking part in inter and intra-cellular signaling pathways (Gregory & Cyr, 2014). Excessive production of ROS can damage the epithelial cells that form the blood-barrier. Oxidative stress weakens the barrier function, making it more susceptible to disruptions. Many studies indicated that basal cells play a role in protecting against free oxygen radical species (Gregory & Cyr, 2014). Basal cells produce some proteins to decrease the level of ROS, including Cu-Zn SOD (SOD1), glutathione-S-transferase (GST), and metallothioneins (MT). In some cases, basal cells may not be sufficient to reduce ROS levels in the lumen, and sperm cells are affected by the high level of ROS (Gregory & Cyr, 2014).

Exposure to environmental toxins such as heavy metals, pesticides, and endocrine disruptors can impair the structure and function of the BEB. Toxins such as cadmium and diazinon can cause the disruption of cell junctions and increase permeability, leading to changes in the morphology of epididymal tissue (Adamkovicova et al., 2014).

Genetic mutations affecting the expression of proteins involved in maintaining the blood-barrier integrity can predispose individuals to barrier dysfunction. Variations in the expression of tight junction proteins or transporters can cause changes in BEB and epididymal luminal contents (Kim et al., 2022; Manfrevola et al., 2021).

Conclusion

The BEB is critical for male reproduction health; it affects many factors that disrupt the exchange of substances between the blood and the epididymal tissue. Understanding the factors that affect this barrier and implementing strategies to preserve its integrity are essential for maintaining reproductive health and fertility in men.

References

Adamali, H. I., & Hermo, L. (1996). Apical and Narrow Cells Are Distinct Cell Types Differing in Their Structure, Distribution, and Functions in the Adult Rat Epididymis. *Journal of Andrology*, *17*(3), 208–222. https://doi.org/10.1002/J.1939-4640.1996.TB01776.X.

Adamkovicova, M., Toman, R., Cabaj, M., Massanyi, P., Martiniakova, M., Omelka, R., Krajcovicova, V., & Duranova, H. (2014). Effects of Subchronic Exposure to Cadmium and Diazinon on Testis and Epididymis in Rats. *The Scientific World Journal*, *2014*(1), 632581. https://doi.org/10.1155/2014/632581.

Akbarsha, M. A., Faisal, K., & Radha, A. (2015). The Epididymis: Structure and Function. In *Mammalian Endocrinology and Male Reproductive Biology* (pp. 132–183). CRC Press. https://doi.org/10.1201/B18900-10.

Barrachina, F., Battistone, M. A., Castillo, J., Mallofré, C., Jodar, M., Breton, S., & Oliva, R. (2022). Sperm acquire epididymis-derived proteins through epididymosomes. *Human Reproduction (Oxford, England)*, *37*(4), 651. https://doi.org/10.1093/HUMREP/DEAC015.

Barrachina, F., Ottino, K., Tu, L. J., Soberman, R. J., Brown, D., Breton, S., & Battistone, M. A. (2023). CX3CR1 deficiency leads to impairment of immune surveillance in the epididymis. *Cellular and Molecular Life Sciences: CMLS*, *80*(1). https://doi.org/10.1007/S00018-022-04664-W.

Belleannée, C., Da Silva, N., Shum, W. W. C., Brown, D., & Breton, S. (2010). Role of purinergic signaling pathways in V-ATPase recruitment to apical membrane of acidifying epididymal clear cells. *American Journal of Physiology. Cell Physiology*, *298*(4). https://doi.org/10.1152/AJPCELL.00460.2009.

Breton, S., Nair, A. V., & Battistone, M. A. (2019). Epithelial dynamics in the epididymis: role in the maturation, protection, and storage of spermatozoa. *Andrology*, *7*(5), 631–643. https://doi.org/10.1111/ANDR.12632.

Carvelli, L., Hermo, L., O'Flaherty, C., Oko, R., Pshezhetsky, A. V., & Morales, C. R. (2023). Effects of Heparan sulfate acetyl-CoA: Alpha-glucosaminide N-acetyltransferase (HGSNAT) inactivation on the structure and function of epithelial and immune cells of the testis and epididymis and sperm parameters in adult mice. *PLOS ONE*, *18*(9). https://doi.org/10.1371/JOURNAL.PONE.0292157.

Dilsiz, N. (2022). Hallmarks of exosomes. *Future Science OA*, *8*(1). https://doi.org/10.2144/FSOA-2021-0102.

Dubé, E., Hermo, L., Chan, P. T. K., & Cyr, D. G. (2008). Alterations in gene expression in the caput epididymides of nonobstructive azoospermic men. *Biology of Reproduction*, *78*(2), 342–351. https://doi.org/10.1095/BIOLREPROD.107.062760.

Elbashir, S., Magdi, Y., Rashed, A., Henkel, R., & Agarwal, A. (2021). Epididymal contribution to male infertility: An overlooked problem. *Andrologia*, *53*(1). https://doi.org/10.1111/AND.13721.

Esteves, S. C., & Miyaoska, R. (2015). Sperm Physiology and Assessment of Spermatogenesis Kinetics In Vivo. *Handbook of Fertility: Nutrition, Diet, Lifestyle and Reproductive Health*, 383–396. https://doi.org/10.1016/B978-0-12-800872-0.00034-2.

Fang, F., Ni, K., Cai, Y., Zhao, Q., Shang, J., Zhang, X., Shen, S., & Xiong, C. (2017). Busulfan administration produces toxic effects on epididymal morphology and inhibits the expression of ZO-1 and vimentin in the mouse epididymis. *Bioscience Reports*, *37*(6). https://doi.org/10.1042/BSR20171059.

Friend, D. S., & Gilula, N. B. (1972). Variations in tight and gap junctions in mammalian tissues. *The Journal of Cell Biology*, *53*(3), 758–776. https://doi.org/10.1083/JCB.53.3.758.

Gregory, M., & Cyr, D. G. (2014). The blood-epididymis barrier and inflammation. *Spermatogenesis*, *4*(2), e979619. https://doi.org/10.4161/21565562.2014.979619.

Hinton, B. T. (1985). The blood-epididymis barrier. In *Male Fertility and Its Regulation* (pp. 371–382). Springer, Dordrecht. https://doi.org/10.1007/978-94-009-4894-5_25.

James, E. R., Carrell, D. T., Aston, K. I., Jenkins, T. G., Yeste, M., & Salas-Huetos, A. (2020). The Role of the Epididymis and the Contribution of Epididymosomes to Mammalian Reproduction. *International Journal of Molecular Sciences*, *21*(15), 1–17. https://doi.org/10.3390/IJMS21155377.

Kim, S. W., Jeong, Y. Da, Lee, G. Y., Lee, J., Lee, J. Y., Kim, C. L., Ko, Y. G., Lee, S. S., & Kim, B. (2022). Differential expression and localization of tight junction proteins in the goat epididymis. *Journal of Animal Science and Technology*, *64*(3), 500. https://doi.org/10.5187/JAST.2022.E13.

Kohane, A. C., Garberi, J. C., Cameo, M. S., & Blaquier, J. A. (1979). Quantitative Determination of Specific Proteins in Rat Epididymis. *Hormonal Steroids*, 671–674. https://doi.org/10.1016/B978-0-08-023796-1.50098-0.

Lin, J. B., & Troyer, D. (2014). Testicular Anatomy and Physiology. In *Pathobiology of Human Disease: A Dynamic Encyclopedia of Disease Mechanisms* (pp. 2464–2475). Academic Press. https://doi.org/10.1016/B978-0-12-386456-7.05102-9.

Liu, Y., Zhang, C., Wang, S., Hu, Y., Jing, J., Ye, L., Jing, R., & Ding, Z. (2020). Dependence of sperm structural and functional integrity on testicular calcineurin isoform PPP3R2 expression. *Journal of Molecular Cell Biology*, *12*(7), 515. https://doi.org/10.1093/JMCB/MJZ115.

Lotti, F., Baldi, E., Corona, G., Lombardo, F., Maseroli, E., Degl'Innocenti, S., Bartoli, L., & Maggi, M. (2018). Epididymal more than testicular abnormalities are associated with the occurrence of antisperm antibodies as evaluated by the MAR test. *Human Reproduction*, *33*(8), 1417–1429. https://doi.org/10.1093/HUMREP/DEY235.

Luo, J., Tan, X., Li, H., & Ding, X. (2022). sncRNAs in Epididymosomes: The Contribution to Embryonic Development and Offspring Health. *International Journal of Molecular Sciences 2022, Vol. 23, Page 10851*, *23*(18), 10851. https://doi.org/10.3390/IJMS231810851.

Manfrevola, F., Martinez, G., Coutton, C., Rocco, D., Reynaud, K., Le Vern, Y., Froment, P., Beauclair, L., Aubert, D., Pierantoni, R., Chianese, R., & Guillou, F. (2021). Ankrd31 in Sperm and Epididymal Integrity. *Frontiers in Cell and Developmental Biology*, *9*, 741975. https://doi.org/10.3389/FCELL.2021.741975/BIBTEX.

Marty, M. S., Chapin, R. E., Parks, L. G., & Thorsrud, B. A. (2003). Development and maturation of the male reproductive system. *Birth Defects Research. Part B, Developmental and Reproductive Toxicology*, *68*(2), 125–136. https://doi.org/10.1002/BDRB.10015.

Meng, F., Hao, H., Guo, Z., Liu, W., Zhang, S., Tang, W., Ma, W., & Shang, X. (2023). Silica nanoparticles induces sperm granuloma formation and blood-epididymal barrier disruption via the p38 MAPK pathway in mice. *Food and Chemical Toxicology*, *182*, 114113. https://doi.org/10.1016/J.FCT.2023.114113.

Orgebin-Crist, M. C. (1967). Sperm maturation in rabbit epididymis. *Nature*, *216*(5117), 816–818. https://doi.org/10.1038/216816A0.

Picut, C. A., & Remick, A. K. (2016). Male Reproductive System. *Atlas of Histology of the Juvenile Rat*, 227–256. https://doi.org/10.1016/B978-0-12-802682-3.00008-2.

Plant, T. M., Ramaswamy, S., & De Gendt, K. (2016). Endocrine Control of Spermatogenesis. In *Encyclopedia of Endocrine Diseases* (pp. 684–691). Academic Press. https://doi.org/10.1016/B978-0-12-801238-3.98871-8.

Ramírez-González, J. A., & Sansone, A. (2022). Male reproductive system. In *Fertility, Pregnancy, and Wellness*. https://doi.org/10.1016/B978-0-12-818309-0.00006-X.

Rehfeld, A., Nylander, M., & Karnov, K. (2017). The Male Reproductive System. In *Compendium of Histology*. https://doi.org/10.1007/978-3-319-41873-5_26.

Roberts, K. P., & Chauvin, T. R. (2018). Gene Regulation in the Epididymis. In *Encyclopedia of Reproduction* (pp. 298–304). Academic Press. https://doi.org/10.1016/B978-0-12-801238-3.64370-2.

Roy, J. W., Hill, E., Ruan, Y. C., Vedovelli, L., Păunescu, T. G., Brown, D., & Breton, S. (2013). Circulating aldosterone induces the apical accumulation of the proton pumping V-ATPase and increases proton secretion in clear cells in the caput epididymis. *American Journal of Physiology - Cell Physiology*, *305*(4), C436. https://doi.org/10.1152/AJPCELL.00410.2012.

Suede, S. H., Malik, A., & Sapra, A. (2023). Histology, Spermatogenesis. In *StatPearls*. StatPearls Publishing. https://www.ncbi.nlm.nih.gov/books/NBK553142/.

Sullivan, R., & Belleannée, C. (2018). Cell Biology of the Epididymis. In *Encyclopedia of Reproduction* (pp. 286–291). Academic Press. https://doi.org/10.1016/B978-0-12-801238-3.64368-4.

Sullivan, R., Frenette, G., & Girouard, J. (2007). Epididymosomes are involved in the acquisition of new sperm proteins during epididymal transit. *Asian Journal of Andrology*, *9*(4), 483–491. https://doi.org/10.1111/J.1745-7262.2007.00281.X.

Yanagimachi, R., Kamiguchi, Y., Mikamo, K., Suzuki, F., & Yanagimachi, H. (1985). Maturation of spermatozoa in the epididymis of the Chinese hamster. *The American Journal of Anatomy*, *172*(4), 317–330. https://doi.org/10.1002/AJA.1001720406.

Yazğan, B., Yazğan, Y., Üniversitesi, S., Fakültesi, T., Demirel Üniversitesi, S., Adresi, Y., Yazğan Selçuk Üniversitesi, B., Fakültesi Blok, T. E., & Anabilim Dalı, F. (n.d.). *Antioksidan redoks sistemi üzerinde metallotionin ve çinko i lişkisinin önemi Importance of relationship metallothioneins and zinc on the antioxidant redox system*.

Zhang, M., Li, H., Ma, J., Yang, C., Yang, Y., Zhao, B., Tie, Y., & Wang, S. (2024). Effects of Zinc Combined with Metformin on Zinc Homeostasis, Blood-Epididymal Barrier, and Epididymal Absorption in Male Diabetic Mice. *Biological Trace Element Research*, 1–14. https://doi.org/10.1007/S12011-024-04171-Y/FIGURES/5.

Zhao, H., Yu, C., He, C., Mei, C., Liao, A., & Huang, D. (2020). The Immune Characteristics of the Epididymis and the Immune Pathway of the Epididymitis Caused by Different Pathogens. *Frontiers in Immunology*, *11*, 576472. https://doi.org/10.3389/FIMMU.2020.02115/BIBTEX.

Chapter 4

The Blood-Urine Barrier

Muhammet Volkan Bulbul[1,*], PhD
and Semiha Mervenur Kalender[2], MS
[1]Department of Histology and Embryology, Agri İbrahim Cecen University, Agri, Turkiye
[2]Department of Histology and Embryology, Istanbul Medipol University, Istanbul, Turkiye

Abstract

In addition to storing urine, the bladder prevents the diffusion of toxic components it contains. It performs this task thanks to the urothelium added to its structure. Urothelium is a multilayered epithelial structure that covers the inner surface of the bladder. The blood-urine barrier function of the bladder is directly related to the function of the urothelium, which consists of basal, intermediate and superficial cells. Superficial cells of the urothelium have tight junction structures that are the basis of the paracellular permeability barrier of the bladder. Tight junctions play a critical role in maintaining the urine-blood barrier by functioning as a barrier to the passage of various chemicals between urine and blood. In this section, bladder histology, urothelium histology, expression products of the cells that form the blood-urine barrier, and the functions of tight junction proteins are discussed.

Keywords: urothelium, tight junction, urine, bladder, permeability

---

* Corresponding Author's Email: mvbulbul@agri.edu.tr

In: A Histological Approach to Human Body Barriers
Editor: İlknur Keskin
ISBN: 979-8-89530-738-0

Introduction

The urinary system (US) consists of kidneys, renal pelvis, ureters, urinary bladder, urethra structures, and its main function is to create urine by providing filtration of blood. US plays a critical role in fluid removal of urea and other liquid wastes. In addition, liquid and electrolyte balance in the body is maintained with chemicals such as sodium and potassium. Although low levels of urea are produced by various tissues, it is primarily produced by urea cycle enzymes in the liver (Wang et al., 2014). Urea is then transported through the bloodstream to the kidneys, where it is removed in the form of urine along with water and other wastes (Yu et al., 2019). Following a series of complex filtration processes that take place in the nephrons and glomerulus structures, which are the functional units of the kidneys, urine is transferred to the urinary bladder (UB) via the ureters. UB serves as a storage and elimination organ for urine (Shen et al., 2021).

UB is located in the extraperitoneal space of the pelvis behind the pubic bones and extends into the abdomen when filled with urine. Anatomically, the upper part above the ureteral openings consists of the apex and body, and the lower part consists of the fundus, trigone and neck. It simulates afferent signals when the bladder is full. Efferent signals then cause the bladder musculature to contract, followed by relaxation of the urethral sphincter (Bolla et al., 2019).

Histologically, the UB consists of epithelium, lamina propria, muscularis propria, serosa/adventitia sections. The epithelium of the urinary bladder is of a specialized multilayered epithelium type and known as urothelium. Urothelium is found in structures that communicate with urine, such as the ureter, bladder and proximal urethra (Abelson et al., 2018; Walz et al., 1995). According to the polarity of the cells in the urothelium structure, it is divided into three layers: apical, intermediate and basal. When the bladder is empty, the urothelium thickens by five to seven structural layers. When the bladder fills with urine, the bladder wall stretches to accommodate the increased volume. The urothelium can rearrange into three layers in the dilated bladder without structural damage. Because of this ability, urothelium is also known as transitional epithelium (Bolla et al., 2023).

Considering that the bladder stores urine with potentially harmful levels of urea, ammonia, and other toxic metabolites for long periods of time, the impermeability of the urothelium is essential for the functioning of normal physiological processes in all mammals (Lasič et al., 2015). Urothelium can respond to chemical and mechanical stimuli, secreting chemical mediators (nitric oxide (NO), adenosine triphosphate (ATP) and prostaglandins) (Birder et al., 2003; Birder et al., 2001; Birder et al., 2002; Burnstock, 2001; Ferguson et al., 1997). Urothelium is a multifunctional epithelium that also plays a role in sensory transmission, and its most important function is to form the blood-urine barrier (Lasič et al., 2015).

The blood-urine barrier, formed during the differentiation of the superficial cells of the urothelium, is the tightest and most impermeable barrier in the body. The barrier in the bladder must resist large changes in surface area during stretching and contraction of the organ. The tight junctions of the superficial cells of the urothelium and the apical plasma membrane play a critical role in maintaining the barrier. Most urinary tract diseases are caused by changes in blood-urine barrier function (Kreft et al., 2010).

The mammalian bladder maintains high electrochemical exchanges between urine and blood, allowing the kidney to alter body chemistry through urinary excretion. To fulfill this function, the urothelium provides a tight permeability barrier (Lavelle et al., 2002). When this barrier is damaged, urine components may leak into the underlying bladder layers and mix with the blood, resulting in various diseases. Additionally, the urothelium prevents overactivity, inflammation, and fibrosis of the bladder detrusor muscle. Disrupted urothelium leads to common urological diseases such as bladder cancer, overactive bladder, urinary tract infections, interstitial cystitis, urethral injuries or strictures (Akkad et al., 2007; Wan et al., 2018).

In this section, bladder histology and especially the urothelium, which plays a critical role in the establishment of the blood-urine barrier, are examined in detail. The connection proteins participating in the barrier structure and the expression products of the cells in the barrier were mentioned by histochemical staining. Additionally, the functioning of paracellular and transcellular pathways related to barrier permeability was mentioned.

Bladder Histology and Urothelium

Histologically, it can be said that the bladder wall is divided into five layers. These are listed from outside to inside as serosa/adventitia, muscularis propria, lamina propria, lining epithelium (urothelium). Adventitia is the loose connective tissue layer in the outer layer of the bladder that is not continuous with any tissue and does not contain serosa. Serosa is the outer layer consisting of thin connective tissue that covers the upper part of the bladder and continues with the peritoneum and contains blood vessels of various sizes (Sánchez Freire et al., 2011).

Muscularis propria is the muscle layer. It may also be called the Detrusor muscle. Muscularis propria is divided into three parts. The inner and outer parts consist of longitudinal muscle cells, and the middle part consists of circular muscle cells. This distinction between inner, middle and outer layers can be clearly distinguished in the neck region of the bladder. However, a random arrangement is seen in other parts of the bladder wall. In the body part of the bladder, more dense smooth muscle content and a well-developed myofibroblast network are found than in the trigone part (Bolla et al., 2019).

The lamina propria, also called as the suburothelial layer, is a loose connective tissue layer located between the urothelium and the muscularis propria. The overlying urothelium cells are separated from the lamina propria by the basal membrane. The lamina propria is a highly heterogeneous layer consisting of adipocytes, interstitial cells of Cajal or telocytes, capillaries, immune cells, elastic fibers, lymphatics, fibroblasts, myofibroblasts and afferent and efferent nerve endings. Interstitial cells of Cajal form a syncytium with smooth muscle cells and nerve endings. They also serve as nerve signal transmitters to the smooth muscle cells of the bladder (Andersson et al., 2014).

Urothelium, also called uroepithelium, is a transitional and stratified type of epithelium (Winder et al., 2014). Almost all epithelial cells are responsible for basic functions such as repair, cleaning, secretion, transport and sensation. They also form diffusion barriers with different permeabilities, either leaky or tight (Shashikanth et al., 2017) (Figure 1).

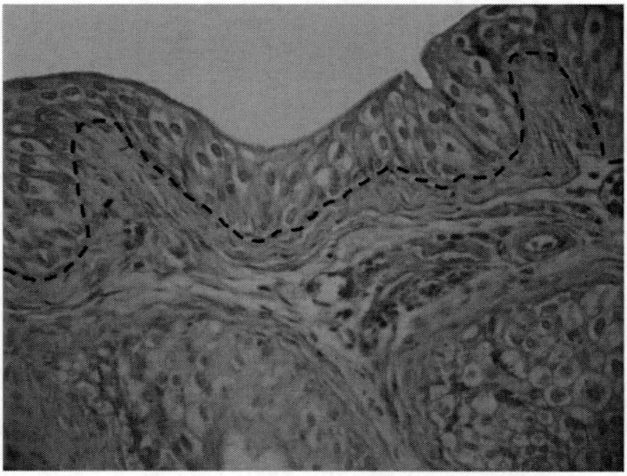

Figure 1. Transitional epithelium in mouse bladder. (Black dashed lines delineate the area, H-E staining, and 40X magnification).

The reason why it is defined as transitional is due to the ability of the urothelium to transition into different forms when the bladder is full or empty. This layer provides a barrier function by preventing the absorption of toxic substances such as urea and acid in the urine and the entry of pathogens from the environment (Hicks, 1975; Song & Abraham, 2008; Yu & Hill, 2011). Urothelium consists of three different cell types and layers: basal, intermediate, and superficial. Basal cells on the basement membrane are the least differentiated cells that essentially play the role of progenitor cells. Intermediate cells are cells with high proliferative properties and may consist of more than one layer, depending on the species. In various pathological conditions, intermediate cells are responsible for the regeneration of the urothelium (Jafari & Rohn, 2022). Superficial cells are the cells located apically in contact with urine. They can also be described as umbrella cells, cap cells and superficial urotheliocytes. Umbrella cells are the principal cells that provide a resistant barrier function by ensuring the high impermeability of the urothelium (Jaimes-Parra et al., 2016; Osborn & Kurzrock, 2015; Winder et al., 2014).

Although basal cells are the smallest cells of the urothelium, with a diameter of 5-10 μm, they outnumber other cells in the adult urothelium (Balsara & Li, 2017). They are located along the basement membrane and are connected directly to the basement membrane by hemidesmosomes and to the upper intermediate cells by desmosomes (Borradori & Sonnenberg, 1999; Jones, 2001; Owaribe et al., 1990). They exhibit stem cell potential that enables regeneration of the urothelium throughout life (Osborn & Kurzrock, 2015).

The thickness of the intermediate cell layer varies depending on the species.(Hicks, 1975). While humans have five intermediate cell layers, rodents have a single layer (Jost et al., 1989; Wu et al., 2009). Intermediate cells are significantly larger than basal cells, with a diameter of approximately 20 μm (Jost et al., 1989). They are connected to the lower basal cells, the upper umbrella cells, and each other through desmosomes (Jost et al., 1989). In some studies, it has been stated that intermediate cells may have the potential of undifferentiated precursor cells that have the ability to differentiate into umbrella cells, just like basal cells (Yamany et al., 2014; Yu & Hill, 2011).

Highly differentiated superficial umbrella cells form the layer directly communicating with the lumen (Yamany et al., 2014). They are hexagonal-shaped polarized cells whose diameters can vary from 25 to 250 μm depending on the distension state of the bladder (Khandelwal et al., 2009). They may be multinucleated in some rodent species such as rats and guinea pigs. (Apodaca,

2004). Umbrella cells are long-lived and can regenerate rapidly when the uroepithelium is damaged. Regeneration can result from cell division in any of the three cell layers (Hicks, 1975; Petry & Amon, 1966). In the relaxed state where the bladder is empty, they are called umbrella cells because they can form a dome at the apical pole and cover the intermediate cells in the lower layer (Jost et al., 1989). When the bladder is full, they expand and flatten. Umbrella cells essentially form a highly resistant blood-urine barrier by connecting to the cells in the lower layer through desmosomes and to each other through tight junctions, closing the intercellular space (Acharya et al., 2004; Khandelwal et al., 2009). Umbrella cells are the only urothelial layer that forms tight, adherent junctions (Dalghi et al., 2020). They contain ZO-1, occludin, claudin-4, 8 and 12 as tight junction proteins (Acharya et al., 2004; Smith et al., 2015). The barrier includes the apical membrane, tight junctions, and an active traffic mechanism (Negrete et al., 1996; Truschel et al., 1999; Zeidel, 1996). The apical membrane consists of four interrelated transmembrane proteins. These are uroplakins, which exhibit low permeability to water thanks to their lipid structure; small non-electrolytes; and protons (Wu et al., 1990; Yu et al., 1990). In a healthy state, umbrella cells express abundant uroplakin. Uroplakin proteins (UPKs) are tetraspanin membrane proteins (Wu et al., 1990). Today, five types are recognized: UPK1A, UPK1B, UPK2, UPK3A and UPK3B (Deng et al., 2002; Wu et al., 1995; Wu et al., 1990; Yu et al., 1994). Uroplakin covers up to 90% of the luminal surface, providing impermeability to water, solutes and toxins (Kachar et al., 1999; Sun et al., 1996). The glycocalyx structure, consisting of uroplakins as well as proteoglycans and glycosaminoglycans (GAG), protects the urothelium from pathogens and toxicants in the urine content (Lilly et al., 1990). GAG contains heparin sulfate, dermatan sulfate, chondroitin sulfate, hyaluronic acid and keratan sulfate. The key ingredients chondroitin sulfate and hyaluronic acid take part in antibacterial defense (Klingler, 2016).

Expression Products of Urothelium Cells

Cells belonging to various layers of the urothelium have common or different proteins, signaling molecules, transcription factors, etc. These differences play a role in determining their specialized functions and distinguishing them from each other at histological and molecular levels. Although numerous markers of urothelial differentiation exist, only a small number have been classified and generally described in mice. Essentially, signaling/transcription factors such as FOX2A, Tp63, Shh, UPK and cytokeratins are included in the classification (Jafari & Rohn, 2022). The increase in lumen surface area due to urothelial distention that occurs with bladder filling requires mechanical support to resist tension (Jafari & Rohn, 2022). Cytokeratins, as cytoskeletal filaments, play a role in protecting urothelial cells against such mechanical stress (Coulombe et al., 2000) (Galou et al., 1997). Cytokeratins differ from other known cytoskeletal filaments in that their flexibility increases in response to tension. When the tension ends and the bladder is emptied, they can quickly return to their previous form (Coulombe et al., 2000). Although many different types of cytokeratins are expressed in the urothelium, expression levels are variable and vary depending on location (Alonso et al., 2009; Erman et al., 2006; Liang et al., 2005; Riedel et al., 2005; Troyanovsky et al., 1989; Veranic & Jezernik, 2006; Veranič et al., 2002). CK7, CK8, CK18 and CK19 expression is present in all parts of the urothelium in adult humans (Moll et al., 1982). CK20 expression is specifically associated with umbrella cells (Achtstätter et al., 1985; Moll et al., 1988). In addition, although CK13 is found in intermediate and basal cells, it can be used as a marker of transitional cells differentiated from basal cells (Fishwick et al., 2017).

Basal cells located in the basal layer express high levels of Sonic hedgehog, p63, cytokeratin-5 (CK5), CK17, while being negative for CK20 and UPKs (Gandhi et al., 2013; Romih et al., 1998; Shin et al., 2011; Yu & Hill, 2011).

Intermediate cells are similar to umbrella cells in that, unlike basal cells, they are negative for CK5 and positive for UPK (Wu et al., 2009; Wu et al., 1994). They can also express p63, unlike umbrella cells (Balsara & Li, 2017). Additionally, intermediate cells have been shown to express junctional proteins such as clauidins and E-cadherins (Khandelwal et al., 2009). However, when evaluated histologically, it is not obvious that they form functionally tight or adhesive connections between each other (Dalghi et al., 2020).

Umbrella cells are highly positive for CK20 and UPKs and negative for CK5, CK14, p63, and Shh (Jafari & Rohn, 2022). As mentioned before, mammalian superficial umbrella cells synthesize UPK1A, UPK1B, UPK2, UPK3A and form a crystal lattice in the apical membrane (Jackson et al., 2020; LIANG et al., 2001). These are the basic components of the unit membrane (AUM) that form the characteristic apical membrane (Wu et al., 2009). UPK1A dimerizes with UPK2 and forms heterodimers with UPK1B, UPK3A, and UPK3B (Deng et al., 2002; Wu et al., 1995; Wu et al., 1990; Yu et al., 1994). Organized as a result of processes in the endoplasmic reticulum and

Golgi complex, six heterotetradimers in the inner and outer rings are packaged into discoidal/fusiform shaped vesicles and form a 16 nm AUM particle directed to the apical membrane (Min et al., 2006; Tu et al., 2002). AUM particles enable the formation of urothelial plaque. Junction complexes and the urothelial plate are the basic elements that ensure the high resistance of the barrier. A recent transcriptomic study of mouse urothelium revealed a new cell population rich in the Plxna4 gene (Li et al., 2021). Although this cell cluster also exhibited UPK3 expression, causing them to be considered umbrella cells, the fact that they were negative for CK20 eliminated this hypothesis and enabled them to be defined as a different urothelial cell group (Li et al., 2021). Another feature that distinguishes umbrella cells from basal and intermediate cells is their subapical discoidal/fusiform vesicles (DFVs) (Jost et al., 1989). DFVs contribute to plasticity in the cell surface area through endocytosis and exocytosis (Khandelwal et al., 2008; Yu et al., 2009). DFVs fuse with the apical membranes of umbrella cells and play a role in the release of UPK and other proteins in response to bladder filling. Thus, expansion of the urothelium is achieved (Khandelwal et al., 2013; Truschel et al., 2002; Zhou et al., 2012). When the bladder empties, the opposite mechanism occurs and the urothelial surface area decreases. CK20 cells trigger the directing of DVFs to the surface (Veranič et al., 2002).

Tight Junction Organization of the Barrier

The barrier structure essentially consists of three parts: apical, lateral and basal barrier. The apical membrane barrier is the part where AUM particles combine in the form of hexagonal plates to form UPK. At the molecular level, the tight junction structure consists of three groups with different functions: integral proteins, peripheral proteins (ZO-1, ZO-2, ZO-3, AF6, MUPP-1) and tight junction-associated proteins (Haynes et al., 2005). Occludin, claudins and JAMs (junctional adhesion molecules) belong to the group of integral proteins and cover the plasma membrane, forming complexes with the same proteins of neighboring cells (Martin & Jiang, 2001). Tight junctions between umbrella cells form lateral barriers. The basal membrane is provided by a group of proteins including laminins, claudins, and cadherins (Klingler, 2016). Apical connections also contain three complexes; the first is the apical tight junction or zonula occludens, formed by claudins and associated with the actin cytoskeleton and other cytoplasmic proteins; the second is the zonula adherens, consisting of cadherins and catenins; the third consists of desmosomes or macula adherens (Franke, 2009; Garcia et al., 2018; Pinheiro & Bellaiche, 2018).

Tight junctions (TJs) are critical in establishing the blood-urine barrier by controlling the passage of substances between urine and blood. TJs play a role in separating different functional parts of the plasma membrane, cell signalling, cell-cell adhesion, preventing cell migration, and controlling cell permeability (Martin & Jiang, 2001). TJs are located at the most apical part of the lateral plasma membrane and provide the distinction between the apical plasma membrane and lateral plasma membrane (Haynes et al., 2005) (Figure 1). Freeze-fracture electron microscopy micrographs reveal that TJs are characterized by 4–6 interrelated protein junctions located between adjacent umbrella cells of the urothelium (Peter & research, 1978). TJs between adjacent umbrella cells separate the plasma membrane from the basolateral membrane, creating a zone of resistance for transcellular ion permeation along with uroplakins (Clausen et al., 1979).

In addition to restricting the lateral diffusion of lipids and proteins by separating the apical-basolateral membranes, TJs have a second function (Lewis & Diamond, 1976; Lewis, 2000; Zihni et al., 2016). This is to regulate the intracellular diffusion of other molecules and ions (Claude, 1978; Easter et al., 1983; Madara & Pappenheimer, 1987; Schneeberger & McCormack, 1984). TJs have two different transmembrane proteins, claudins and occludins, and these form homotypic occludin-occludin, clauidin-clauidin complexes (Van Itallie & Anderson, 2014).

Different isoforms of clauidin exist. Their combination regulates the permeability of ions of different charges and sizes, allowing the separation of claudins into barrier-forming and pore-forming (Van Itallie & Anderson, 2006). Claudin 1 is the type that is expressed in many tissue types (Saitou et al., 1998), has a barrier-forming function (Inai et al., 1999; McCarthy et al., 2000) and is located along the basal and intermediate cell membranes (Freire et al., 2010; Sánchez Freire et al., 2011). Claudin 2 provides a cation-selective pore (Amasheh et al., 2002; Hou et al., 2006; Van Itallie et al., 2008) structure called leaky epithelium in the proximal tubule and intestinal crypts (Enck et al., 2001; Holmes et al., 2006; Muto et al., 2010). Claudin 3 is especially necessary for the formation of tight junctions at the terminals of umbrella cells in the human urothelium (Smith et al., 2015). Different studies have shown that claudin 4 participates in the barrier structure (Lejeune et al., 2011; Michikawa et al., 2008) and is expressed higher in the umbrella and intermediate layers than in basal cells (Törzsök et al., 2011). Claudin 5 is localized at the boundaries between the plasma membranes of umbrella cells

(Törzsök et al., 2011; Varley et al., 2006). Claudin 7 is expressed in the plasma membrane of all cells in the three layers of the urothelium (Nakanishi et al., 2008). Also, Claudin 7 participates in the barrier structure in humans by showing a claudin 4-like distribution outside the umbrella cells (Alan et al., 2003; Boireau et al., 2007; Varley et al., 2006). Claudin 8 is another claudin type that participates in the barrier structure by localizing to the TJs of umbrella cells (Carattino et al., 2013; Hu & Song, 2019). Apart from these, it has been reported that Claudin 11 is found in RT112/84 cells (Awsare et al., 2011), Clauidin 12, 14, and 16 are found in TEU-2 cells (Rickard et al., 2008), and Clauidin 13 is found in mRNA form in mouse bladder tissue (Acharya et al., 2004).

The Transcellular and Paracellular Pathway

In the cells of the urothelium, two parallel resistance transcellular pathways extend in series across the apical and basolateral plasma membranes (Claude, 1978; Powell & Physiology, 1981). The intracellular cytoplasm is part of the transcellular pathway. It has a resistance of up to 150,000 Ωcm^2, which is negligible (Lewis & Diamond, 1976). Transcellular transport is accomplished by transporters and channels. While it can be passive or active, it has direction and is energy dependent (Anderson, 2001). Electrodiffusion occurs through conductive channels, while electroneutral and electrogenic primary and secondary active transport occur(Frings et al., 1990).

Although paracellular transport is passive, it occurs by diffusion and osmosis and has no directional discrimination (Anderson, 2001). The paracellular resistance of the urothelium consists of two resistances in series: the cell-cell junctions and the intercellular cleft (Claude, 1978; Powell & Physiology, 1981). The resistance of the intercellular space is less than 10% of the total intracellular resistance (Claude, 1978). The length of the lateral intercellular space provides resistance in series with the lateral plasma membrane. This gap is very small (0.68 nm) (Clausen et al., 1979). The current of the paracellular pathway depends on the ratio of its two pathways per unit area of the epithelial surface, as well as the resistance of the pathway. The amount of connectivity per unit area of epithelium depends on the size and packing of the cells. The diameters of superficial urothelium cells vary between 25 and 250 μm (Fadda et al., 1998). Within 24 hours after injury, some superficial urothelium cells have been shown to flatten and stretch. Their length may be three times greater than that of normal-sized superficial urothelium cells (150-300 μm) (Kreft et al., 2005). Superficial urothelium cells have fewer cell-cell contacts per unit area and are arranged hexagonally (Anderson & Van Itallie, 2009; Claude, 1978; Jerman et al., 2014). Adjacent cells connect to each other, increasing the amount of connections per unit area. Interdigitations, which act as membrane zippers at the borders of superficial urothelium cells, contribute to the barrier function. Membrane overlap connects two cells by providing more apical membrane surface contact because it does not involve tight junctions. Additionally, these overlaps can stabilize tight connections by increasing the electrical resistance of the connection (Kreplak et al., 2007; Višnjar et al., 2012; Višnjar et al., 2013).

The main pathway for passive ion permeability is through cell junctions, and transepithelial resistance is a measure of ion permeability. The pithelium is classified according to the magnitude of transepithelial resistance and its relative resistance to transcellular and paracellular pathways. According to epithelium transepithelial resistance values, the epithelium is classified into four categories: leaky (6-133 Ωcm^2), medium firm (300-600 Ωcm^2), tight (365-2,000 Ωcm^2), and very tight (1,000-2,000 Ωcm^2) (Claude & Goodenough, 1973; Fromter & Diamond, 1972; Lewis, 2000). Based on this classification, the urothelium is a tight epithelium. Tight epithelium is able to maintain electrochemical gradients produced by active intracellular transport because it reduces passive leakage of ions. High-resistance epithelium has tight junctions with more filaments than low-resistance epithelium (Fromter & Diamond, 1972). This shows that there is a relationship between the number of tight junction strands and passive resistance (Claude, 1978; Furuse et al., 2001). It is known that Clauidins in the tight junction structure play an important role in the size of transepithelial conductance (Lasič et al., 2015).

Conclusion

Urothelium is a specialized epithelial layer composed of different cell layers. It has the ability to change size and shape depending on the change in urine volume. However, its most important function is to create a unique blood-urine barrier structure by preventing the passage of toxic substances and various pathogenic microorganisms. The causes of chronic urinary tract diseases and various dysfunctions can be closely associated with deterioration or damage in the urothelium structure. In previous studies, studies were carried out on the structure and function of the blood-urine barrier, specifically the urothelium. However, the changes that occur in the urothelium structure with age, its role in the pathogenesis of urinary tract diseases, structural changes caused by gender differences, and changes between species need to be revealed in more comprehensive studies. In the coming years, with the development of integrated organoid technologies, the urothelium structures to be mimicked will enable us to deeply understand the histology and physiology of the normal blood-urine barrier.

References

Abelson, B., Sun, D., Que, L., Nebel, R. A., Baker, D., Popiel, P.,…DiSanto, M. J. B. o. s. d. (2018). Sex differences in lower urinary tract biology and physiology. *9*, 1-13. doi:10.1186/s13293-018-0204-8.

Acharya, P., Beckel, J., Ruiz, W. G., Wang, E., Rojas, R., Birder, L., & Apodaca, G. J. A. J. o. P.-R. P. (2004). Distribution of the tight junction proteins ZO-1, occludin, and claudin-4,-8, and-12 in bladder epithelium. *287*(2), F305-F318. doi: 10.1152/ajprenal.00341.2003.

Achtstätter, T., Moll, R., Moore, B., Franke, W. W. J. J. o. H., & Cytochemistry. (1985). Cytokeratin polypeptide patterns of different epithelia of the human male urogenital tract: immunofluorescence and gel electrophoretic studies. *33*(5), 415-426. doi: 10.1177/33.5.2580881.

Akkad, T., Pelzer, A. E., Mitterberger, M., Rehder, P., Leonhartsberger, N., Bartsch, G., & Strasser, H. J. B. i. (2007). Influence of intravesical potassium on pelvic floor activity in women with recurrent urinary tract infections: comparative urodynamics might lead to enhanced detection of dysfunctional voiding. *100*(5), 1071-1074. doi: 10.1111/j.1464-410X.2007.07120.x.

Alan, S., Enck, A. H., Lencer, W. I., & Schneeberger, E. E. J. J. o. B. C. (2003). Claudin-8 expression in Madin-Darby canine kidney cells augments the paracellular barrier to cation permeation. *278*(19), 17350-17359. doi: 10.1074/jbc.M213286200.

Alonso, A., Ikinger, U., Kartenbeck, J. J. H., & histopathology. (2009). Staining patterns of keratins in the human urinary tract. doi: 10.14670/HH-24.1425.

Amasheh, S., Meiri, N., Gitter, A. H., Schöneberg, T., Mankertz, J., Schulzke, J. r. D., & Fromm, M. J. J. o. c. s. (2002). Claudin-2 expression induces cation-selective channels in tight junctions of epithelial cells. *115*(24), 4969-4976. doi: 10.1242/jcs.00165.

Anderson, J. M., & Van Itallie, C. M. J. C. S. H. p. i. b. (2009). Physiology and function of the tight junction. *1*(2), a002584. doi: 10.1101/cshperspect.a002584.

Anderson, J. M. J. P. (2001). Molecular structure of tight junctions and their role in epithelial transport. *16*(3), 126-130. doi: 10.1152/physiologyonline.2001.16.3.126.

Andersson, K. E., McCloskey, K. D. J. N., & urodynamics. (2014). Lamina propria: the functional center of the bladder? , *33*(1), 9-16. doi: 10.1002/nau.22465.

Apodaca, G. J. T. (2004). The uroepithelium: not just a passive barrier. *5*(3), 117-128. doi: 10.1046/j.1600-0854.2003.00156.x.

Awsare, N. S., Martin, T. A., Haynes, M. D., Matthews, P. N., & Jiang, W. G. J. O. r. (2011). Claudin-11 decreases the invasiveness of bladder cancer cells. *25*(6), 1503-1509. doi: 10.3892/or.2011.1244.

Balsara, Z. R., & Li, X. J. A. J. o. P.-R. P. (2017). Sleeping beauty: awakening urothelium from its slumber. *312*(4), F732-F743. doi: 10.1152/ajprenal.00337.2016.

Birder, L., Barrick, S., Roppolo, J., Kanai, A., De Groat, W., Kiss, S., & Buffington, C. J. A. J. o. P.-R. P. (2003). Feline interstitial cystitis results in mechanical hypersensitivity and altered ATP release from bladder urothelium. *285*(3), F423-F429. doi: 10.1152/ajprenal.00056.2003.

Birder, L. A., Kanai, A. J., De Groat, W. C., Kiss, S., Nealen, M. L., Burke, N. E.,…Caterina, M. J. J. P. o. t. N. A. o. S. (2001). Vanillcid receptor expression suggests a sensory role for urinary bladder epithelial cells. *98*(23), 13396-13401. doi: 10.1073/pnas.231243698.

Birder, L. A., Nealen, M. L., Kiss, S., De Groat, W. C., Caterina, M. J., Wang, E.,…Kanai, A. J. J. J. o. N. (2002). β-Adrenoceptor agonists stimulate endothelial nitric oxide synthase in rat urinary bladder urothelial cells. *22*(18), 8063-8070. doi: 10.1523/JNEUROSCI.22-18-08063.2002.

Boireau, S., Buchert, M., Samuel, M. S., Pannequin, J., Ryan, J. L., Choquet, A.,…Ernst, M. J. C. (2007). DNA-methylation-dependent alterations of claudin-4 expression in human bladder carcinoma. *28*(2), 246-258. doi: 10.1093/carcin/bgl120.

Bolla, S. R., Odeluga, N., Amraei, R., & Jetti, R. (2023). *Histology, Bladder*. StatPearls Publishing, Treasure Island (FL). http://europepmc.org/abstract/MED/31082007. http://europepmc.org/books/NBK540963. https://www.ncbi.nlm.nih.gov/books/NBK540963.

Bolla, S. R., Odeluga, N., & Jetti, R. (2019). Histology, bladder.

Borradori, L., & Sonnenberg, A. J. J. o. i. d. (1999). Structure and function of hemidesmosomes: more than simple adhesion complexes. *112*(4), 411-418. doi: 10.1046/j.1523-1747.1999.00546.x.

Burnstock, G. J. T. i. p. s. (2001). Purine-mediated signalling in pain and visceral perception. *22*(4), 182-188. doi: 10.1016/s0165-6147(00)01643-6.

Carattino, M. D., Prakasam, H. S., Ruiz, W. G., Clayton, D. R., McGuire, M., Gallo, L. I., & Apodaca, G. J. A. J. o. P.-R. P. (2013). Bladder filling and voiding affect umbrella cell tight junction organization and function. *305*(8), F1158-F1168. doi: 10.1152/ajprenal.00282.2013.

Claude, P., & Goodenough, D. A. J. T. J. o. c. b. (1973). Fracture faces of zonulae occludentes from" tight" and" leaky" epithelia. *58*(2), 390-400. doi: 10.1083/jcb.58.2.390.

Claude, P. J. T. J. o. m. b. (1978). Morphological factors influencing transepithelial permeability: a model for the resistance of the zonula occludens. *39*, 219-232. doi: 10.1007/BF01870332.

Clausen, C., Lewis, S. A., & Diamond, J. M. J. B. j. (1979). Impedance analysis of a tight epithelium using a distributed resistance model. *26*(2), 291-317. doi: 10.1016/S0006-3495(79)85250-9.

Coulombe, P. A., Bousquet, O., Ma, L., Yamada, S., & Wirtz, D. J. T. i. c. b. (2000). The 'ins' and 'outs' of intermediate filament organization. *10*(10), 420-428. doi: 10.1016/s0962-8924(00)01828-6.

Dalghi, M. G., Montalbetti, N., Carattino, M. D., & Apodaca, G. J. P. r. (2020). The urothelium: life in a liquid environment. *100*(4), 1621-1705 doi: 10.1152/physrev.00041.2019.

Deng, F.-M., Liang, F.-X., Tu, L., Resing, K. A., Hu, P., Supino, M.,…Kreibich, G. J. T. J. o. c. b. (2002). Uroplakin IIIb, a urothelial differentiation marker, dimerizes with uroplakin Ib as an early step of urothelial plaque assembly. *159*(4), 685-694. doi: 10.1083/jcb.200204102.

Easter, D. W., Wade, J. B., & Boyer, J. L. J. T. J. o. c. b. (1983). Structural integrity of hepatocyte tight junctions. *96*(3), 745-749. doi: 10.1083/jcb.96.3.745.

Enck, A. H., Berger, U. V., & Yu, A. S. J. A. J. o. P.-R. P. (2001). Claudin-2 is selectively expressed in proximal nephron in mouse kidney. *281*(5), F966-F974. doi: 10.1152/ajprenal.2001.281.5.F966.

Erman, A., Veranič, P., Pšeničnik, M., Jezernik, K. J. T., & Cell. (2006). Superficial cell differentiation during embryonic and postnatal development of mouse urothelium. *38*(5), 293-301. doi: 10.1016/j.tice.2006.07.001.

Fadda, L., Turriziani, P., Carlesimo, G. A., Nocentini, U., & Caltagirone, C. J. E. J. o. N. (1998). Selective proper name anomia in a patient with asymmetric cortical degeneration. *5*(4), 417-422.

Ferguson, D., Kennedy, I., & Burton, T. J. T. J. o. p. (1997). ATP is released from rabbit urinary bladder epithelial cells by hydrostatic pressure changes--a possible sensory mechanism? , *505*(Pt 2), 503. doi: 10.1111/j.1469-7793.1997.503bb.x.

Fishwick, C., Higgins, J., Percival-Alwyn, L., Hustler, A., Pearson, J., Bastkowski, S.,…Differentiation. (2017). Heterarchy of transcription factors driving basal and luminal cell phenotypes in human urothelium. *24*(5), 809-818. doi: 10.1038/cdd.2017.10.

Franke, W. W. J. C. S. H. p. i. b. (2009). Discovering the molecular components of intercellular junctions—a historical view. *1*(3), a003061. doi: 10.1101/cshperspect.a003061.

Freire, V. S., Burkhard, F. C., Kessler, T. M., Kuhn, A., Draeger, A., & Monastyrskaya, K. J. T. A. j. o. p. (2010). MicroRNAs may mediate the down-regulation of neurokinin-1 receptor in chronic bladder pain syndrome. *176*(1), 288-303. doi: 10.2353/ajpath.2010.090552.

Frings, S., Purves, R. D., Macknight, A. D. J. K., & Research, B. P. (1990). Ion channels in urinary bladder. *13*(1-2), 112-128. doi: 10.1159/000173352.

Fromter, E., & Diamond, J. J. N. N. B. (1972). Route of passive ion permeation in epithelia. *235*(53), 9-13.

Furuse, M., Furuse, K., Sasaki, H., & Tsukita, S. J. T. J. o. c. b. (2001). Conversion of zonulae occludentes from tight to leaky strand type by introducing claudin-2 into Madin-Darby canine kidney I cells. *153*(2), 263-272. doi: 10.1083/jcb.153.2.263.

Galou, M., Gao, J., Humbert, J., Mericskay, M., Li, Z., Paulin, D., & Vicart, P. J. B. o. t. C. (1997). The importance of intermediate filaments in the adaptation of tissues to mechanical stress: evidence from gene knockout studies. *89*(2), 85-97.

Gandhi, D., Molotkov, A., Batourina, E., Schneider, K., Dan, H., Reiley, M.,…Liao, Y. J. D. c. (2013). Retinoid signaling in progenitors controls specification and regeneration of the urothelium. *26*(5), 469-482. doi: 10.1016/j.devcel.2013.07.017.

Garcia, M. A., Nelson, W. J., & Chavez, N. J. C. S. H. p. i. b. (2018). Cell–cell junctions organize structural and signaling networks. *10*(4), a029181. doi: 10.1101/cshperspect.a029181.

Haynes, M. D., Martin, T. A., Jenkins, S. A., Kynaston, H. G., Matthews, P. N., & Jiang, W. G. J. I. j. o. m. m. (2005). Tight junctions and bladder cancer. *16*(1), 3-9.

Hicks, R. M. J. B. R. (1975). The mammalian urinary bladderan accommodating organ. *50*(2), 215-246. doi: 10.1111/j.1469-185x.1975.tb01057.x.

Holmes, J. L., Van Itallie, C. M., Rasmussen, J. E., & Anderson, J. M. J. G. E. P. (2006). Claudin profiling in the mouse during postnatal intestinal development and along the gastrointestinal tract reveals complex expression patterns. *6*(6), 581-588. doi: 10.1016/j.modgep.2005.12.001.

Hou, J., Gomes, A. S., Paul, D. L., & Goodenough, D. A. J. J. o. B. C. (2006). Study of claudin function by RNA interference. *281*(47), 36117-36123. doi: 10.1074/jbc.M608853200.

Hu, A., & Song, B.-L. J. C. o. i. c. b. (2019). The interplay of Patched, Smoothened and cholesterol in Hedgehog signaling. *61*, 31-38. doi: 10.1016/j.ceb.2019.06.008.

Inai, T., Kobayashi, J., & Shibata, Y. J. E. j. o. c. b. (1999). Claudin-1 contributes to the epithelial barrier function in MDCK cells. *78*(12), 849-855. doi: 10.1016/S0171-9335(99)80086-7.

Jackson, A. R., Ching, C. B., McHugh, K. M., & Becknell, B. J. N. R. U. (2020). Roles for urothelium in normal and aberrant urinary tract development. *17*(8), 459-468. doi: 10.1038/s41585-020-0348-2.

Jafari, N. V., & Rohn, J. L. J. M. I. (2022). The urothelium: a multi-faceted barrier against a harsh environment. *15*(6), 1127-1142. doi: 10.1038/s41385-022-00565-0.

Jaimes-Parra, B. D., Valle-Díaz de la Guardia, F., Arrabal-Polo, M. Á., Herrera-Imbroda, B., Lara, M. F., Machuca-Santa-Cruz, F. J.,…Garzón, I. J. I. J. o. U. (2016). Ex vivo construction of a novel model of bioengineered bladder mucosa: A preliminary study. *23*(1), 85-92. doi: 10.1111/iju.12963.

Jerman, U. D., Veranič, P., & Kreft, M. E. J. T. E. P. C. M. (2014). Amniotic membrane scaffolds enable the development of tissue-engineered urothelium with molecular and ultrastructural properties comparable to that of native urothelium. *20*(4), 317-327. doi: 10.1089/ten.TEC.2013.0298.

Jones, J. J. U. (2001). Hemidesmosomes in bladder epithelial cells. *57*(6), 103. doi: 10.1016/s0090-4295(01)01025-1.

Jost, S. P., Gosling, J. A., & Dixon, J. S. J. J. o. a. (1989). The morphology of normal human bladder urothelium. *167*, 103.

Kachar, B., Liang, F., Lins, U., Ding, M., Wu, X.-R., Stoffler, D ,…Sun, T.-T. J. J. o. m. b. (1999). Three-dimensional analysis of the 16 nm urothelial plaque particle: luminal surface exposure, preferential head-to-head interaction, and hinge formation. *285*(2), 595-608. doi: 10.1006/jmbi.1998.2304.

Khandelwal, P., Abraham, S. N., & Apodaca, G. J. A. J. o. P.-R. P. (2009). Cell biology and physiology of the uroepithelium. *297*(6), F1477-F1501. doi: 10.1152/ajprenal.00327.2009.

Khandelwal, P., Prakasam, H. S., Clayton, D. R., Ruiz, W. G., Gallo, L. I., van Roekel, D.,…Apodaca, G. J. M. b. o. t. c. (2013). A Rab11a-Rab8a-Myo5B network promotes stretch-regulated exocytosis in bladder umbrella cells. *24*(7), 1007-1019. doi: 10.1091/mbc.E12-08-0568.

Khandelwal, P., Ruiz, W. G., Balestreire-Hawryluk, E., Weisz, O. A., Goldenring, J. R., & Apodaca, G. J. P. o. t. N. A. o. S. (2008). Rab11a-dependent exocytosis of discoidal/fusiform vesicles in bladder umbrella cells. *105*(41), 15773-15778. doi: 10.1073/pnas.0805636105.

Klingler, C. H. J. U. J. (2016). Glycosaminoglycans: how much do we know about their role in the bladder? , *83*(1_suppl), 11-14. doi: 10.5301/uro.5000184.

Kreft, M. E., Hudoklin, S., Jezernik, K., & Romih, R. J. P. (2010). Formation and maintenance of blood–urine barrier in urothelium. *246*, 3-14. doi: 10.1007/s00709-010-0112-1.

Kreft, M. E., Sterle, M., Veranič, P., Jezernik, K. J. H., & biology, c. (2005). Urothelial injuries and the early wound healing response: tight junctions and urothelial cytodifferentiation. *123*, 529-539. doi: 10.1007/s00418-005-0770-9.

Kreplak, L., Wang, H., Aebi, U., & Kong, X.-P. J. J. o. m. b. (2007). Atomic force microscopy of mammalian urothelial surface. *374*(2), 365-373. doi: 10.1016/j.jmb.2007.09.040.

Lasič, E., Višnjar, T., Kreft, M. E. J. R. o. p., biochemistry, & pharmacology. (2015). Properties of the urothelium that establish the blood–urine barrier and their implications for drug delivery. 1-29. doi: 10.1007/112_2015_22.

Lavelle, J., Meyers, S., Ramage, R., Bastacky, S., Doty, D., Apodaca, G., & Zeidel, M. L. J. A. J. o. P.-R. P. (2002). Bladder permeability barrier: recovery from selective injury of surface epithelial cells. *283*(2), F242-F253. doi: 10.1152/ajprenal.00307.2001.

Lejeune, M., Moreau, F., & Chadee, K. J. T. A. j. o. p. (2011). Prostaglandin E2 produced by Entamoeba histolytica signals via EP4 receptor and alters claudin-4 to increase ion permeability of tight junctions. *179*(2), 807-818. doi: 10.1016/j.ajpath.2011.05.001.

Lewis, S. A., & Diamond, J. M. J. T. J. o. m. b. (1976). Na+ transport by rabbit urinary bladder, a tight epithelium. *28*, 1-40. doi: 10.1007/BF0186968.

Lewis, S. A. J. A. J. o. P.-R. P. (2000). Everything you wanted to know about the bladder epithelium but were afraid to ask. *278*(6), F867-F874. doi: 10.1152/ajprenal.2000.278.6.F867.

Li, Y., Liu, Y., Gao, Z., Zhang, L., Chen, L., Wu, Z.,…Chai, T. C. J. C. P. (2021). Single-cell transcriptomes of mouse bladder urothelium uncover novel cell type markers and urothelial differentiation characteristics. *54*(4), e13007. doi: 10.1111/cpr.13007.

Liang, F.-X., Bosland, M. C., Huang, H., Romih, R., Baptiste, S., Deng, F.-M.,…Sun, T.-T. J. T. J. o. c. b. (2005). Cellular basis of urothelial squamous metaplasia: roles of lineage heterogeneity and cell replacement. *171*(5), 835-844. doi: 10.1083/jcb.200505035.

Liang, F.-X., Riedel, I., Deng, F.-M., Zhou, G., Xu, C., Wu, X.-R.,…Sun, T.-T. J. B. J. (2001). Organization of uroplakin subunits: transmembrane topology, pair formation and plaque composition. *355*(1), 13-18. doi: 10.1042/0264-6021:3550013.

Lilly, J. D., Parsons, C. L. J. S., gynecology, & obstetrics. (1990). Bladder surface glycosaminoglycans is a human epithelial permeability barrier. *171*(6), 493-496.

Madara, J., & Pappenheimer, J. J. T. J. o. m. b. (1987). Structural basis for physiological regulation of paracellular pathways in intestinal epithelia. *100*, 149-164. doi: 10.1007/BF02209147.

Martin, T. A., & Jiang, W. G. (2001). Tight junctions and their role in cancer metastasis.

McCarthy, K., Francis, S., McCormack, J., Lai, J., Rogers, R., Skare, I.,…Schneeberger, E. J. J. o. c. s. (2000). Inducible expression of claudin-1-myc but not occludin-VSV-G results in aberrant tight junction strand formation in MDCK cells. *113*(19), 3387-3398. doi: 10.1242/jcs.113.19.3387.

Michikawa, H., Fujita-Yoshigaki, J., Sugiya, H. J. C., & research, t. (2008). Enhancement of barrier function by overexpression of claudin-4 in tight junctions of submandibular gland cells. *334*(2), 255-264. doi: 10.1007/s00441-008-0689-2.

Min, G., Wang, H., Sun, T.-T., & Kong, X.-P. J. T. J. o. c. b. (2006). Structural basis for tetraspanin functions as revealed by the cryo-EM structure of uroplakin complexes at 6-A resolution. *173*(6), 975-983. doi: 10.1083/jcb.200602086.

Moll, R., Achtstätter, T., Becht, E., Balcarova-Ständer, J., Ittensohn, M., & Franke, W. J. T. A. j. o. p. (1988). Cytokeratins in normal and malignant transitional epithelium. Maintenance of expression of urothelial differentiation features in transitional cell carcinomas and bladder carcinoma cell culture lines. *132*(1), 123.

Moll, R., Franke, W. W., Schiller, D. L., Geiger, B., & Krepler, R. J. C. (1982). The catalog of human cytokeratins: patterns of expression in normal epithelia, tumors and cultured cells. *31*(1), 11-24. doi: 10.1016/0092-8674(82)90400-7.

Muto, S., Hata, M., Taniguchi, J., Tsuruoka, S., Moriwaki, K., Saitou, M.,…Imai, M. J. P. o. t. N. A. o. S. (2010). Claudin-2–deficient mice are defective in the leaky and cation-selective paracellular permeability properties of renal proximal tubules. *107*(17), 8011-8016. doi: 10.1073/pnas.0912901107.

Nakanishi, K., Ogata, S., Hiroi, S., Tominaga, S., Aida, S., & Kawai, T. J. A. j. o. c. p. (2008). Expression of occludin and claudins 1, 3, 4, and 7 in urothelial carcinoma of the upper urinary tract. *130*(1), 43-49. doi: 10.1309/U77A6ETEXVCA5D0E.

Negrete, H., Lavelle, J., Berg, J., Lewis, S., & Zeidel, M. J. A. J. o. P.-R. P. (1996). Permeability properties of the intact mammalian bladder epithelium. *271*(4), F886-F894. doi: 10.1152/ajprenal.1996.271.4.F886.

Osborn, S. L., & Kurzrock, E. A. J. C. u. r. (2015). Production of urothelium from pluripotent stem cells for regenerative applications. *16*, 1-7. doi: 10.1007/s11934-014-0466-6.

Owaribe, K., Kartenbeck, J., Stumpp, S., Magin, T. M., Krieg, T., Diaz, L. A., & Franke, W. W. J. D. (1990). The hemidesmosomal plaque: I. Characterization of a major constituent protein as a differentiation marker for certain forms of epithelia. *45*(3), 207-220. doi: 10.1111/j.1432-0436.1990.tb00475.x.

Peter, S. J. C., & research, t. (1978). The junctional connections between the cells of the urinary bladder in the rat. *187*, 439-448. doi: 10.1007/BF00229608.

Petry, G., & Amon, H. J. Z. f. Z. u. M. A. (1966). Licht und elektronenmikroskopische Studien über Struktur und Dynamik des Übergangsepithels. *69*, 587-612.

Pinheiro, D., & Bellaiche, Y. J. D. c. (2018). Mechanical force-driven adherens junction remodeling and epithelial dynamics. *47*(1), 3-19. doi: 10.1016/j.devcel.2018.09.014.

Powell, D. J. A. J. o. P.-G., & Physiology, L. (1981). Barrier function of epithelia. *241*(4), G275-G288. doi: 10.1152/ajpgi.1981.241.4.G275.

Rickard, A., Dorokhov, N., Ryerse, J., Klumpp, D. J., McHowat, J. J. I. V. C., & Biology-Animal, D. (2008). Characterization of tight junction proteins in cultured human urothelial cells. *44*, 261-267. doi: 10.1007/s11626-008-9116-y.

Riedel, I., Liang, F.-X., Deng, F.-M., Tu, L., Kreibich, G., Wu, X.-R.,…Moll, R. J. E. j. o. c. b. (2005). Urothelial umbrella cells of human ureter are heterogeneous with respect to their uroplakin composition: different degrees of urothelial maturity in ureter and bladder? , *84*(2-3), 393-405. doi: 10.1016/j.ejcb.2004.12.011.

Romih, R., Jezernik, K., Mašera, A. J. H., & biology, c. (1998). Uroplakins and cytokeratins in the regenerating rat urothelium after sodium saccharin treatment. *109*(3), 263-269. doi: 10.1007/s004180050226.

Saitou, M., Fujimoto, K., Doi, Y., Itoh, M., Fujimoto, T., Furuse, M.,…Tsukita, S. J. T. J. o. c. b. (1998). Occludin-deficient embryonic stem cells can differentiate into polarized epithelial cells bearing tight junctions. *141*(2), 397-408. doi: 10.1083/jcb.141.2.397.

Sánchez Freire, V., Burkhard, F. C., Schmitz, A., Kessler, T. M., & Monastyrskaya, K. J. B. i. (2011). Structural differences between the bladder dome and trigone revealed by mRNA expression analysis of cold-cut biopsies. *108*(2b), E126-E135. doi: 10.1111/j.1464-410X.2010.09934.x.

Schneeberger, E., & McCormack, J. J. T. A. R. (1984). Intercellular junctions in upper airway submucosal glands of the rat: a tracer and freeze fracture study. *210*(3), 421-433. doi: 10.1002/ar.1092100303.

Shashikanth, N., Yeruva, S., Ong, M., Odenwald, M. A., Pavlyuk, R., & Turner, J. R. J. C. P. (2017). Epithelial organization: the gut and beyond. *7*(4), 1497-1518. doi: 10.1002/cphy.c170003.

Shen, J.-D., Chen, S.-J., Chen, H.-Y., Chiu, K.-Y., Chen, Y.-H., & Chen, W.-C. J. B. (2021). Review of animal models to study urinary bladder function. *10*(12), 1316. doi: 10.3390/biology10121316.

Shin, K., Lee, J., Guo, N., Kim, J., Lim, A., Qu, L.,…Beachy, P. A. J. N. (2011). Hedgehog/Wnt feedback supports regenerative proliferation of epithelial stem cells in bladder. *472*(7341), 110-114. doi: 10.1038/nature09851.

Smith, N. J., Hinley, J., Varley, C. L., Eardley, I., Trejdosiewicz, L. K., & Southgate, J. J. B. (2015). The human urothelial tight junction: claudin 3 and the ZO-1α+ switch. *2*(1), e9. doi: 10.14440/bladder.2015.33.

Song, J., & Abraham, S. N. J. C. o. i. m. (2008). TLR-mediated immune responses in the urinary tract. *11*(1), 66-73. doi: 10.1016/j.mib.2007.12.001.

Sun, T.-T., Zhao, H., Provet, J., Aebi, U., & Wu, X.-R. J. M. b. r. (1996). Formation of asymmetric unit membrane during urothelial differentiation. *23*, 3-11. doi: 10.1007/BF00357068.

Törzsök, P., Riesz, P., Kenessey, I., Székely, E., Somorácz, Á., Nyirády, P.,…Cytochemistry. (2011). Claudins and ki-67: potential markers to differentiate low-and high-grade transitional cell carcinomas of the urinary bladder. *59*(11), 1022-1030. doi: 10.1369/0022155411424606.

Troyanovsky, S., Guelstein, V., Tchipysheva, T., Krutovskikh, V., & Bannikov, G. J. J. o. c. s. (1989). Patterns of expression of keratin 17 in human epithelia: dependency on cell position. *93*(3), 419-426. doi: 10.1242/jcs.93.3.419.

Truschel, S. T., Ruiz, W. G., Shulman, T., Pilewski, J., Sun, T.-T., Zeidel, M. L., & Apodaca, G. J. J. o. B. C. (1999). Primary uroepithelial cultures: a model system to analyze umbrella cell barrier function. *274*(21), 15020-15029. doi: 10.1074/jbc.274.21.15020.

Truschel, S. T., Wang, E., Ruiz, W. G., Leung, S.-M., Rojas, R., Lavelle, J.,…Apodaca, G. J. M. b. o. t. c. (2002). Stretch-regulated exocytosis/endocytosis in bladder umbrella cells. *13*(3), 830-846. doi: 10.1091/mbc.01-09-0435.

Tu, L., Sun, T.-T., & Kreibich, G. J. M. b. o. t. c. (2002). Specific heterodimer formation is a prerequisite for uroplakins to exit from the endoplasmic reticulum. *13*(12), 4221-4230. doi: 10.1091/mbc.e02-04-0211.

Van Itallie, C. M., & Anderson, J. M. (2014). Architecture of tight junctions and principles of molecular composition. Seminars in cell & developmental biology, doi: 10.1016/j.semcdb.2014.08.011.

Van Itallie, C. M., & Anderson, J. M. J. A. R. P. (2006). Claudins and epithelial paracellular transport. *68*, 403-429. doi: 10.1146/annurev.physiol.68.040104.131404.

Van Itallie, C. M., Holmes, J., Bridges, A., Gookin, J. L., Coccaro, M. R., Proctor, W.,…Anderson, J. M. J. J. o. c. s. (2008). The density of small tight junction pores varies among cell types and is increased by expression of claudin-2. *121*(3), 298-305. doi: 10.1242/jcs.021485. Epub 2008 Jan 15.

Varley, C. L., Garthwaite, M. A., Cross, W., Hinley, J., Trejdosiewicz, L. K., & Southgate, J. J. J. o. c. p. (2006). PPARγ-regulated tight junction development during human urothelial cytodifferentiation. *208*(2), 407-417. doi: 10.1002/jcp.20676.

Veranic, P., & Jezernik, K. J. A. J. C. B. (2006). The cytokeratins of urinary bladder epithelial cells. *1*(1), 1-8.

Veranič, P., Jezernik, K. J. C. m., & cytoskeleton, t. (2002). Trajectorial organisation of cytokeratins within the subapical region of umbrella cells. *53*(4), 317-325. doi: 10.1002/cm.10077.

Višnjar, T., Kocbek, P., Kreft, M. E. J. H., & biology, c. (2012). Hyperplasia as a mechanism for rapid resealing urothelial injuries and maintaining high transepithelial resistance. *137*, 177-186. doi: 10.1007/s00418-011-0893-0.

Višnjar, T., Kreft, M. E. J. I. V. C., & Biology-Animal, D. (2013). Air–liquid and liquid–liquid interfaces influence the formation of the urothelial permeability barrier in vitro. *49*, 196-204. doi: 10.1007/s11626-013-9585-5.

Walz, T., Häner, M., Wu, X.-R., Henn, C., Engel, A., Sun, T.-T., & Aebi, U. J. J. o. m. b. (1995). Towards the molecular architecture of the asymmetric unit membrane of the mammalian urinary bladder epithelium: a closed “twisted ribbon” structure. *248*(5), 887-900. doi: 10.1006/jmbi.1995.0269.

Wan, Q., Xiong, G., Liu, G., Shupe, T. D., Wei, G., Zhang, D.,…therapy. (2018). Urothelium with barrier function differentiated from human urine-derived stem cells for potential use in urinary tract reconstruction. *9*, 1-13. doi: 10.1186/s13287-018-1035-6.

Wang, H., Ran, J., & Jiang, T. J. U. T. (2014). Urea. 7-29.

Winder, M., Tobin, G., Zupančič, D., & Romih, R. J. B. r. i. (2014). Signalling molecules in the urothelium. *2014*. doi: 10.1155/2014/297295.

Wu, X.-R., Kong, X.-P., Pellicer, A., Kreibich, G., & Sun, T.-T. J. K. i. (2009). Uroplakins in urothelial biology, function, and disease. *75*(11), 1153-1165. doi: 10.1038/ki.2009.73.

Wu, X.-R., Lin, J.-H., Walz, T., Häner, M., Yu, J., Aebi, U., & Sun, T.-T. J. J. o. B. C. (1994). Mammalian uroplakins. A group of highly conserved urothelial differentiation-related membrane proteins. *269*(18), 13716-13724.

Wu, X.-R., Medina, J. J., & Sun, T.-T. J. J. o. B. C. (1995). Selective interactions of UPIa and UPIb, two members of the transmembrane 4 superfamily, with distinct single transmembrane-domained proteins in differentiated urothelial cells. *270*(50), 29752-29759. doi: 10.1074/jbc.270.50.29752.

Wu, X., Manabe, M., Yu, J., & Sun, T.-T. J. J. o. B. C. (1990). Large scale purification and immunolocalization of bovine uroplakins I, II, and III. Molecular markers of urothelial differentiation. *265*(31), 19170-19179.

Yamany, T., Van Batavia, J., & Mendelsohn, C. J. C. o. i. o. t. (2014). Formation and regeneration of the urothelium. *19*(3), 323-330. doi: 10.1097/MOT. 0000000000000084.

Yu, J., Lin, J.-H., Wu, X.-R., & Sun, T.-T. J. T. J. o. c. b. (1994). Uroplakins Ia and Ib, two major differentiation products of bladder epithelium, belong to a family of four transmembrane domain (4TM) proteins. *125*(1), 171-182. doi: 10.1083/jcb.125.1.171.

Yu, J., Manabe, M., Wu, X.-R., Xu, C., Surya, B., & Sun, T.-T. J. T. J. o. c. b. (1990). Uroplakin I: a 27-kD protein associated with the asymmetric unit membrane of mammalian urothelium. *111*(3), 1207-1216. doi: 10.1083/jcb.111.3.1207.

Yu, L., Liu, T., Fu, S., Li, L., Meng, X., Su, X.,…Lv, X. J. P. A.-E. J. o. P. (2019). Physiological functions of urea transporter B. *471*, 1359-1368. doi: 10.1007/s00424-019-02323-x.

Yu, W., & Hill, W. G. J. A. J. o. P.-R. P. (2011). Defining protein expression in the urothelium: a problem of more than transitional interest. *301*(5), F932-F942. doi: 10.1152/ajprenal.00334.2011.

Yu, W., Khandelwal, P., & Apodaca, G. J. M. b. o. t. c. (2009). Distinct apical and basolateral membrane requirements for stretch-induced membrane traffic at the apical surface of bladder umbrella cells. *20*(1), 282-295. doi: 10.1091/mbc.e08-04-0439.

Zeidel, M. J. A. J. o. P.-R. P. (1996). Low permeabilities of apical membranes of barrier epithelia: what makes watertight membranes watertight? , *271*(2), F243-F245. doi: 10.1152/ajprenal.1996.271.2.F243.

Zhou, G., Liang, F.-X., Romih, R., Wang, Z., Liao, Y., Ghiso, J.,…Alonso, M. A. J. M. b. o. t. c. (2012). MAL facilitates the incorporation of exocytic uroplakin-delivering vesicles into the apical membrane of urothelial umbrella cells. *23*(7), 1354-1366. doi: 10.1091/mbc.E11-09-0823.

Zihni, C., Mills, C., Matter, K., & Balda, M. S. J. N. r. M. c. b. (2016). Tight junctions: from simple barriers to multifunctional molecular gates. *17*(9), 564-580. doi: 10.1038/nrm.2016.80.

Chapter 5

The Blood-Follicle Barrier

Oya Korkmaz*, PhD
Department of Histology and Embryology, Faculty of Medicine,
Malatya Turgut Özal University, Malatya, Türkiye

Abstract

Oocyte and granulosa cells engage in tight and intricate communication during the process of follicular formation. Insufficient signalling between these two cell types leads to infertility. Follicular fluid is an intricate fluid that makes up the environment in which follicles form. It contains substances generated by the surrounding cells and compounds from the blood plasma that pass over the blood-follicle barrier (BFB). The BFB is a type of blood-tissue barrier found throughout the mammalian body and serves to maintain the balance of the oocyte environment by separating blood from follicular fluid. The BFB functions as a molecular sieve, selectively allowing molecules to pass through based on their size and charge within the ovarian follicles. The BFB is primarily formed by the tight junction-permeability barrier of the endothelial cells in the microvessels surrounding the developing follicle. Additionally, the basement membrane of the developing follicle plays a significant role in the BFB by undergoing rapid changes in its composition during follicle development. The pharmacodynamics of the BFB are intricate, and there is difficulty in overcoming physiological barriers that impact different local and systemic methods of delivery. Although the BFB and its ultrastructure were explained over sixty years ago, there are few reports in the literature that specifically explore the biology, regulation, and function of the BFB in both healthy and diseased states. The objective of this chapter is to offer the latest information on the crucial BFB. To

* Corresponding Author's Email: oya.korkmaz@ozal.edu.tr

In: A Histological Approach to Human Body Barriers
Editor: İlknur Keskin
ISBN: 979-8-89530-738-0

improve ovarian function, it is important to comprehensively understand the blood follicle barrier and to investigate this area further.

Keywords: blood–follicle barrier, ovary, oocyte, follicular fluid, permeability

Introduction

The ovary is a bilateral pair of almond-shaped structures situated laterally in the pelvic cavity, adjacent to the uterus. The organ is classified as an exocrine organ due to its role in producing gametes (specifically, oocyte development or oogenesis). Additionally, it is classified as an endocrine organ since it synthesises and releases steroid hormones (a process known as steroidogenesis). Ovarian folliculogenesis and oogenesis take place within the ovary.

Folliculogenesis refers to the process of development that encompasses all the stages from the initial primordial follicle to the production of the tertiary follicle, ultimately resulting in ovulation. During this stage, the size of the follicle increases, and its cellular features undergo changes. Throughout the process of folliculogenesis, there is continuous interaction between the granulosa cells (mural and cumulus) and the oocyte. These two types of cells exchange nutrients in both directions and communicate through paracrine signalling (Wigglesworth et al., 2013; Coticchio et al., 2015; Russell et al., 2016). Intercellular communication is crucial for the growth of the follicular compartment, maturation of oocytes, and acquisition of competence (Gilchrist et al., 2008; Kidder & Vanderhyden, 2010; Dumesic et al., 2015). After the oocyte finishes the process of meiosis, specifically from prophase I to metaphase II, it attains full competence and is capable of being fertilised to develop into a viable embryo (Eppig et al., 1994). Granulosa cells in antral follicles provide metabolic support and help maintain meiotic arrest in the developing oocyte (Wigglesworth et al., 2013; Coticchio et al., 2015; Monniaux, 2016). Simultaneously, several substances released by the oocyte, facilitate the metabolic activity, maturation, and viability of granulosa cells (Gilchrist et al., 2008).

Oogenesis is a lengthy and intricate process that relies on both elements within the ovary itself and factors outside of the ovary (Matzuk et al., 2002; Gosden, 2013). Upon birth, all oocytes are in a state of dormancy within primordial follicles, existing as primary oocytes in the prophase I stage of the initial meiotic division. The oocytes are enveloped by a layer of somatic cells known as granulosa cells. The primary oocyte, which has initiated meiosis I but has halted division, undergoes further growth within the secondary and tertiary follicles. Within the tertiary follicle, the first division of the cell is completed and immediately followed by the second division, which occurs approximately 6-12 hours prior to ovulation. During this phase, it has transformed into a secondary oocyte. The division of the secondary oocyte ceases during the metaphase phase, approximately 2-3 hours before ovulation. In this scenario, the division of the ovulatory egg ceases during the metaphase phase approximately 2-3 hours prior to ovulation. The oocyte that is released during ovulation is referred to as the secondary oocyte. An optimal environment within the follicle promotes the development of oocytes via the combined efforts of granulosa cells and follicular fluid (Eppig et al., 1994; Dumesic et al., 2015). An oocyte is deemed competent when it has the ability to undergo meiosis, fertilisation, embryo creation, and stage development (Eppig et al., 1994).

During folliculogenesis, the ovarian follicle undergoes significant growth as the oocyte matures within the follicular fluid, which is a complicated metabolic environment (Leroy et al., 2004). Follicular fluid is a combination of serum exudate and locally generated chemicals resulting from the metabolic activity of follicular cells (Gérard et al., 2002). The process involves the passage of blood plasma components via the "blood-follicle" barrier, facilitated by the secretory activity of the granulosa, and teca cells in the surrounding area. The follicular fluid plays a crucial role in providing a specialised environment that is essential for the maturation and growth of the oocyte (Fortune et al., 2004; Baka et al., 2006; Revelli et al., 2009; Rodgers et al., 2010; Kranc et al., 2017). The substance consists of essential nutrients, hormones, enzymes, growth factors, lipids, albumin, glycoproteins, and other complex solutes such as immunoglobulins (Mantzavinos et al., 1993; Leroy et al., 2004; Hsieh et al., 2009; Siu et al., 2012; Ambekar et al., 2013; O'Gorman et al., 2013; Dunning et al., 2014). Hence, the constituents of the follicular fluid accurately mirror the various phases of oocyte growth and the level of follicle maturation (Eppig et al., 2005; Sugiura et al., 2005). Therefore, specific constituents of the follicular fluid can serve as markers for the maturity and, consequently, the quality of the follicle (Mihm et al., 2000; Anahory et al., 2002; Mendoza et al., 2002).

The ovary is composed of diverse cells and membranes that regulate the intake of nutrients into the growing follicles and prevent the entry of external substances and toxins. Research has established clear disparities in the protein makeup and levels between follicular fluid and blood plasma, resulting in the development of the blood-follicle barrier (BFB) (Zachariae, 1958; Shalgi et al., 1973). The BFB is a crucial barrier that separates the follicle from the blood. It is composed of several biofilms and a gap matrix (Zhou et al., 2007; Siu & Cheng, 2012). It exhibits selective permeability and is referred to as a 'molecular sieve' that regulates the exchange of molecules between follicular fluid and blood (Zachariae, 1958; Shalgi et al., 1973). The BFB is composed of the vascular endothelium, subendothelial basement membrane, interstitial layer, follicular basement membrane, and granulosa membrane (Figure 1). The BFB functions as a selective filter, allowing the passage of only large molecules and particles with a size of less than 500 kDa (Cheng, 2014).

Follicular fluid is generated by granulosa cells in the later stages of secondary follicle development. It is in close proximity to the cumulus-oocyte complex and consists of a plasma exudate and secretory substances from granulosa cells (mural and cumulus) and thecal cells. The primary constituents of follicular fluid consist of steroid hormones, metabolites, polysaccharides, proteins, reactive oxygen species (ROS), and antioxidants (Ambekar et al., 2013). Hormonal, paracrine, and autocrine signalling mechanisms can directly modify the constituents of folicular fluid, whereas systemic circumstances can indirectly modify them (Von Wald et al., 2010; Chattopadhayay et al., 2010; Liu et al., 2012; Prieto et al., 2012; Moreno et al., 2015). Alterations in the composition of follicular fluid have been proposed to impact the quality of oocytes, including their maturation and fertilisation, as well as the early development of embryos and eventual pregnancy (Gode et al., 2011; Liu et al., 2012; Yang et al., 2015). The folicular fluid also contains metabolites that build up inside the oocyte and supply the essential components needed for oocyte differentiation (Hennet & Combelles, 2012). The metabolites mentioned consist of lipids, nucleotides, amino acids, and various other tiny molecules. These substances are produced from the serum and metabolic processes of follicular cells (Edwards, 1974). Metabolic activity and characteristics of the "barrier" follicular wall vary considerably during ovarian follicular maturation (Gérard et al., 2002). Imbalances in hormones and metabolism, as well as different types of oxidative stressors, might result in the creation and upkeep of ovarian follicles, which can contribute to infertility issues (El-Badry et al., 2020). This chapter will specifically examine the blood-follicle barrier, which is one of the several barriers present in the human body.

The Blood-Follicle Barrier (BFB)

Concept

In an ovarian follicle, the follicular fluid is located in the follicular antrum, and it surrounds the ovum to protect it from external influences. This creates a specific microenvironment that is beneficial to the development of the follicle as well as the maturation of the oocyte (Rodgers & Irving-Rodgers, 2010). The BFB has been proposed as a result of previous research that has revealed distinct differences in the protein composition and levels of blood plasma and follicular fluid. These findings have led to the proposition that a BFB exists (Zachariae, 1958; Shalgi et al., 1973). It has been proven via morphological studies carried out in the 1950s and 1960s that the ovarian follicles are surrounded by a network of capillaries in the theca interna. While the follicular compartment itself does not include any blood vessels, a unique basement membrane serves to isolate each individual follicle from the microvessels located in close proximity to it. It is clear from this that there is a barrier between the blood and the tissue at this particular place, which was referred to as the "blood-liquor barrier" in the year 1958 (Bjersing & Cajander, 1951; Burr & Davis, 1951; Zachariae, 1958; Byskov, 1969). In spite of this, the acronym BFB was first presented in the scientific literature in 1973. This was in response to the fact that researchers had observed differences in the protein content and concentration of follicular fluid in comparison to blood serum or plasma. The results of a second study that examined follicular fluids and serum samples taken from women undergoing in vitro fertilisation (IVF) helped to provide additional evidence in support of this discovery (Shalgi et al., 1973; Schweigert et al., 2006). A proteomic method was utilised in order to widen the scope of the investigation. This method indicated that human follicular fluid contains a number of proteins that are associated with the acute inflammatory phase. These proteins include hemopexin, transferrin, haptoglobin, afamin, ceruloplasmin, and plasma amyloid protein. At the same time, it was discovered that the amounts of these proteins in the plasma were different from those in the follicular fluid.

Ovulation is akin to an inflammatory reaction, according to Angelucci et al. (2006), and this finding gives additional evidence that this is the case. Additionally, a number of antioxidant enzymes were found in the research. These enzymes include glutathione transferase (GST), superoxide dismutase (SOD), paraoxonase (PON), catalase (CAT), and heat shock protein 27 (HSP27). According to Angelucci et al. (2006), these enzymes have the capacity to protect human follicles from the potentially damaging effects of oxidative stress. It is believed that the proteins present in the follicular fluid are comparable to those found in the plasma level of the blood. Specifically, Angelucci et al. (2006) found that these proteins play a significant part in the process of fostering the development of follicles and the maturation of oocytes. The constituents of follicular fluid closely resemble those present in blood plasma, particularly in terms of proteins with a low molecular weight (Shalgi et al., 1973; Gosden et al., 1988). The selective BFB, which functions as a "molecular sieve," is responsible for the fact that the protein composition of human follicular fluid is distinct from that of human blood plasma (Zachariae, 1958; Shalgi et al., 1973). Ferritin, which has a molecular weight of 500 kDa, and colloidal gold, which has a molecular weight of 1000 kDa, were utilised as tracers in a research investigation in order to measure the permeability of the BFB. Based on the findings of the study, it was discovered that the BFB can function as a selective filter, enabling proteins with a molecular weight of less than 500 kDa to pass through (Cran et al., 1976). After some time had passed, it was found that the BFB displayed selectivity in mouse ovaries with regard to both charge and size (Hess et al., 1988).

Structure

The BFB is composed of the vascular endothelium, subendothelial basement membrane, thecal interstitium, follicular basement membrane, and granulosa membrane (Siu & Cheng, 2012) (Figure 1). This barrier, along with other blood-tissue barriers, restricts the passage of macromolecules and solutes (including proteins and peptides, carbohydrates, electrolytes, and ions) across cells on the basis of the molecular sizes of these substances. It is of critical importance in the ovary since it has the ability to block external chemicals and hazardous substances from accessing the follicles that are developing. Additionally, it produces two distinct compartments, which enables the follicular fluid and serum to have distinct compositions according to their respective needs (Von Wald et al., 2010; Siu & Cheng, 2012; Prieto et al., 2012; Da Broi et al., 2016).

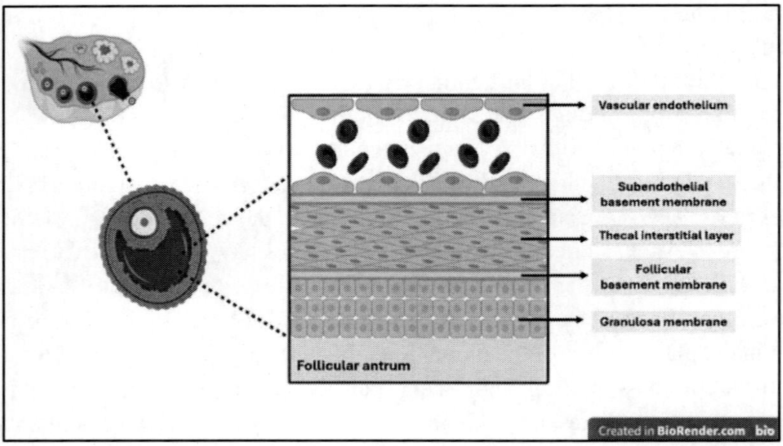

Figure 1. Components of the blood-follicle barrier (BFB).

Selective-Permeability Function

There are two basic mechanisms that are responsible for intercellular communication. These mechanisms are gap junctions and paracrine signals (Monniaux, 2016). Connexins are the components that make up gap junctions, which are intercellular membrane channels. Whenever these channels are connected to connexins in nearby cells, they make it possible for solutes to pass through (Winterhager & Kidder, 2015). Connexin 37 (Cx37) is responsible for the formation of gap junctions, which are responsible for facilitating the interaction between the granulosa cells and the oocyte that occurs within the follicle. The granulosa cells and the oocyte are able to communicate with one another thanks to the gap junctions that extend across the zona pellucida. In addition to this, the granulosa cells are connected to one another through gap junctions that are created by connexin 43 (Cx43) (Kidder & Mhawi, 2002; Winterhager & Kidder, 2015). It is possible for gap junctions to promote the movement of a number of small molecules from granulosa cells to the oocyte. These molecules include ions, cyclic nucleotides (cAMP and cGMP), metabolites, amino acids, and RNA transcripts. Meiosis, the production of ATP, and the preservation of the pH balance in the oocyte are all processes that are significantly influenced by these molecules (Kidder & Mhawi, 2002; FitzHarris et al., 2007; Monniaux, 2016). The differentiation between granulosa cells is also dependent on this communication, which is quite important (Simon et al., 1997). In the process of oogenesis, there is a process known as intrafollicular paracrine signalling, which involves active communication between cells that are contained within the follicle. It is essential for the development and maturation of the follicle that this process takes place (Coticchi et al., 2015). In addition to being controlled by circulating endocrine hormones, such as follicle stimulating hormone (FSH), the process is also influenced by growth factors, which include members of the transforming growth factor beta (TGF-β) superfamily. The process occurs through a variety of receptors and signalling pathways (Joyce et al., 1999; Williams & Erickson, 2000; Thomas et al., 2005; Thomas & Vanderhyden, 2006; Sugiura et al., 2007; Su et al., 2008). The paracrine signalling that originates from cumulus cells and is directed towards the oocyte helps to facilitate the process of meiotic restart, increases the maturation of both the nucleus and the cytoplasm, and regulates the activity of transcriptional genes (Albertini et al., 2001; Monniaux, 2016).

Like the blood-brain barrier and the blood-testis barrier, the BFB is not just a "molecular sieve" in the ovary. It does this by preventing solutes and macromolecules from moving freely across the various membrane structures in order to reach the growing follicles when they are needed. A constraint like this one is imposed because of the size of the molecules. IαI, which is an inter-α-trypsin inhibitor with a molecular weight of 240 kilodaltons, and pre-α-trypsin inhibitor, which has a molecular weight of 125 kilodaltons, were shown to be absent from the follicular fluid until an ovulatory stimulus in the form of an LH surge was administered. After that, both of these proteins were discovered in the antrum of mature follicles, typically within minutes, and they were revealed to have a close connection to the freshly created hyaluronic acid-rich cumulus extracellular matrix (Chen et al., 1992; Chen et al., 1994). Researchers have discovered that when conditions are normal, BFB allows low- and medium-sized proteins such as albumin (69 kDa) and immunoglobulin G1 (IgG1; 150 kDa) to enter the follicular fluid. However, it prevents higher-sized components such as IgM (900 kDa) or larger particles from entering the follicular fluid (Shalgi et al., 1973; Cran et al., 1976; Zhou et al., 2007).

Nitric oxide (NO) has been shown to modulate both vascular function and permeability, as well as the permeability function of the Sertoli cell tight junction-barrier, according to additional research that has shown that the alterations in permeability function at the BFB are also controlled by NO. This finding is in line with the findings of previous research that demonstrated that NO governs both of these functions (Moncada et al., 1991; Powers et al., 1995; Gu et al., Lee et al., 2003; 2011; Oberleithner et al., 2010). In a study that was conducted not too long ago by Zhou et al. (2007), the 'in vivo cryotechnique' (IVCT) was utilised to investigate the morphological and immunohistochemical changes that occurred in mouse ovaries. Albumin, a protein with a molecular size of roughly 69 kDa, was discovered in the blood vessels, interstitium, and growing follicles, according to the findings of the study. Given this information, it appears that proteins with a tiny molecular size are able to cross the BFB and make their way to the developing follicles. In ovarian follicles, the immunostaining of molecules with a molecular weight of around 150 kilodaltons (kDa), inter-α-trypsin inhibitor (IαI) with a molecular weight of 220 kDa, and fibrinogen with a molecular weight of 340 kDa revealed a noteworthy decrease. In light of this, it appears that proteins with a molecular size that is intermediate can travel through blood vessels and reach the interstitium; however, the follicular basement membranes prevent these molecules from moving freely through the blood vessels. Immunostaining of high-molecular-weight proteins, typically IgM (with a molecular weight of around 900 kilodaltons), was largely seen in the blood vessels. Consequently, this suggests that the endothelial tight junction barrier of blood arteries acts as a barrier that prevents proteins with high molecular sizes from passing through. Based on the findings, it can be concluded that the BFB is present during the beginning stages of folliculogenesis and that it plays specific functions in the development of follicles up until the time of ovulation (Zhou et al., 2007).

Administration of hCG in mice results in a 15% increase in the radius of the pores in the capillaries of ovarian follicles (Mitsube et al., 2013). It is possible to find NO in the preovulatory follicular secretions of equines, and the concentration of this substance increases after the administration of hCG (Pinto et al., 2003). As a result, this suggests that hCG stimulates the production of NO within the ovarian follicle (Da Broi et al., 2018). Furthermore, it is anticipated that hCG will influence the BFB by increasing the permeability of capillaries. The mice that had the endothelial NO synthase gene (eNOS), which is responsible for producing NO in the endothelium, knocked out showed a decrease in the number of ovulated oocytes, a lower rate of MII oocytes, a decrease in the number of pups born per litter, and an increased incidence of pup mortality in comparison to the mice that were of the wild-type (Jablonka-Shariff & Olson, 1998). Therefore, it is thought that alterations in the production of NO and endothelial nitric oxide synthase (eNOS) can potentially lead to infertility by changing the composition of follicular fluid through disruptions in capillary permeability. This is because these alterations have the potential to cause changes in the follicular fluid composition. This, in turn, can make it more difficult for oocytes to mature and for the process of ovulation to take place (Da Broi et al., 2018).

The growth of the antrum and the follicular fluid is influenced by the presence of an osmotic gradient and the level of vascular permeability. Granulosa cells are hypothesised to be responsible for the formation of cavities as a consequence of their production of hyaluronan and versican, which results in the formation of an osmotic gradient (Rodgers & Irving-Rodgers, 2010). Aquaporins, which are found on the basal and apical surfaces of granulosa cells, are responsible for facilitating the passage of water between cells, which ultimately leads to the creation of a plasma transudate within follicles (McConnell et al., 2002; Skowronski et al., 2009).

PCOS, also known as polycystic ovary syndrome, is a hormonal illness that is commonly found in women. It is distinguished by anovulation, which leads to irregular menstruation, infertility, and the development of polycystic ovaries (Legro, 2001; Ehrmann, 2005). Follicle formation is interrupted in patients with PCOS during the early stages of development (Franks, 1989). The permselectivity of the BFB has the potential to alter PCOS by influencing the composition of the follicular fluid and the proteins that make up the fluid, which in turn has an effect on the production of follicles. Prior research has shown that people with PCOS have abnormal modulation of soluble Fas ligand, insulin-like growth factor-binding proteins, and inhibins A and B in their follicular fluids (San Roman & Magoffin, 1992; Onalan et al., 2005; Welt et al., 2005).

According to Zhou et al. (2008), the in vivo cryotechnique (IVCT) was utilised in order to evaluate the morphology and permselectivity of the BFB in mouse ovaries that had been stimulated with mifepristone. According to the findings of the study, the blood vessels in the ovaries were found to be larger and their blood flow was found to be enhanced. In addition, the development of follicular cysts was seen, which was accompanied by a membrane granulosa that was thinner in the blood vessels, interstitium, and growing follicles (Zhou et al., 2008). The immunostaining analysis of low- and high-molecular-weight proteins, namely albumin and IgM, respectively, in the ovaries of mice with PCOS, exhibited resemblances to the immunostaining patterns reported in healthy animals. According to Zhou et al. (2008), albumin was discovered in multiple locations, including the interstitium, developing follicles, and blood vessels. On the other hand, IgM was largely discovered within the blood vessels. Moreower, the immunostaining of molecules of a medium size, such as fibrinogen, IgG, and ITI, displayed unique patterns in the PCOS model. The follicular basement membranes in the PCOS model hindered the movement of both IgG and ITI from the interstitium to the follicles. This restriction was observed in the PCOS model. Furthermore, fibrinogen was predominantly restricted to the blood vessels and protected by the endothelial cells in the mouse that were affected by PCOS (Zhou et al., 2008). According to the findings, the selective permeability of the BFB, which is controlled by the endothelial cells of the microvessels and the basement membrane of the follicles, may have a substantial influence on the development of PCOS (Zhou et al., 2008).

When it comes to cancers that affect the female reproductive system, ovarian cancer is the most lethal of all the different varieties (Siu et al., 2009; Siu et al., 2010). Approximately 90% of malignant ovarian tumours are believed to arise from alterations in the surface epithelium or surface epithelial inclusion cysts of the ovary (Feeley & Wells, 2001; Bell, 2005). It is possible that the dysregulation of the BFB is responsible for two primary factors: (a) the abnormal modifications that occur in the epithelium, and (b) the formation of surface epithelial inclusion cysts in the ovaries. On the other hand, these elements could potentially contribute to the progression of cancer. Future research must be conducted in order to further investigate the potential impact that BFB could have on ovarian cancer.

Endothelial Cells of Blood Vessels

There is a capillary network that surrounds the follicle, which is made up of somatic follicular cells and the oocyte. This network is responsible for supplying the follicle with blood vessels. This vasculature, in addition to follicular cells, is responsible for the formation of the BFB, which is an essential component in the process of oocyte protection and the facilitation of the production of follicular fluid (Siu & Cheng, 2012).

The process of angiogenesis in the ovarian cortex is linked to the formation of follicles and is regulated in a manner that is distinct for each individual follicle (Tamanini & De Ambrogi, 2004). Utilising a process known as passive diffusion, primary and primordial follicles are able to acquire nutrients and oxygen from blood veins located in the stroma. On the other hand, as the development of the follicles continues, the granulosa and the thecal cells generate vascular endothelial growth factor (VEGF), which drives the formation of a network of blood capillaries between the layers of the thecal cells (Berisha et al., 2000). The nutrient resources are directed precisely to the follicle as a result of this (Figure 2).

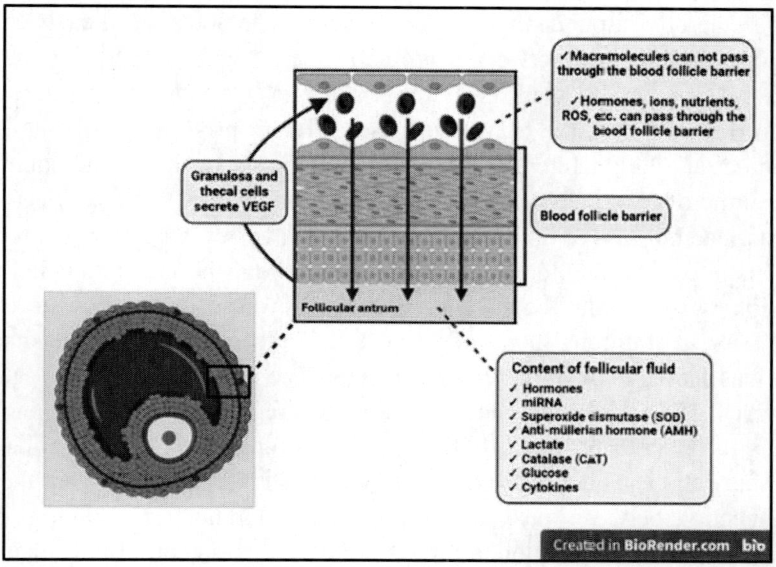

Figure 2. Role of the blood-follicle barrier and granulosa cells in follicular physiology. During follicular development, VEGF is secreted by these cells, and a vascular network is formed. The BFB limits the transcellular transport of molecules between blood and follicular fluid according to molecular size.

It was through the injection of radioactive microspheres into the ovarian artery that the researchers were able to investigate the flow of blood to the preovulatory follicles in sheep. They made the discovery that the blood supply to the follicles increased during the preovulatory surge of luteinizing hormone (LH), but it dropped around the time that the follicle went through rupture (Murdoch et al., 1983). The progesterone receptor influences VEGF expression by affecting the development of thecal cells, endothelial cell proliferation, the recruitment of perivascular mural cells and vascularization, according to the findings of a study that investigated the effect of a progesterone receptor antagonist (RU486) on the expression of VEGF in follicular cells (Mauro et al., 2014). There is a regulation of VEGF by BMP-7. The cytokine known as BMP-7 is largely expressed in the cells of the respiratory system. Through the induction of VEGF expression in granulosa cells and the enhancement of endothelial cells' responsiveness to VEGF, it encourages the formation of blood vessels in the follicle by endothelial cells.

An important part of the BFB is played by endothelial cells, which are most commonly seen in capillaries. By performing the function of a filter, this barrier regulates the passage of serum proteins from blood arteries to the tissue that is directly around them. The dynamic character of the junctional complexes that exist between endothelial cells, which include tight and adherent junctions as well as desmosomes, plays a significant role in the careful regulation of the transit of these different proteins (Bazzoni, 2006; Dejana et al., 2009). Intercellular junctional complexes between endothelial cells in the ovary, such as those found in mouse ovaries, have not been well investigated because of their lack of research. However, previous research has demonstrated that the blocking of mid-sized proteins by the endothelial tight junction-barrier in this context is regulated by nitric oxide (Powers et al., 1995). As an additional point of interest, it is essential to point out that the BFB was shown to be impaired as a consequence of a decrease in the activity of ovarian SOD in diabetic mouse, leading to irregularities in ovulation. This highlights the crucial role of ROS in the functioning of the BFB.

Many studies have been conducted to investigate whether or not there is a connection between vascularity and the development of follicles or the quality of oocytes. Doppler ultrasonography was used in a study that was carried out on cows to establish that follicles that had perifollicular blood flow had a much higher probability of generating high-quality cumulus oophorus complexes in contrast to follicles that did not have perifollicular blood flow (Pancarci et al., 2012). Women were shown to have a direct connection between the Doppler index of their ovarian follicles and the quality of their oocytes, in addition to seeing improvements in their reproductive results (Nargund et al., 1996a; Nargund et al., 1996b; Huey et al., 1999; Coulam et al., 1999). In addition, research conducted by Monteleone et al. (2008) and Vural et al. (2016) has demonstrated that there is a correlation between the levels of VEGF in follicular fluid and the blood flow surrounding the follicles in patients undergoing controlled ovarian stimulation (COS) for IVF.

Subendothelial Basement Membranes

On the basis of the size of its holes and the selective charge of its components, such as laminin, heparan sulphate proteoglycans and Type IV collagen, the basement membrane of blood vessels has the potential to function as a molecular sieve (Holmquist et al., 2004).

Follicular Basement Membranes

It is an essential component of BFB that makes a major contribution to permselectivity. Permselectivity is a term that describes the selective permeability of molecules, notably soluble plasma proteins (Powers et al , 1995; Zhou et al., 2007). It has been hypothesised that the existence of different extracellular matrix components is the reason of the differential in permselectivity that exists between the follicular basement membranes and the subendothelial basement membranes. There are continual modifications that take place in the components of the follicular basement membrane throughout the process of folliculogenesis. These changes take place at a rapid pace throughout the course of time (Rodgers et al., 2003). It is possible to find collagen IV alpha 1–6 throughout the early stages of development, more specifically during the primordial and pre-antral stages. On the other hand, in cows and mice, the follicular basement membrane only contains alpha 1 and alpha 2 chains at the later stages of the antral and attretic stages (Rodgers et al., 1998). On the other hand, perlecan, nidogen 1, and nidogen 2 are the primary components of the follicular basement membrane in cows during the pre-antral stage and afterwards (McArthur et al., 2000; Irving-Rodgers et al., 2006). Laminin alpha 1, beta 2, and gamma 1 have been observed to be present in the follicular basement membrane within cows throughout the process of follicle development (Rodgers et al., 2003). There is a possibility that differences in the permeability of the basement membrane can occur during folliculogenesis as a result of dynamic changes that occur in the components of the follicular basement membrane.

Conclusion

The blood-follicle barrier (BFB) is a crucial barrier in the ovary that restricts the passage of exogenous chemicals and toxic substances into developing follicles. It has a strong connection with the growth of follicles and controls the makeup of follicular fluid by making small adjustments to the composition of the basement membrane throughout the development of follicles. Therefore, various constituents, such as electrolytes, ions, proteins, peptides, and carbohydrates, can be efficiently and swiftly absorbed into the follicular fluid in accordance with the requirements of the growing follicles. Granulosa cells have a crucial role in protecting the oocyte and ensuring its competence. They operate as a connection and a barrier between the oocyte and the surrounding milieu outside the follicle. Granulosa cells and follicular fluid play a direct role in determining the quality of the oocyte. They also create a protective environment that shields the gamete from any local or systemic diseases that could hinder its ability to develop. Disruption of this specific habitat leads to a disturbance in the BFB, which in turn affects the metabolism of the barrier and has a detrimental impact on the development of oocytes. Changes in the permselectivity of the BFB are recognised as significant factors in the development and progression of polycystic ovary syndrome (PCOS) and ovarian malignancies. There is a scarcity of research on the biology and control of the BFB. Conducting thorough investigations on this topic is crucial. To effectively treat and cure ovarian problems, it is essential to get a comprehensive understanding of the BFB and conduct additional research in this area.

References

Akiyama, I., Yoshino, O., Osuga, Y., Shi, J., Harada, M., Koga, K., Hirota, Y., Hirata, T., Fujii, T., Saito, S., & Kozuma, S. (2014). Bone morphogenetic protein 7 increased vascular endothelial growth factor (VEGF)-a expression in human granulosa cells and VEGF receptor expression in endothelial cells. *Reproductive sciences (Thousand Oaks, Calif.),* 21(4), 477–482. https://doi.org/10.1177/1933719113503411.

Albertini, D. F., Combelles, C. M., Benecchi, E., & Carabatsos, M. J. (2001). Cellular basis for paracrine regulation of ovarian follicle development. *Reproduction (Cambridge, England),* 121(5), 647–653. https://doi.org/10.1530/rep.0.1210647.

Ambekar, A. S., Nirujogi, R. S., Srikanth, S. M., Chavan, S., Kelkar, D. S., Hinduja, I., Zaveri, K., Prasad, T. S., Harsha, H. C., Pandey, A., & Mukherjee, S. (2013). Proteomic analysis of human follicular fluid: a new perspective towards understanding folliculogenesis. *Journal of proteomics,* 87, 68–77. https://doi.org/10.1016/j.jprot.2013.05.017.

Anahory, T., Dechaud, H., Bennes, R., Marin, P., Lamb, N. J. & Laoudj, D. (2002). Identification of new proteins in follicular fluid of mature human follicles. *Electrophoresis,* 23(7-8), 1197–1202. https://doi.org/10.1002/1522-2683(200204)23:7/8<1197::AID-ELPS1197>3.0.CO;2-2.

Angelucci, S., Ciavardelli, D., Di Giuseppe, F., Eleuterio, E., Sulpizio, M., Tiboni, G. M., Giampietro, F., Palumbo, P., & Di Ilio, C. (2006). Proteome analysis of human follicular fluid. *Biochimica et biophysica acta,* 1764(11), 1775–1785. https://doi.org/10.1016/j.bbapap.2006.09.001.

Baka, S., & Malamitsi-Puchner, A. (2006). Novel follicular fluid factors influencing oocyte developmental potential in IVF: a review. *Reproductive biomedicine online,* 12(4), 500–506. https://doi.org/10.1016/s1472-6483(10)62005-6.

Bazzoni G. (2006). Endothelial tight junctions: permeable barriers of the vessel wall. *Thrombosis and haemostasis,* 95(1), 36–42.

Bell D. A. (2005). Origins and molecular pathology of ovarian cancer. *Modern pathology : an official journal of the United States and Canadian Academy of Pathology, Inc,* 18(2), 19–32. https://doi.org/10.1038/modpathol.3800306.

Berisha, B., Schams, D., Kosmann, M., Amselgruber, W., & Einspanier, R. (2000). Expression and localisation of vascular endothelial growth factor and basic fibroblast growth factor during the final growth of bovine ovarian follicles. *The Journal of endocrinology,* 167(3), 371–382. https://doi.org/10.1677/joe.0.1670371.

Bjersing, L., & Cajander, S. (1974). Ovulation and the mechanism of follicle rupture. I. Light microscopic changes in rabbit ovarian follicles prior to induced ovulation. *Cell and tissue research,* 149(3), 287–300. https://doi.org/10.1007/BF00226764.

Burr JH, Davis JR. (1951). The vascular system of the rabbit ovary and its relationship to ovulation. *The Anatomical record,* 111(3), 273–297. https://doi.org/10.1002/ar.1091110302.

Byskov A. G. (1969). Ultrastructural studies on the preovulatory follicle in the mouse ovary. *Zeitschrift fur Zellforschung und mikroskopische Anatomie (Vienna, Austria : 1948),* 100(2), 285–299. https://doi.org/10.1007/BF00343884.

Chattopadhayay, R., Ganesh, A., Samanta, J., Jana, S. K., Chakravarty, B. N., & Chaudhury, K. (2010). Effect of follicular fluid oxidative stress on meiotic spindle formation in infertile women with polycystic ovarian syndrome. *Gynecologic and obstetric investigation,* 69(3), 197–202. https://doi.org/10.1159/000270900.

Chen, L., Mao, S. J. T., Larsen, W. J. (1992). Identification of a factor in fetal bovine serum that stabilizes the cumulus extracellular matrix. *J Biol Chem,* 1992; 267(17): 12380–12386. https://doi.org/10.1016/S0021-9258(19)49851-7.

Chen, L., Mao, S. J. T., McLean, L. R., Powers, R. W., Larsen, W. J. (1994). Proteins of the inter-α-trypsin family stabilize the cumulus extracellular matrix through direct binding with hyaluronic acid. *J Biol Chem,* 269(45): 28282– 28287. https://doi.org/10.1016/s0021-9258(18)46925-6.

Cheng, C. Y. (Ed.). (2014). Biology and Regulation of Blood-Tissue Barriers (Vol. 763). Springer Science & Business Media.

Cheng, C. Y., & Mruk, D. D. (2012). The blood-testis barrier and its implications for male contraception. *Pharmacological reviews,* 64(1), 16–64. https://doi.org/10.1124/pr.110.002790.

Coticchio, G., Dal Canto, M., Mignini Renzini, M., Guglielmo, M. C., Brambillasca, F., Turchi, D., Novara, P. V., & Fadini, R. (2015). Oocyte maturation: gamete-somatic cells interactions, meiotic resumption, cytoskeletal dynamics and cytoplasmic reorganization. *Human reproduction update,* 21(4), 427–454. https://doi.org/10.1093/humupd/dmv011.

Coulam, C. B., Goodman, C., & Rinehart, J. S. (1999). Colour Doppler indices of follicular blood flow as predictors of pregnancy after in-vitro fertilization and embryo transfer. *Human reproduction (Oxford, England),* 14(8), 1979–1982. https://doi.org/10.1093/humrep/14.8.1979.

Cran, D. G., Moor, R. M., & Hay, M. F. (1976). Permeability of ovarian follicles to electron-dense macromolecules. *Acta endocrinologica,* 82(3), 631–636. https://doi.org/10.1530/acta.0.0820631.

Da Broi, M. G., de Albuquerque, F. O., de Andrade, A. Z., Cardoso, R. L., Jordão Junior, A. A., Navarro, P. A. (2016). Increased concentration of 8-hydroxy-2′-deoxyguanosine in follicular fluid of infertile women with endometriosis. *Cell Tissue Res,* 366(1):231-242. https://doi.org/10.1007/s00441-016-2428-4.

Da Broi, M. G., Giorgi, V. S. I., Wang, F., Keefe, D. L., Albertini, D., Navarro, P. A. (2018). Influence of follicular fluid and cumulus cells on oocyte quality: clinical implications. *J Assist Reprod Genet,* 35(5):735-751. https://doi.org/10.1007/s10815-018-1143-3.

Dejana, E., Tournier-Lasserve, E., & Weinstein, B. M. (2009). The control of vascular integrity by endothelial cell junctions: molecular basis and pathological implications. *Developmental cell,* 16(2), 209–221. https://doi.org/10.1016/j.devcel.2009.01.004.

Dumesic, D. A., Meldrum, D. R., Katz-Jaffe, M. G., Krisher, R. L., & Schoolcraft, W. B. (2015). Oocyte environment: follicular fluid and cumulus cells are critical for oocyte health. *Fertility and sterility,* 103(2), 303–316. https://doi.org/10.1016/j.fertnstert. 2014.11.015.

Dunning, K. R., Russell, D. L., & Robker, R. L. (2014). Lipids and oocyte developmental competence: the role of fatty acids and β-oxidation. *Reproduction* (Cambridge, England), 148(1), R15–R27. https://doi.org/10.1530/REP-13-0251.

Edwards R. G. (1974). Follicular fluid. *Journal of reproduction and fertility,* 37(1), 189–219. https://doi.org/10.1530/jrf.0.0370189.

Ehrmann D. A. (2005). Polycystic ovary syndrome. *The New England journal of medicine,* 352(12), 1223–1236. https://doi.org/10.1056/NEJMra041536.

El-Badry, D. A., Maha, A. I. & Amal, Z. L. (2020). Hormonal and biochemical studies on female dromedary camels affected with multiple ovarian cysts. *Small Ruminant Res.,* 188: 106138. https://doi.org/10.1016/j.smallrumres.2020.106138.

Eppig, J. J., Schultz, R. M., O'Brien, M., & Chesnel, F. (1994). Relationship between the developmental programs controlling nuclear and cytoplasmic maturation of mouse oocytes. *Developmental biology,* 164(1), 1–9. https://doi.org/10.1006/dbio. 1994.1175.

Eppig, J. J., Pendola, F. L., Wigglesworth, K., & Pendola, J. K. (2005). Mouse oocytes regulate metabolic cooperativity between granulosa cells and oocytes: amino acid transport. *Biology of reproduction,* 73(2), 351–357. https://doi.org/10.1095/ biolreprod.105.041798.

Feeley, K. M., & Wells, M. (2001). Precursor lesions of ovarian epithelial malignancy. *Histopathology,* 38(2), 87–95. https://doi.org/10.1046/j.1365-2559.2001.01042.x.

FitzHarris, G., Siyanov, V., & Baltz, J. M. (2007). Granulosa cells regulate oocyte intracellular pH against acidosis in preantral follicles by multiple mechanisms. *Development (Cambridge, England),* 134(23), 4283–4295. https://doi.org/10.1242/ dev.005272.

Fortune, J. E., Rivera, G. M., & Yang, M. Y. (2004). Follicular development: the role of the follicular microenvironment in selection of the dominant follicle. *Animal reproduction science,* 82-83, 109–126. https://doi.org/10.1016/j.anireprosci. 2004.04.031.

Franks S. (1989). Polycystic ovary syndrome: a changing perspective. *Clinical endocrinology,* 31(1), 87–120. https://doi.org/10.1111/j.1365-2265.1989.tb00457.x.

Gérard, N., Loiseau, S., Duchamp, G., & Seguin, F. (2002). Analysis of the variations of follicular fluid composition during follicular growth and maturation in the mare using proton nuclear magnetic resonance (1H NMR). *Reproduction* (Cambridge, England), 124(2), 241–248. https://doi.org/10.1530/rep.0.1240241.

Gilchrist, R. B., Lane, M., & Thompson, J. G. (2008). Oocyte-secreted factors: regulators of cumulus cell function and oocyte quality. *Human reproduction update,* 14(2), 159–177. https://doi.org/10.1093/humupd/dmm040.

Gode, F., Gulekli, B., Dogan, E., Korhan, P., Dogan, S., Bige, O., Cimrin, D., & Atabey, N. (2011). Influence of follicular fluid GDF9 and BMP15 on embryo quality. *Fertility and sterility*, 95(7), 2274–2278. https://doi.org/10.1016/j.fertnstert.2011.03.045.

Gosden, R. G., Hunter, R. H., Telfer, E., Torrance, C., & Brown, N. (1988). Physiological factors underlying the formation of ovarian follicular fluid. *Journal of reproduction and fertility,* 82(2), 813–825. https://doi.org/10.1530/jrf.0.0820813.

Gosden R. G. (2013). Oocyte development and loss. *Seminars in reproductive medicine,* 31(6), 393–398. https://doi.org/10.1055/s-0033-1356475.

Gu, Y., Dee, C. M., & Shen, J. (2011). Interaction of free radicals, matrix metalloproteinases and caveolin-1 impacts blood-brain barrier permeability. *Frontiers in bioscience (Scholar edition),* 3(4), 1216–1231. https://doi.org/10.2741/222.

Hawkins, B. T., & Davis, T. P. (2005). The blood-brain barrier/neurovascular unit in health and disease. *Pharmacological reviews,* 57(2), 173–185. https://doi.org/10.1124/pr.57.2.4.

Hennet, M. L., & Combelles, C. M. (2012). The antral follicle: a microenvironment for oocyte differentiation. *The International journal of developmental biology,* 56(10-12), 819–831. https://doi.org/10.1387/ijdb.120133cc.

Hess, K. A., Chen, L., & Larsen, W. J. (1998). The ovarian blood follicle barrier is both charge- and size-selective in mice. *Biology of reproduction,* 58(3), 705–711. https://doi.org/10.1095/biolreprod58.3.705.

Holmquist, P., Sjoblad, S., Torffvit, O. (2004). Pore size and charge selectivity of the glomerular membrane at the time of diagnosis of diabetes. *Pediatr Nephrol,* 19:1361–1366. https://doi.org/10.1007/s00467-004-1610-1.

Hsieh, M., Zamah, A. M., & Conti, M. (2009). Epidermal growth factor-like growth factors in the follicular fluid: role in oocyte development and maturation. *Seminars in reproductive medicine,* 27(1), 52–61. https://doi.org/10.1055/s-0028-1108010.

Huey, S., Abuhamad, A. Z., Barroso, G., Hsu, M., Kolm, P., Mayer, J. F., & Oehninger, S. (1999). Perifollicular blood flow Doppler indices, but not follicular pO2, pCO2, or pH, predict oocyte developmental competence in in vitro fertilization. *Fertility and sterility,* 72(4), 707-12 . https://doi.org/10.1016/S0015-0282%2899%2900327-1.

Irving-Rodgers, H. F., & Rodgers, R. J. (2006). Extracellular matrix of the developing ovarian follicle. *Seminars in reproductive medicine,* 24(4), 195–203. https://doi.org/10.1055/s-2006-948549.

Jablonka-Shariff, A., & Olson, L. M. (1998). The role of nitric oxide in oocyte meiotic maturation and ovulation: meiotic abnormalities of endothelial nitric oxide synthase knock-out mouse oocytes. *Endocrinology,* 139(6), 2944–2954. https://doi.org/10.1210/endo.139.6.6054.

Joyce, I. M., Pendola, F. L., Wigglesworth, K., & Eppig, J. J. (1999). Oocyte regulation of kit ligand expression in mouse ovarian follicles. *Developmental biology,* 214(2), 342–353. https://doi.org/10.1006/dbio.1999.9437.

Kidder, G. M., & Vanderhyden, B. C. (2010). Bidirectional communication between oocytes and follicle cells: ensuring oocyte developmental competence. *Canadian journal of physiology and pharmacology,* 88(4), 399–413. https://doi.org/10.1139/y10-009.

Kidder, G. M., & Mhawi, A. A. (2002). Gap junctions and ovarian folliculogenesis. *Reproduction* (Cambridge, England), 123(5), 613–620. https://doi.org/10.1530/rep.0.1230613.

Kranc, W., Budna, J., Kahan, R., Chachuła, A., Bryja, A., Ciesiółka, S., Borys, S., Antosik, M. P., Bukowska, D., Brussow, K. P., Bruska, M., Nowicki, M., Zabel, M. and Kempisty, B. (2017). Molecular basis of growth, proliferation, and differentiation of mammalian follicular granulosa cells. *J. Biol. Regul. Homeost. Agents,* 31(1): 1–8.

Lee, N. P., & Cheng, C. Y. (2003). Regulation of Sertoli cell tight junction dynamics in the rat testis via the nitric oxide synthase/soluble guanylate cyclase/3',5'-cyclic guanosine monophosphate/protein kinase G signaling pathway: an in vitro study. *Endocrinology,* 144(7), 3114–3129. https://doi.org/10.1210/en.2002-0167.

Legro, R. S. (2001). Polycystic ovary syndrome: the new millenium. *Mol Cell Endocrinol,* 184(1-2): 87–93. https://doi.org/10.1016/S0303-7207(01)00640-2.

Leroy, J. L., Vanholder, T., Delanghe, J. R., Opsomer, G., Van Soom, A., Bols, P. E., & de Kruif, A. (2004). Metabolite and ionic composition of follicular fluid from different-sized follicles and their relationship to serum concentrations in dairy cows. *Animal reproduction science,* 80(3-4), 201–211. https://doi.org/10.1016/S0378-4320(03)00173-8.

Liu, N., Ma, Y., Li, R., Jin, H., Li, M., Huang, X., Feng, H. L., & Qiao, J. (2012). Comparison of follicular fluid amphiregulin and EGF concentrations in patients undergoing IVF with different stimulation protocols. *Endocrine,* 42(3), 708–716. https://doi.org/10.1007/s12020-012-9706-z.

Mantzavinos, T., Dalamanga, N., Hassiakos, D., Dimitriadou, F., Gregoriou, O., & Zourlas, P. A. (1993). Immunoglobulins IgG, IgA, IgM, complement C3, C4 and ferritin and transferrin levels in serum and follicular fluid in IVF patients. *Clinical and experimental obstetrics & gynecology,* 20(1), 32–36.

Matzuk, M. M., Burns, K. H., Viveiros, M. M., & Eppig, J. J. (2002). Intercellular communication in the mammalian ovary: oocytes carry the conversation. *Science (New York, N.Y.),* 296(5576), 2178–2180. https://doi.org/10.1126/science.1071965.

Mauro, A., Martelli, A., Berardinelli, P., Russo, V., Bernabò, N., Di Giacinto, O., Mattioli, M., & Barboni, B. (2014). Effect of antiprogesterone RU486 on VEGF expression and blood vessel remodeling on ovarian follicles before ovulation. *PLoS One,* 9(4): e95910. https://doi.org/10.1371/journal.pone.0095910.

McConnell, N. A., Yunus, R. S., Gross, S. A., Bost, K. L., Clemens, M. G., & Hughes, F. M., Jr (2002). Water permeability of an ovarian antral follicle is predominantly transcellular and mediated by aquaporins. *Endocrinology,* 143(8), 2905–2912. https://doi.org/10.1210/endo.143.8.8953.

McArthur, M. E., Irving-Rodgers, H. F., Byers, S., & Rodgers, R. J. (2000). Identification and immunolocalization of decorin, versican, perlecan, nidogen, and chondroitin sulfate proteoglycans in bovine small-antral ovarian follicles. *Biology of reproduction,* 63(3), 913–924. https://doi.org/10.1095/biolreprod63.3.913.

Mendoza, C., Ruiz-Requena, E., Ortega, E., Cremades, N., Martinez, F., Bernabeu, R., Greco, E., & Tesarik, J. (2002). Follicular fluid markers of oocyte developmental potential. *Human reproduction* (Oxford, England), 17(4), 1017–1022. https://doi.org/10.1093/humrep/17.4.1017.

Mihm, M., Austin, E. J., Good, T. E., Ireland, J. L., Knight, P. G., Roche, J. F., & Ireland, J. J. (2000). Identification of potential intrafollicular factors involved in selection of dominant follicles in heifers. *Biology of reproduction,* 63(3), 811–819. https://doi.org/10.1095/biolreprod63.3.811.

Miller, D. S., Bauer, B., & Hartz, A. M. (2008). Modulation of P-glycoprotein at the blood-brain barrier: opportunities to improve central nervous system pharmacotherapy. *Pharmacological reviews,* 60(2), 196–209. https://doi.org/10.1124/pr.107.07109.

Mitsube, K., Brännström, M., & Haraldsson, B. (2013). Modulation of microvascular permeability in the preovulatory rat ovary by an ovulatory gonadotropin stimulus. *Fertility and sterility,* 99(3), 903–909. https://doi.org/10.1016/j.fertnstert.2012.11.017.

Moncada, S., Palmer, R. M., & Higgs, E. A. (1991). Nitric oxide: physiology, pathophysiology, and pharmacology. *Pharmacological reviews,* 43(2), 109–142.

Monniaux D. (2016). Driving folliculogenesis by the oocyte-somatic cell dialog: Lessons from genetic models. *Theriogenology,* 86(1), 41–53. https://doi.org/10.1016/j.theriogenology.2016.04.017.

Monteleone, P., Giovanni Artini, P., Simi, G., Casarosa, E., Cela, V., & Genazzani, A. R. (2008). Follicular fluid VEGF levels directly correlate with perifollicular blood flow in normoresponder patients under- going IVF. *J Assist Reprod Genet,* 25(5): 183–6. https://doi.org/10.1007/s10815-008-9218-1.

Moreno, J. M., Núñez, M. J., Quiñonero, A., Martínez, S., de la Orden, M., Simón, C., Pellicer, A., Díaz-García, C., & Domínguez, F. (2015). Follicular fluid and mural granulosa cells microRNA profiles vary in in vitro fertilization patients depending on their age and oocyte maturation stage. *Fertil Steril,* 104(4), 1037–46.e1. https://doi.org/10.1016/j.fertnstert.2015.07.001.

Murdoch, W. J., Nix, K. J., & Dunn, T. G. (1983). Dynamics of ovarian blood supply to periovulatory follicles of the ewe. *Biology of reproduction,* 28(4), 1001–1006. https://doi.org/10.1095/biolreprod28.4.1001.

Nargund, G., Bourne, T., Doyle, P., Parsons, J., Cheng, W., Campbell, S., & Collins, W. (1996a). Associations between ultrasound indices of follicular blood flow, oocyte recovery and preimplantation embryo quality. *Human reproduction (Oxford, England),* 11(1), 109– https://doi.org/113. 10.1093/oxfordjournals.humrep.a019000.

Nargund, G., Doyle, P. E., Bourne, T. H., Parsons, J. H., Cheng, W. C., Campbell, S., & Collins, W. P. (1996b). Ultrasound derived indices of follicular blood flow before HCG administration and the prediction of oocyte recovery and preimplantation embryo quality. *Hum Reprod,* 11(11): 2512–7. https://doi.org/10.1093/oxfordjournals.humrep.a019150.

Oberleithner, H., Kusche-Vihrog, K., & Schillers, H. (2010). Endothelial cells as vascular salt sensors. *Kidney international,* 77(6), 490–494. https://doi.org/10.1038/ki.2009.490.

O'Gorman, A., Wallace, M., Cottell, E., Gibney, M. J., McAuliffe, F. M., Wingfield, M., & Brennan, L. (2013). Metabolic profiling of human follicular fluid identifies potential biomarkers of oocyte developmental competence. *Reproduction* (Cambridge, England), 146(4), 389–395. https://doi.org/10.1530/REP-13-0184.

Onalan, G., Selam, B., Baran, Y., Cincik, M., Onalan, R., Gündüz, U., Ural, A. U., & Pabuccu, R. (2005). Serum and follicular fluid levels of soluble Fas, soluble Fas ligand and apoptosis of luteinized granulosa cells in PCOS patients undergoing IVF. *Human reproduction* (Oxford, England), 20(9), 2391–2395. https://doi.org/10.1093/humrep/dei068.

Pancarci, S. M., Ari, U. Ç., Atakisi, O., Güngör, O., Ciğremiş, Y., & Bollwein, H. (2012). Nitric oxide concentrations, estradiol-17β progesterone ratio in follicular fluid, and COC quality with respect to perifollicular blood flow in cows. *Animal reproduction science,* 130(1-2), 9–15. https://doi.org/10.1016/j.anireprosci.2011.12.013.

Pelletier, R. M. (2011). The blood-testis barrier: the junctional permeability, the proteins and the lipids. *Prog Histochem Cytochem,* 46(2): 49–127. https://doi.org/10.1016/j.proghi.2011.05.001.

Pinto, C., Paccamonti, D., Eilts, B., Venugopal, C., Short, C., Gentry, L., Thompson, D., & Godke, R. (2003). Concentrations of nitric oxide in equine preovulatory follicles before and after administration of human chorionic gonadotropin. *Theriogenology,* 60 (5), 819-827. https://doi.org/10.1016/S0093-691X(03)00096-7.

Prieto, L., Quesada, J. F., Cambero, O., Pacheco, A., Pellicer, A., Codoceo, R., & Garcia-Velasco, J. A. (2012). Analysis of follicular fluid and serum markers of oxidative stress in women with infertility related to endometriosis. *Fertility and sterility,* 98(1), 126–130. https://doi.org/10.1016/j.fertnstert.2012.03.052.

Powers, R. W., Chen, L., Russell, P. T., & Larsen, W. J. (1995). Gonadotropin-stimulated regulation of blood-follicle barrier is mediated by nitric oxide. *The American journal of physiology,* 269(2 Pt 1), E290–E298. https://doi.org/10.1152/ajpendo.1995.269.2.E290.

Revelli, A., Delle Piane, L., Casano, S., Molinari, E., Massobrio, M., & Rinaudo, P. (2009). Follicular fluid content and oocyte quality: from single biochemical markers to metabolomics. *Reproductive biology and endocrinology:RB&E,* 7, 40. https://doi.org/10.1186/1477-7827-7-40.

Russell, D. L., Gilchrist, R. B., Brown, H. M., & Thompson, J. G. (2016). Bidirectional communication between cumulus cells and the oocyte: Old hands and new players?. *Theriogenology,* 86(1), 62–68. https://doi.org/10.1016/j.theriogenology.2016.04.019.

Rodgers, H. F., Irvine, C. M., van Wezel, I. L., Lavranos, T. C., Luck, M. R., Sado, Y., Ninomiya, Y., & Rodgers, R. J. (1998). Distribution of the alpha1 to alpha6 chains of type IV collagen in bovine follicles. *Biology of reproduction,* 59(6), 1334–1341. https://doi.org/10.1095/biolreprod59.6.1334.

Rodgers, R. J., Irving-Rodgers, H. F., & Russell, D. L. (2003). Extracellular matrix of the developing ovarian follicle. *Reproduction* (Cambridge, England), 126(4), 415–424. https://doi.org/10.1530/rep.0.1260415.

Rodgers, R. J., & Irving-Rodgers, H. F. (2010). Formation of the ovarian follicular antrum and follicular fluid. *Biology of reproduction,* 82(6), 1021–1029. https://doi.org/10.1095/biolreprod.109.082941.

San Roman, G. A., & Magoffin, D. A. (1992). Insulin-like growth factor binding proteins in ovarian follicles from women with polycystic ovarian disease: cellular source and levels in follicular fluid. *The Journal of clinical endocrinology and metabolism,* 75(4), 1010–1016. https://doi.org/10.1210/jcem.75.4.1383254.

Schweigert, F. J., Gericke, B., Wolfram, W., Kaisers, U., & Dudenhausen, J. W. (2006). Peptide and protein profiles in serum and follicular fluid of women undergoing IVF. *Human reproduction (Oxford, England),* 21(11), 2960–2968. https://doi.org/10.1093/humrep/del257.

Shalgi, R., Kraicer, P., Rimon, A., Pinto, M., & Soferman, N. (1973). Proteins of human follicular fluid: the blood-follicle barrier. *Fertility and sterility,* 24(6), 429–434.

Shimasaki, S., Moore, R. K., Otsuka, F., & Erickson, G. F. (2004). The bone morphogenetic protein system in mammalian reproduction. *Endocrine reviews,* 25(1), 72–101. https://doi.org/10.1210/er.2003-0007.

Simon, A. M., Goodenough, D. A., Li, E., & Paul, D. L. (1997). Female infertility in mice lacking connexin 37. *Nature,* 385(6616), 525–529. https://doi.org/10.1038/385525a0.

Siu, M. K., Wong, O. G., & Cheung, A. N. (2009). TrkB as a therapeutic target for ovarian cancer. *Expert opinion on therapeutic targets,* 13(10), 1169–1178. https://doi.org/10.1517/14728220903196787.

Siu, M. K., Chan, H. Y., Kong, D. S., Wong, E. S., Wong, O. G., Ngan, H. Y., Tam, K. F., Zhang, H., Li, Z., Chan, Q. K., Tsao, S. W., Strömblad, S., & Cheung, A. N. (2010). p21-activated kinase 4 regulates ovarian cancer cell proliferation, migration, and invasion and contributes to poor prognosis in patients. *Proceedings of the National Academy of Sciences of the United States of America,* 107(43), 18622–18627. https://doi.org/10.1073/pnas.0907481107.

Siu, M. K., & Cheng, C. Y. (2012). The blood-follicle barrier (BFB) in disease and in ovarian function. *Advances in experimental medicine and biology,* 763, 186–192. https://doi.org/10.1007/978-1-4614-4711-5_9.

Skowronski, M. T., Kwon, T. H., & Nielsen, S. (2009). Immunolocalization of aquaporin 1, 5, and 9 in the female pig reproductive system. *The journal of histochemistry and cytochemistry: official journal of the Histochemistry Society,* 57(1), 61–67. https://doi.org/10.1369/jhc.2008.952499.

Sugiura, K., Pendola, F. L., & Eppig, J. J. (2005). Oocyte control of metabolic cooperativity between oocytes and companion granulosa cells: energy metabolism. *Developmental biology,* 279(1), 20–30. https://doi.org/10.1016/j.ydbio.2004.11.027.

Tamanini, C., De Ambrogi, M. (2004). Angiogenesis in developing follicle and corpus luteum. *Reprod Domest Anim,* 39(4): 206–16. https://doi.org/10.1111/j.1439-0531.2004.00505.x.

Thomas, F. H., Ethier, J. F., Shimasaki, S., & Vanderhyden, B. C. (2005). Follicle-stimulating hormone regulates oocyte growth by modulation of expression of oocyte and granulosa cell factors. *Endocrinology,* 146(2), 941–949. https://doi.org/10.1210/en.2004-0826.

Thomas, F. H., & Vanderhyden, B. C. (2006). Oocyte-granulosa cell interactions during mouse follicular development: regulation of kit ligand expression and its role in oocyte growth. *Reproductive biology and endocrinology:RB&E,* 4, 19. https://doi.org/10.1186/1477-7827-4-19.

Von Wald, T., Monisova, Y., Hacker, M. R., Yoo, S. W., Penzias, A. S., Reindollar, R. R., & Usheva, A. (2010). Age-related variations in follicular apolipoproteins may influence human oocyte maturation and fertility potential. *Fertility and sterility,* 93(7), 2354–2361. https://doi.org/10.1016/j.fertnstert.2008.12.129.

Vural, F., Vural, B., Doğer, E., Çakıroğlu, Y., & Çekmen, M. (2016). Perifollicular blood flow and its relationship with endometrial vascularity, follicular fluid EG-VEGF, IGF-1, and inhibin-a levels and IVF outcomes. *Journal of assisted reproduction and genetics,* 33(10), 1355–1362. https://doi.org/10.1007/s10815-016-0780-7.

Welt, C. K., Taylor, A. E., Fox, J., Messerlian, G. M., Adams, J. M., & Schneyer, A. L. (2005). Follicular arrest in polycystic ovary syndrome is associated with deficient inhibin A and B biosynthesis. *The Journal of clinical endocrinology and metabolism,* 90(10), 5582–5587. https://doi.org/10.1210/jc.2005-0695.

Wigglesworth, K., Lee, K. B., O'Brien, M. J., Peng, J., Matzuk, M. M., & Eppig, J. J. (2013). Bidirectional communication between oocytes and ovarian follicular somatic cells is required for meiotic arrest of mammalian oocytes. *Proceedings of the National Academy of Sciences of the United States of America,* 110(39), E3723–E3729. https://doi.org/10.1073/pnas.1314829110.

Williams, C. J., & Erickson, G. F. (2012). Morphology and Physiology of the Ovary. In K. R. Feingold (Eds.) et al., *Endotext.* MDText.com, Inc. South Dartmouth (MA).

Winterhager, E., & Kidder, G. M. (2015). Gap junction connexins in female reproductive organs: implications for women's reproductive health. *Human reproduction update,* 21(3), 340–352. https://doi.org/10.1093/humupd/dmv007.

Yang, W. J., Liu, F. C., Hsieh, J. S., Chen, C. H., Hsiao, S. Y., & Lin, C. S. (2015). Matrix metalloproteinase 2 level in human follicular fluid is a reliable marker of human oocyte maturation in in vitro fertilization and intracytoplasmic sperm injection cycles. *Reproductive biology and endocrinology: RB&E,* 13, 102. https://doi.org/10.1186/s12958-015-0099-8.

Zachariae, F. (1958). Studies on the mechanism of ovulation: permeability of the blood-liquor barrier. *Acta Endocrinol,* 27(3): 339-42. https://doi.org/10.1530/acta.0.0270339.

Zhou, H., Ohno, N., Terada, N., Saitoh, S., Fujii, Y., & Ohno, S. (2007). Involvement of follicular basement membrane and vascular endothelium in blood follicle barrier formation of mice revealed by 'in vivo cryotechnique'. *Reproduction* (Cambridge, England), 134(2), 307–317. https://doi.org/10.1530/REP-07-0062.

Zhou, H., Ohno, N., Terada, N., Saitoh, S., Naito, I., & Ohno, S. (2008). Permselectivity of blood follicle barriers in mouse ovaries of the mifepristone-induced polycystic ovary model revealed by in vivo cryotechnique. *Reproduction (Cambridge, England),* 136(5), 599–610. https://doi.org/10.1530/REP-08-0022.

Chapter 6

The Placenta-Blood Barrier

Seda Karabulut*, PhD
Department of Histology and Embryology, International School of Medicine, İstanbul Medipol University, İstanbul, Turkiye

Abstract

The placenta is a fetomaternal organ that forms during pregnancy and acts as a connection and an exchange organ between the mother and the fetus. It provides the foetus with nourishment and oxygen, and also produces hormones. An important factor in achieving efficient targeting of drugs to the placenta is to prevent particles from crossing the placenta and reaching the foetus when it is not wanted. Coordination in the placenta is achieved through maternal-fetal interfaces called the blood-placental barrier (BPB), which receives signals from both maternal and fetal circulation. BPB consists of a multilayer interface that separates maternal and fetal blood. BPB undertakes a regulatory role that allocates and even synthesizes hormones, nutrients and growth factors necessary for the fetal development and pregnancy, carries out gas exchange, removes waste from the fetal circulation and limits fetal toxicity.

Keywords: placenta, placenta-blood barrier, fetus, embryo

Introduction

The placenta is a fetomaternal organ that forms during pregnancy and acts as a connection and an exchange organ between the mother and the fetus. It

* Corresponding Author's Email: sedakarabulut@medipol.edu.tr

In: A Histological Approach to Human Body Barriers
Editor: İlknur Keskin
ISBN: 979-8-89530-738-0

provides the foetus with nourishment and oxygen, and also produces hormones (Burton & Fowden, 2015). The placenta originates from the blastocyst after attachment of the blastocyst to the endometrium (the inner lining of the uterus) 7-10 days after fertilization. The placenta structure consists of 3 compartments: 1. basal plate, 2. intervillous site, and 3. chorionic plate. The basal plate develops from the endometrium and consists of trophoblastic cells (outer cells of blastocyst) and decidual cells which are modified stromal cells of endometrium. Trophoblast cells establishe the initial layer that separates maternal structures from fetal structures. The chorionic plate consists of the primary stem villi, as well as the arteries and veins of the chorion that stretch from the basal plate into the intervillous site (Jansen et al., 2020). The arteries of the umbilical cord bifurcate into chorionic arteries and terminate as capillaries. Maternal blood flows via the intervillous area and enters the arteries of the umbilical cord, ultimately reaching the foetal blood. Substances present in the mother's bloodstream encounter multiple layers of cellular barriers before they can potentially get into the bloodstream of the foetus. Drugs and nanoparticles present in the mother's bloodstream have the potential to pass through the placenta, depending on their physicochemical properties. This can have either positive or negative effects on the developing foetus (Griffiths & Campbell, 2015). The biology of placentation and the anatomy of the placenta differ among different species.

Delivery to the Placenta

An important factor in achieving efficient targeting of drugs to the placenta is to prevent particles from crossing the placenta and reaching the foetus when it is not wanted. Extensive research has been conducted to investigate the influence of particle size, charge, and material composition on the buildup of particles in the placenta and foetal tissue. Liposomes, being one of the initial delivery methods designed for targeted drug distribution throughout the body, have been the subject of substantial research. (Barzago et al., 1996). Encapsulating valproic acid in neutrally charged liposomes with a diameter of 230 nm resulted in a decrease in transfer to the foetus compared to free valproic acid (Barzago et al., 1996). Another study reported the same placenta model to examine the impact of liposome size on its ability to traverse the placenta. The transplacental transfer of fluorescently labelled liposomes of varying sizes, which contained equal quantities of phosphatidylcholine (PC) and cholesterol, was investigated (Bajoria & Contractor,1997a). The researchers employed a technique called thin film hydration to create multilamellar liposomes measuring 296 nm in diameter. They then subjected the liposomes to sonication for 2 and 30 minutes, resulting in smaller liposomes measuring 147 and 74 nm in diameter, respectively. Comparatively, the liposomes with a size of 74 nm exhibited enhanced placental uptake and transplacental transfer compared to the larger liposomes (Bajoria & Contractor,1997a). The impact of the surface charge of liposomes, with a size of around 70 nm, was examined outside of a living organism using the perfused human placenta model (Bajoria & Contractor,1997b). Liposomes with a neutral charge were created using PC and cholesterol. Liposomes with a negative charge were created using dicetylphosphate (DCP), PC, and cholesterol. Liposomes with a positive charge were created by substituting DCP with stearyl amine. Placental uptake of neutral and anionic liposomes containing carboxyfluorescein was 6-9 times greater compared to cationic liposomes, which exhibited similar uptake to free dye (Bajoria & Contractor, 1997b). This phenomenon can be explained by the selective absorption of negatively and neutrally charged liposomes of trophoblasts (Bajoria et al., 1997a). The transfer of carboxyfluorescein through the placenta was greatly enhanced by neutral and anionic liposomes, with an increase of 2.5-3%. On the other hand, cationic liposomes only showed a slight increase of 0.4% (Bajoria & Contractor, 1997b). Subsequently, these discoveries were utilised to explore the feasibility of employing liposomal drug carriers for delivering drugs to the foetus. The transplacental transfer of thyroxine was evaluated by testing anionic liposomes loaded with the medication in a perfused placenta model (Bajoria et al., 1997b). The findings demonstrated that the inclusion of thyroxine into anionic liposomes enhanced the medicine's ability to cross the placenta, in comparison to the substance administered alone. In its free form, the drug is quickly metabolised in blood-based media before crossing the placenta. However, drugs in soluble form generally can cross the placenta. An in vivo study was conducted to investigate the impact of liposome composition on the transplacental transport of different medicines to the rat placenta (Tüzel-Kox et al., 1995). Liposomes with neutral, negative, and positive charges were synthesised using the method described before. The liposomes were loaded with radiolabeled inulin and subsequent sonication to create particles with a size range of around 30 nm. The rat placenta and uterus rats contained up to double the quantity of inulin when it was encapsulated in negatively charged liposomes, compared to when it was in its free form. Additionally, after intravenous injection into maternal blood, the amount of inulin was approximately 1.5 times higher when encapsulated in negatively charged liposomes compared to neutral or positively charged ones.

While no free inulin was found in the foetuses, this may be because it has a low ability to cross the foetal side. However, other radioactive drugs including methotrexate, penicillin, and riboflavin were loaded in liposomes, were taken up 2-5 times more than the free drugs (Tüzel-Kox et al., 1995). Therefore, although smaller and negatively charged liposomes are more easily taken up by the placenta, their usage should be approached with more care due to the possibility of their transferring from the placenta to the foetus. It is crucial to emphasise that various nanomaterials exhibited distinct size thresholds for passing the placenta. Gold nanoparticles ranging from 10 to 30 nanometers in size were taken up by trophoblasts, but could not be detected on the foetal side of the human placenta after 6 hours of perfusion (Myllynen et al., 2008). Nevertheless, research has demonstrated that polystyrene nanoparticles with a size of up to 240 nm can pass through the human placenta during a period of 3 hours after perfusion. It is important to conduct specific toxicological tests on both the foetus and the mother for each new nanomedicine before determining its safety during pregnancy.

The addition of polyethylene glycol (PEG) to the surface of liposomes has been demonstrated to decrease the uptake of liposomes by the placenta and hinder their transfer across the placenta by preventing interactions with cell surfaces (Soininen et al., 2015). The absorption and cytotoxicity of liposomal doxorubicin were dramatically reduced in human placental choriocarcinoma cells compared to the unencapsulated drug. Using a human placenta perfusion model, it was observed that up to 12% of the doxorubicin dose passed the placenta after 4 hours of perfusion when administered in the free or non-PEGylated liposome form. However, no transport was observed with the PEGylated liposome (Soininen et al., 2015). Animal models were used to conduct additional tests on PEGylated liposomes (Kaga et al., 2012). PEGylated liposomes were utilised as carriers for haemoglobin to potentially treat foetal hypoxia. Liposomes with a neutral charge were created using PC, cholesterol, and PEG–lipid with a 5 kDa PEG chain. These liposomes had a size of 250 nm. Following intravenous administration, the liposomes were detected in maternal organs such as the liver, spleen, kidney, and placenta, but were not observed in the tissues of the rat foetus. Although the study showed that this medication is well-tolerated during pregnancy, additional research is needed to assess the therapeutic effects in hypoxic models (Kaga et al., 2012). The inclusion of gadolinium within liposomes, which were approximately 120 nm in size and coated with polyethylene glycol (PEG), consisting of phosphatidylcholine (PC), cholesterol, and PEG-lipid, resulted in a decrease in its ability to penetrate the placenta in pregnant mice (Shetty et al., 2016). The authors introduced this technique as a novel approach to visualise placental dysfunction using magnetic resonance imaging (MRI), particularly in cases where it is challenging to observe the attachment of placental villi to the myometrium using noncontrast MRI (Shetty et al., 2016).

Blood-Placenta Barrier (BPB)

The placenta is an important fetomaternal organ that plays a role in maintaining fetal life throughout pregnancy, consisting of the fetal and maternal face, with a diameter of 12-25 cm, a thickness of 3 cm, and a weight of approximately 500-600 g. Research on the placenta has increased due to the 'Human Placenta Project' initiated by the National Institutes of Health in 2014 (Guttmacher et al.,2014; Guttmacher & Spong, 2015). But there is still limited data on how the placenta facilitates a healthy intrauterine environment.

Coordination in the placenta is achieved through maternal-fetal interfaces called the blood-placental barrier (BPB), which receive signals from both maternal and fetal circulation (Griffiths & Campbell, 2015). BPB undertakes a regulatory role that allocates and even synthesizes hormones, nutrients and growth factors necessary for the fetal development and pregnancy, carries out gas exchange, removes waste from the fetal circulation and limits fetal toxicity. Dysfunction in BPB and placental insufficiency may cause intrauterine growth restriction (Baschat & Hecher, 2004; Krishna & Bhalerao, 2011). Therefore, proper functioning of BPB is important for a healthy fetal development (Griffiths & Campbell, 2015; Garnica & Chan, 1996; Jansson, 2016). Modeling BPB has been an active research area in terms of determining which substances can reach the fetus and learning whether they affect fetal development (Al-Enazy et al., 2017). In the literature, there are hydrogel (Nishiguchi et al., 2018; Levkovitz et al., 2013; Arumugasaamy et al., 2019a), bioreactor (Ma et al., 1999; McConkey et al., 2016), organ-on-chip (Zhu et al., 2018; Lee et al., 2015; Pemathilaka et al., 2019) and bioprinting (Mandt et al., 2018)-based models developed to mimic the placental barrier. These models, developed in terms of placenta biology, the understanding of placental transport mechanism, fetal development and new drug discovery, are promising.

Transition from BPB is achieved by simple diffusion or through carrier proteins, such as the oxygen transfer (Watson & Cross, 2005). Most substances, including antibodies, small molecules and drugs (Al-Enazy et al., 2017; Palmeira et al., 2012), require membrane proteins for passage, which is achieved by protein-dependent transport, facilitated diffusion or active transport. Thus, communication is allowed by bidirectional passage through the placenta (Nugent & Bale, 2015). Biological barriers' apical and basal sides are structurally distinct, giving them a semi-permeable nature permitting the uptake of useful substances while restricting harmful and toxic substances. The apical side of the BPB includes a brush-border membrane to increase the surface area, thus facilitating higher contact with maternal blood. Carrier proteins are abundant in this apical membrane (Watson & Cross, 2005). Various maternal and fetal cell types are essential for the proper development and function of the placental barrier. However, syncytiotrophoblasts are the main cell population that regulate the placental transport and exchange (Wang & Zhao, 2010). For a healthy fetal development, it is necessary to examine BPB and placental transport mechanism.

Development and Structure of the Blood Placenta Barrier

The human placenta develops from the trophoblast cells, the outer layer of the embryo during the preimplantation process, approximately 5 days after fertilization. At the preimplantation stage, the embryonic embryo is called the blastocyst (the zonna pellucida has disappeared) and consists of 2 cell populations: the inner cell mass or embryoblast; It is in the form of an outer cell mass or trophoblast. Approximately on the 6th day of development, with the implantation of the blastocyst from the embryoblast pole into the uterus, trophoblast cells rapidly proliferate and give rise to cytotrophoblasts and syncytiotophoblasts. Cytotrophoblasts and syncytiotophoblasts have a key role in placenta development after the embryo implants the uterus (Cindrova-Davies & Sferruzzi-Perri, 2022). The first uteroplacental circulation through the fetal and maternal interfaces is observed at approximately the 9th day of development, with the formation of trophoblastic lacunae within the syncytiotrophoblasts and the anastomosis of trophoblastic lacunae with maternal blood vessels. In the future, with the proliferation of cytotrophoblasts, the growth of extraembryonic mesoderm and the blood vessel development, primary, secondary and tertiary chorionic villi will participate in the establishement of BPD. Primary chorionic villi appear on 11th and 13th days of development due to the inductive effect of the extraembryonic mesoderm on the cytotrophoblasts. Here, rapidly proliferating cytotrophoblasts send cell cords towards the syncytiotrophoblasts, in which lacunae are observed. Secondary chorionic villi will develop with the observation of extraembryonic mesoderm-derived mesenchyme in the center of these cell cords. Here, secondary chorionic villi cover the chorionic sac surface. At the end of the 3rd week, tertiary chorionic villi will be observed with the formation of blood vessels in the mesenchyme of secondary chorionic villi. As the tertiary chorionic villi develop, the cytotrophoblastic cells in the villi will continue to grow outward, passing through the syncytiotrophoblasts, and thus a trophoblastic shell consisting of cytotrophoblasts will form around the syncytiotrophoblasts. The trophoblastic shell plays a role in the advanced development of the placenta and in maintaining the connection of the fetal part with the endometrium (Kojima et al., 2022). After ~8 weeks of pregnancy, the basic structure of the placenta is formed and maternal blood starts to flow through the villi. The placenta and villi will continue to change and grow for suppliying the necessary nutrition throughout the pregnancy. The thickness of the placental barrier in the first trimester is ~ 20–30 μm, and the thickness will decrease significantly at the end of the third trimester (to ~ 5 μm) to allow increased exchange between mother and the fetus (Jauniaux et al., 2003; Knöfler et al., 2019).

BPB consists of a multilayer interface that separates maternal and fetal blood. Fetal section from chorion frondosum; The maternal part consists of decidua basalis. BPB is a cellular-rich structure. Here, there are villous cytotrophoblasts, syncytiotrophoblasts, extravillous trophoblasts and trophoblast giant cells, which are of trophoblast origin. Cells that participate in the formation of the placenta but are not of trophoblast origin are Hofbauer cells (placental macrophages), fetal endothelial cells and decidual cells (Douglas et al., 2009; Costa, 2016). All of these cells interact with each other and contribute to the functions of the placenta, which is a physical and chemical barrier responsible for immunity and hormone production (Tang et al., 2011; Arumugasaamy et al., 2019b; Tarrade et al., 2001). The elements that make up the BPB are listed below from inside to outside (Figure 1). Here, the desmosomal connections between cytotrophoblasts and syncytiophoblasts and the combined basal lamina of cytotrophoblasts and fetal endothelial cells are important for the formation of BPB (Ravishankar & Redline, 2019).

1) Endothelial cells lining the fetal capillaries
2) Basal lamina of the fetal capillaries
3) Basal lamina where cytotrophoblasts and syncytiotrophoblasts sit
4) Cytotrophoblasts

5) Syncytiotrophoblasts (rich in microvilli)
6) Maternal blood vessels and decidual cells

Subtypes of trophoblast (villous cytotrophoblasts, syncytiotrophoblasts and extravillous trophoblasts) originating from the fetal trophoectoderm constitute the majority of the cells that make up BPB. Villous cytotrophoblasts originating from the cytotrophoblast stem cell population merge to form multi-nucleated syncytiotrophoblasts, which serve as the dominant coordinator of placental transport and hormone production, or can differentiate into extravillous trophoblasts, acquiring invasive properties. In addition, fetal endothelial cells and Hofbauer cells, which are of fetal origin and mesoderm origin and play a role in regulating placental transport and trophoblast function, also participate in the formation of BPB. Decidual cells of maternal origin function as a source of nutrients during placental and fetal development. The basement membrane where villous cytotrophoblasts and syncytiotrophoblasts reside and the extracellular matrix (ECM) in its continuity contribute to the formation of the microenvironment within the BBP and to molecular transport throughout the BPB (Wang & Zhao, 2010; Kao et al., 1988).

At the molecular level, syncytiotrophoblasts have a chemical barrier function that regulates the absorption of endogenous and exogenous substances (Kitano et al., 2004). In addition to participating in the formation of BPB, syncytiotrophoblasts also produce hormones for a healthy pregnancy. Hormones required for the continuation of pregnancy, placental development, trophoblast invasion, placental angiogenesis, embryo implantation, and fetal development include human chorionic gonadotropin (hCG), progesterone, estrogen, and placental lactogens (Costa, 2016; Evain-Brion & Malassine, 2003). Additionally, a model of BPB can be mimicked by in vitro modeling of syncytiotrophoblasts (Haider et al., 2018). Various cell lines can be used as models of syncytiotrophoblasts in vitro, such as primary human trophoblasts and human choriocarcinoma cell line clones (Vähäkangas & Myllynen, 2009). Recent advances allow the derivation of human trophoblast stem cells from PHTs. This enables the investigation of the molecular and functional properties of human trophoblasts and creates a potential application area in the examination of placental pathologies (Haider et al., 2018; Turco et al., 2018).

As villous cytotrophoblasts gain an invasive phenotype, they begin to form cytotrophoblast cells that help anchor the placenta to the uterus. Some of the cytotrophoblasts develop into extravillous trophoblasts. Extravillous trophoblasts exceed the upper syncytiotrophoblast cell layer and invade and reshape the maternal tissue, uterine spiral arteries and uterine glands (Costa, 2016; Pollheimer et al., 2018; Lunghi et al., 2007). Some of the extravillous trophoblast cells help to anchor the placenta to the maternal decidua (cytotrophoblastic shell). Additionally, these cells fuse to form giant multinucleated trophoblastic cell populations, which lose their migration ability, invade, and inhibit deeper penetration to the uterus. It has been stated that trophoblast giant cells may have important roles for regulating blood circulation by releasing vasoactive and angiogenic factors (Hemberger et al., 2003). With the invasive and remodeling properties of extravillous trophoblast cells, increased maternal blood flow to the placenta and nutrients become available for the placenta for the fetus development (Costa, 2016; Lunghi et al., 2007; Tessier et al., 2015).

Decidualization is the name of a process in which endometrial cells undergo functional and morphological changes to prepare for pregnancy. While these changes occur, a lining is formed in the area with the secretion of cytokines, growth factors and proteins, as well as an increase in leukocytes. It is reported that decidual stromal cells and leukocytes initiate remodeling of maternal vasculature. However, it is also reported that the decidua must be occupied by extravillous trophoblasts for extensive remodeling of the maternal spiral arteries (Harris, 2010). Some of the extravillous trophoblasts migrate through the lumen through the walls of the uterine spiral arteries and significantly expand these vessels to change blood flow to the placenta. During the first trimester, extravillous trophoblasts form plugs that partially block maternal blood flow to the placenta. It is stated that this situation is an important physiological process for early placental development and trophoblast differentiation, thus creating a temporary hypoxia state. (James et al., 2015; James et al., 2018). In addition, extravillous trophoblasts also invade the uterine glands and thus provide early access of nutrients to the developing fetus during the period when maternal blood flow to the placenta is restricted (Moser et al., 2015). Extravillous trophoblasts and decidual cells together provide a suitable environment to support early placental development and fetal growth and help placental transport (Lunghi et al., 2007).

Hofbauer cells are macrophages of the placenta, and there is limited data about their role in regulating transport (Wang & Zhao, 2010; Tang et al., 2011). Macrophages have the M1 phenotype, which triggers an inflammatory response to protect from foreign agents such as bacteria, and the M2 phenotype, which plays a role in repair mechanisms, including ECM construction (Reyers & Golos, 2018). Hofbauer cells seem to be more similar to the M2 phenotype. Additionally, it has been stated that these cells may have a role in regulating the expression of growth factors and cytokines, which may affect trophoblast function (Wang & Zhao, 2010; Reyers & Golos, 2018). As a result, the role of these cells is still unknown but they may have a function in immunological transfer or fetus protection (Tang et al., 2011).

Endothelial cells play an important role in BPB. Fetal blood passes through the fetal capillaries and reaches the placenta via the umbilical arteries. Here, after the fetal blood receives oxygen, nutrients and hormones from the mother, clean blood returns to the fetus through the umbilical veins. Fetal endothelial cells forming these capillaries exhibit different phenotypes for the arterial and venous system. It is also stated that, besides acting as vascular cells, they establish an extra barrier to regulate the transport (Cvitic et al., 2018; Lang et al., 2008). It has also been reported that fetal endothelial cells are carriers that allow substrates taken up by the syncytiotrophoblast layer to enter the fetal circulation and remove potentially harmful substances (Elad et al., 2014). In studies trying to model placental transport, it has been reported that human umbilical vein-derived endothelial cells (HUVECs) were used in vitro and that HUVECs contributed to the general phenotype in establishing the CPB architecture (Levkovitz et al., 2013; Arumugasaamy et al., 2018; Blundell et al., 2016). However, it is controversial whether there is a cell type that can best mimic placental transport physiologically (Lang et al., 2008; Sobrevia et al., 2011).

BPB contains ECM and basement membrane proteins, including laminin, fibronectin, and collagen, that help regulate trophoblast behavior (Wang & Zhao, 2010). Thickening and hardness of basement membrane is reported to be associated with placental pathologies (Wong et al., 2018; Fox, 1968). In addition, it has been reported that changes in trophoblastic cell organization, differentiation, and gene expressions are observed depending on the basement membrane content or thickness (Wong et al., 2018; Kuo et al., 2018).

Corrugated junctions are groups of transmembrane channels that include connexin proteins which enable cell-cell communications in all tissue types. Connexins are membrane proteins of a multigene family including more than 20 members in humans. Connexin expression and intracellular and intercellular communication through corrugated junctions play an important role in development and differentiation processes (Bruzzone, 1996). Corrugated connections play a major role in the development and functions of the placenta, which is responsible for the exchange of substances between mother and fetus (Leiser & Kaufmann, 1994; Cronier et al., 2001). Gene knockouts applied in rodent studies provide insight into the role of Cx genes in mouse placental development. Cx26 is involved in transplacental uptake of glucose (Gabriel et al., 1998); Cx31 is involved in the proliferative process of trophoblastic cells (Plum et al., 2001); Cx45 plays a role in placental vascularization (Kruger et al., 2000). In humans, Cx43 is involved in the fusion process of cytotrophoblastic cells while syncytiotrophoblasts are formed (Frendo et al., 2003); It is stated that Cx40 plays a critical role in the transition of trophoblastic cells invading the endometrium to a proliferative phenotype (Hellmann et al., 1996). In addition, the invasive function of trophoblasts is important for placenta development. Erosion of the uterine epithelium and connective tissue causes trophoblasts to come closer to the maternal tissue. Here, cytotrophoblastic cells will differentiate into multinucleated syncytiotrophoblasts by fusion. The existence of corrugated connections between cytotrophoblastic cells and syncytiotrophoblasts has been demonstrated structurally and it has been stated that these connections function in the trophoblastic cell-cell fusion process (Malassine et al., 1984).

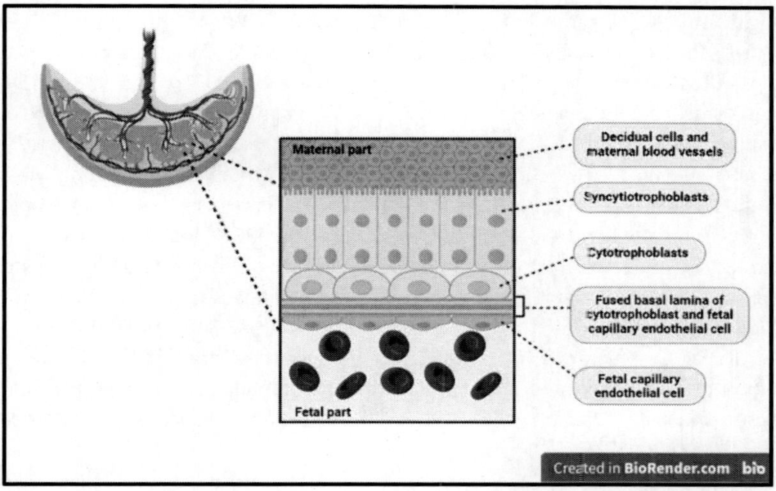

Figure 1. Schematic representation of the placenta-blood barrier.

Conclusion

The placenta is a fetomaternal organ which belongs to both the fetus and the mother. It is an exchange organ between the fetus and the mother and establishes an important barrier between them. The blood-placental barrier (BPB) is the interface that acts as a selectively permeable barrier, which permits many metabolites' passage while limiting the others. This function is strictly controlled by the contributors of this structure. Any perturbations in the system may lead to important problems in embryonic development and the fetal period. Novel research is needed to better understand the structural components and physiology as well as its control mechanisms to reflect its role for potential diseases of fetal development and defects.

References

Al-Enazy, S., Ali, S., Albekairi, N., El-Tawil, M., & Rytting. E. (2017). Placental control of drug delivery. *Adv. Drug Deliv. Rev,* 116, 63-72. https://doi.org/10.1016/j.addr.2016.08.002.

Arumugasaamy, N., Gudelsky, A., Hurley-Novatny, A., Kim, P. C. W., & Fisher, J. P. (2019a). Model placental barrier phenotypic response to fluoxetine and sertraline: a comparative study. *Adv Healthc Mater,* 8 (18), e1900476. https://doi.org/10.1002/adhm.201900476.

Arumugasaamy, N., Navarro, J., Kent Leach, J., Kim, P. C. W., & Fisher, J. P. (2019b). In Vitro Models for Studying Transport Across Epithelial Tissue Barriers. *Annals of biomedical engineering,* 47(1), 1–21. https://doi.org/10.1007/s10439-018-02124-w.

Arumugasaamy, N., Ettehadieh, L. E., Kuo, C. Y., Paquin-Proulx, D., Kitchen, S. M., Santoro, M., Placone, J. K., Silveira, P. P., Aguiar, R. S., Nixon, D. F., Fisher, J. P., & Kim, P. C. W. (2018). Biomimetic Placenta-Fetus Model Demonstrating Maternal-Fetal Transmission and Fetal Neural Toxicity of Zika Virus. *Annals of biomedical engineering,* 46(12), 1963–1974. https://doi.org/10.1007/s10439-018-2090-y.

Bajoria, R., & Contractor, S. F. (1997a). Effect of the size of liposomes on the transfer and uptake of carboxyfluorescein by the perfused human term placenta. *J Pharm Pharmacol,* 49(7), 675-81. https://doi.org/10.1111/j.2042-7158.1997.tb06091.x.

Bajoria, R., & Contractor, S. (1997b). Effect of Surface Charge of Small Unilamellar Liposomes on Uptake and Transfer of Carboxyfluorescein across the Perfused Human Term Placenta. *Pediatr Res,* 42, 520–527. https://doi.org/10.1203/00006450-199710000-00017.

Bajoria, R., Sooranna, S. R., & Contractor, S. F. (1997a). Endocytotic uptake of small unilamellar liposomes by human trophoblast cells in culture. *Hum Reprod,* 12(6), 1343-8. https://doi.org/10.1093/humrep/12.6.1343.

Bajoria, R., Fisk, N. M., & Contractor, S. F. (1997b). Liposomal thyroxine: a noninvasive model for transplacental fetal therapy. *J Clin Endocrinol Metab,* 82(10), 3271-7. https://doi.org/10.1210/jcem.82.10.4301.

Baschat, A. A., & Hecher. K. (2004). Fetal growth restriction due to placental disease. *Semin. Perinatol,* 28(1), 67-80. https://doi.org/10.1053/j.semperi.2003.10.014.

Barzago, M. M., Bortolotti, A., Stellari, F. F., Diomede, L., Algeri, M., Efrati, S., Salmona, M., & Bonati, M. (1996). Placental transfer of valproic acid after liposome encapsulation during in vitro human placenta perfusion. *J Pharmacol Exp Ther,* 277(1), 79-86.

Blundell, C., Tess, E. R., Schanzer, A. S., Coutifaris, C., Su, E. J., Parry, S., & Huh, D. (2016). A microphysiological model of the human placental barrier. *Lab on a chip,* 16(16), 3065–3073. https://doi.org/10.1039/c6lc00259e.

Bruzzone, R., White, T. W., & Paul, D. L. (1996). Connections with connexins: the molecular basis of direct intercellular signaling. *European journal of biochemistry,* 238(1), 1–27. https://doi.org/10.1111/j.1432-1033.1996.0001q x.

Burton, G. J., & Fowden, A. L. (2015). The placenta: a multifaceted, transient organ. *Philos Trans R Soc Lond B Biol Sci,* 370(1663), 20140066. https //doi.org/10.1098/rstb. 2014.0066.

Cindrova-Davies, T., & Sferruzzi-Perri, A. N. (2022). Human placental development and function. *Semin Cell Dev Biol,* 131, 66-77. https://doi.org/10.1016/j.semcdb. 2022.03.039.

Costa, M. A. (2016). The endocrine function of human placenta: an overview. *Reproductive biomedicine online,* 32(1), 14–43. https://doi.org/10.1016/j.rbmo.2015.10.005.

Cronier, L., Bastide, B., Defamie, N., Niger, C., Pointis, G., Gasc, J. M., & Malassiné, A. (2001). Involvement of gap junctional communication and connexin expression in trophoblast differentiation of the human placenta. *Histology and histopathology,* 16(1), 285–295. https://doi.org/10.14670/HH-16.285.

Cvitic, S., Novakovic, B., Gordon, L., Ulz, C. M., Mühlberger, M., Diaz-Perez, F. I., Joo, J. E., Svendova, V., Schimek, M. G., Trajanoski, S., Saffery, R., Desoye, G., & Hiden, U. (2018). Human fetoplacental arterial and venous endothelial cells are differentially programmed by gestational diabetes mellitus, resulting in cell-specific barrier function changes. *Diabetologia,* 61(11), 2398–2411. https://doi.org/10.1007/s00125-018-4699-7.

Douglas, G. C., VandeVoort, C. A., Kumar, P., Chang, T. C., & Golos, T. G. (2009). Trophoblast stem cells: models for investigating trophectoderm differentiation and placental development. *Endocrine reviews,* 30(3), 228–240. https://doi.org/10.1210/er.2009-0001.

Elad, D., Levkovitz, R., Jaffa, A. J., Desoye, G., & Hod, M. (2014). Have we neglected the role of fetal endothelium in transplacental transport?. *Traffic (Copenhagen, Denmark),* 15(1), 122–126. https://doi.org/10.1111/tra.12130.

Evain-Brion, D., & Malassine, A. (2003). Human placenta as an endocrine organ. *Growth Horm IGF Res,* 13, 34–37. https://doi.org/10.1016/s1096-6374(03)00053-4.

Fox H. (1968). Basement membrane changes in the villi of the human placenta. *The Journal of obstetrics and gynaecology of the British Commonwealth,* 75(3), 302–306. https://doi.org/10.1111/j.1471-0528.1968.tb02082.x.

Frendo, J. L., Cronier, L., Bertin, G., Guibourdenche, J., Vidaud, M., Evain-Brion, D. & Malassine, A. (2003). Involvement of connexin 43 in human trophoblast cell fusion and differentiation. *J Cell Sci,* 116(16), 3413–3421. https://doi.org/10.1242/jcs.00648.

Gabriel, H. D., Jung, D., Bützler, C., Temme, A., Traub, O., Winterhager, E., & Willecke, K. (1998). Transplacental uptake of glucose is decreased in embryonic lethal connexin26-deficient mice. *The Journal of cell biology,* 140(6), 1453–1461. https://doi.org/10.1083/jcb.140.6.1453.

Garnica, A. D., & Chan, W. Y. (1996). The role of the placenta in fetal nutrition and growth. *J. Am. Coll. Nutr,* 15(3), 206-222. https://doi.org/10.1080/07315724.1996.10718591.

Griffiths, S., & Campbell, J. P. (2015). Placental structure, function and drug transfer. *Continuing Education in Anaesthesia, Critical Care & Pain,* 15(2), 84-89. https://doi.org/10.1093/bjaceaccp/mku013.

Guttmacher, A. E., Maddox, Y. T., & Spong, C. Y. (2014). The human placenta project: placental structure, development, and function in real time. *Placenta,* 35(5), 303-304. https://doi.org/10.1016/j.placenta.2014.02.012.

Guttmacher, A. E., & Spong, C. Y. (2015). The human placenta project: it's time for real time. *American Journal of Obstetrics & Gynecology,* 213(4), 3-5. https://doi.org/10.1016/j.ajog.2015.08.037.

Haider, S., Meinhardt, G., Saleh, L., Kunihs, V., Gamperl, M., Kaindl, U., Ellinger, A., Burkard, T. R., Fiala, C., Pollheimer, J., Mendjan, S., Latos, P. A., & Knöfler, M. (2018). Self-Renewing Trophoblast Organoids Recapitulate the Developmental Program of the Early Human Placenta. *Stem cell reports,* 11(2), 537–551. https://doi.org/10.1016/j.stemcr.2018.07.004.

Harris L. K. (2010). Review: Trophoblast-vascular cell interactions in early pregnancy: how to remodel a vessel. *Placenta,* 31, 93–98. https://doi.org/10.1016/j.placenta.2009.12.012.

Hellmann, P., Winterhager, E., & Spray, D. C. (1996). Properties of connexin40 gap junction channels endogenously expressed and exogenously overexpressed in human choriocarcinoma cell lines. *Pflugers Archiv: European journal of physiology,* 432(3), 501–509. https://doi.org/10.1007/s004240050162.

Hemberger, M., Nozaki, T., Masutani, M., & Cross, J. C. (2003). Differential expression of angiogenic and vasodilatory factors by invasive trophoblast giant cells depending on depth of invasion. *Dev. Dyn.,* 227 (2), 185-191. https://doi.org/10.1002/dvdy.10291.

James, J. L., Hurley, D. G., Gamage, T. K., Zhang, T., Vather, R., Pantham, P., Murthi, P., & Chamley, L. W. (2015). Isolation and characterisation of a novel trophoblast side-population from first trimester placentae. *Reproduction* (Cambridge, England), 150(5), 449–462. https://doi.org/10.1530/REP-14-0646.

James, J. L., Saghian, R., Perwick, R., & Clark, A. R. (2018). Trophoblast plugs: impact on utero-placental haemodynamics and spiral artery remodelling. *Human reproduction* (Oxford, England), 33(8), 1430–1441. https://doi.org/10.1093/humrep/dey225.

Jansen, C. H. J. R., Kastelein, A. W., Kleinrouweler, C. E., Van Leeuwen, E., De Jong, K. H., Pajkrt, E., & Van Noorden, C. J. F. (2020). Development of placental abnormalities in location and anatomy. *Acta Obstet Gynecol Scand,* 99(8), 983-993. https://doi.org/10.1111/aogs.13834.

Jansson, T. (2016). Placenta plays a critical role in maternal–fetal resource allocation. *Proceedings of the National Academy of Sciences,* 113(40), 11066-11068. https://doi.org/10.1073/pnas.1613437113.

Jauniaux, E., Hempstock, J., Greenwold, N., & Burton, G. J. (2003). Trophoblastic oxidative stress in relation to temporal and regional differences in maternal placental blood flow in normal and abnormal early pregnancies. *The American journal of pathology,* 162(1), 115–125. https://doi.org/10.1016/S0002-9440(10)63803-5.

Kaga, M., Li, H., Ohta, H., Taguchi, K., Ogaki, S., Izumi, H., Inagaki, M., Tsuchiya, S., Okamura, K., Otagiri, M., Sakai, H., & Yaegashi, N. (2012). Liposome-encapsulated hemoglobin (hemoglobin-vesicle) is not transferred from mother to fetus at the late stage of pregnancy in the rat model. *Life Sciences,* 91(11-12), 420-428. https://doi.org/10.1016/j.lfs.2012.08.021.

Kao, L. C., Caltabiano, S., Wu, S., Strauss, J. F., & Kliman, H. J. (1988). The human villous cytotrophoblast: interactions with extracellular matrix proteins, endocrine function, and cytoplasmic differentiation in the absence of syncytium formation. *Dev Biol,* 130(2), 693-702. https://doi.org/10.1016/0012-1606(88)90361-2.

Kitano, T., Iizasa, H., Hwang, I. W., Hirose, Y., Morita, T., Maeda, T., & Nakashima, E. (2004). Conditionally immortalized syncytiotrophoblast cell lines as new tools for study of the blood-placenta barrier. *Biol. Pharm. Bull.,* 27(6), 753-759. https://doi.org/10.1248/bpb.27.753.

Knöfler, M., Haider, S., Saleh, L., Pollheimer, J., Gamage, T. K. J. B., & James, J. (2019). Human placenta and trophoblast development: key molecular mechanisms and model systems. *Cellular and molecular life sciences: CMLS,* 76(18), 3479–3496. https://doi.org/10.1007/s00018-019-03104-6.

Krishna, U., & Bhalerao, S. (2011). Placental insufficiency and fetal growth restriction. *J Obstet Gynaecol India,* 61(5), 505–511. https://doi.org/10.1007/s13224-011-0092-x.

Kojima, J., Ono, M., Kuji, N., & Nishi, H. (2022). Human Chorionic Villous Differentiation and Placental Development. *Int J Mol Sci,* 23(14), 8003. https://doi.org/10.3390/ijms23148003.

Krüger, O., Plum, A., Kim, J. S., Winterhager, E., Maxeiner, S., Hallas, G., Kirchhoff, S., Traub, O., Lamers, W. H., & Willecke, K. (2000). Defective vascular development in connexin 45-deficient mice. *Development* (Cambridge, England), 127(19), 4179–4193. https://doi.org/10.1242/dev.127.19.4179.

Kuo, C. Y., Guo, T., Cabrera-Luque, J., Arumugasaamy, N., Bracaglia, L., Garcia-Vivas, A., Santoro, M., Baker, H., Fisher, J., & Kim, P. (2018). Placental basement membrane proteins are required for effective cytotrophoblast invasion in a three-dimensional bioprinted placenta model. *Journal of biomedical materials research. Part A,* 106(6), 1476–1487. https://doi.org/10.1002/jbm.a.36350.

Lang, I., Schweizer, A., Hiden, U., Ghaffari-Tabrizi, N., Hagendorfer, G., Bilban, M., Pabst, M. A., Korgun, E. T., Dohr, G., & Desoye, G. (2008). Human fetal placental endothelial cells have a mature arterial and a juvenile venous phenotype with adipogenic and osteogenic differentiation potential. *Differentiation; research in biological diversity,* 76(10), 1031–1043. https://doi.org/10.1111/j.1432-0436.2008.00302.x.

Lee, J. S., Romero, R., Han, Y. M., Kim, H. C., Kim, C. J., Hong, J. S., & Huh, D. (2016). Placenta-on-a-chip: a novel platform to study the biology of the human placenta. J. *Matern. Fetal Neonatal Med,* 29(7), 1046-54. https://doi.org/10.3109/14767058.2015.1038518.

Leiser, R., & Kaufmann, P. (1994). Placental structure: in a comparative aspect. *Experimental and clinical endocrinology,* 102(3), 122–134. https://doi.org/10.1055/s-0029-1211275.

Levkovitz, R., Zaretsky, U., Gordon, Z., Jaffa, A. J., & Elad, D. (2013). In vitro simulation of placental transport: part I. biological model of the placental barrier. *Placenta,* 34 (8), 699-707. https://doi.org/10.1016/j.placenta.2013.03.014.

Lunghi, L., Ferretti, M. E., Medici, S., Biondi, C., & Vesce, F. (2007). Control of human trophoblast function. *Reproductive biology and endocrinology: RB&E,* 5, 6. https://doi.org/10.1186/1477-7827-5-6.

Ma, T., Yang, S. T., & Kniss. D. A. (1999). Development of an in vitro human placenta model by the cultivation of human trophoblasts in a fiber-based bioreactor system. *Tissue Eng,* 5(2), 91-102. https://doi.org/10.1089/ten.1999.5.91.

Malassiné, A., & Leiser, R. (1984). Morphogenesis and fine structure of the near-term placenta of Talpa europaea: I. Endotheliochorial labyrinth. *Placenta,* 5(2), 145–158. https://doi.org/10.1016/s0143-4004(84)80058-2.

Mandt, D., Gruber, P., Markovic, M., Tromayer, M., Rothbauer, M., Kratz, S. R. A., Ali, S. F., Van Hoorick, J., Holnthoner, W., Mühleder, S., Dubruel, P., Van Vlierberghe, S., Ertl, P., Liska, R., & Ovsianikov, A. (2018). Fabrication of biomimetic placental barrier structures within a microfluidic device utilizing two-photon polymerization. *Int J Bioprinting,* 4(2), 144. https://doi.org/10.18063/IJB.v4i2.144.

McConkey, C. A., Delorme-Axford, E., Nickerson, C. A., Kim, K. S., Sadovsky, Y., Boyle, J. P., & Coyne, C. B. (2016). A three-dimensional culture system recapitulates placental syncytiotrophoblast development and microbial resistance. *Sci. Adv,* 2(3), e1501462. https://doi.org/10.1126/sciadv.1501462.

Moser, G., Weiss, G., Gauster, M., Sundl, M., & Huppertz, B. (2015). Evidence from the very beginning: endoglandular trophoblasts penetrate and replace uterine glands in situ and in vitro. *Human reproduction* (Oxford, England), 30(12), 2747–2757. https://doi.org/10.1093/humrep/dev266.

Myllynen, P. K., Loughran, M. J., Howard, C. V., Sormunen, R., Walsh, A. A., & Vähäkangas, K. H. (2008). Kinetics of gold nanoparticles in the human placenta. *Reprod Toxicol,* 26(2), 130-7. https://doi.org/10.1016/j.reprotox.2008.06.008.

Nishiguchi, A., Gilmore, C., Sood, A., Matsusaki, M., Collett, G., Tannetta, D., Sargent, I. L., McGarvey, J., Halemani, N. D., Hanley, J., Day, F., Grant, S., Murdoch-Davis, C., Kemp, H., Verkade, P., Aplin, J. D., Akashi, M., & Case. C. P. (2018). In vitro placenta barrier model using primary human trophoblasts, underlying connective tissue and vascular endothelium. *Biomaterials,* 192, 140-148. https://doi.org/10.1016/j.biomaterials.2018.08.025.

Nugent, B. M., & Bale, T. L. (2015). The omniscient placenta: Metabolic and epigenetic regulation of fetal programming. *Front Neuroendocrinol,* 39, 28-37. https://doi.org/10.1016/j.yfrne.2015.09.001.

Pemathilaka, R. L., Reynolds, D. E., & Hashemi, N. N. (2019). Drug transport across the human placenta: review of placenta-on-a-chip and previous approaches. *Interface Focus,* 9(5), 201900319 https://doi.org/10.1098/rsfs.2019.0031.

Pollheimer, J., Vondra, S., Baltayeva, J., Beristain, A. G., & Knöfler, M. (2018). Regulation of Placental Extravillous Trophoblasts by the Maternal Uterine Environment. *Frontiers in immunology,* 9, 2597. https://doi.org/10.3389/fimmu.2018.02597.

Plum, A., Winterhager, E., Pesch, J., Lautermann, J., Hallas, G., Rosentreter, B., Traub, O., Herberhold, C., & Willecke, K. (2001). Connexin31-deficiency in mice causes transient placental dysmorphogenesis but does not impair hearing and skin differentiation. *Developmental biology,* 231(2), 334–347. https://doi.org/10.1006/dbio.2000.0148.

Ravishankar, S., & Redline, R. W. (2019). The placenta. *Handbook of clinical neurology,* 162, 57–66. https://doi.org/10.1016/B978-0-444-64029-1.00003-5.

Reyes, L., & Golos, T. G. (2018). Hofbauer Cells: Their Role in Healthy and Complicated Pregnancy. *Frontiers in immunology,* 9, 2628. https://doi.org/10.3389/fimmu.2018.02628.

Shetty, A. N., Pautler, R., Ghaghada, K., Rendon, D., Gao, H., Starosolski, Z., Bhavane, R., Patel, C., Annapragada, A., Yallampalli, C., & Lee, W. (2016). A liposomal Gd contrast agent does not cross the mouse placental barrier. *Sci Rep,* 6, 27863. https://doi.org/10.1038/srep27863.

Sobrevia, L., Abarzúa, F., Nien, J. K., Salomón, C., Westermeier, F., Puebla, C., Cifuentes, F., Guzmán-Gutiérrez, E., Leiva, A., & Casanello, P. (2011). Review: Differential placental macrovascular and microvascular endothelial dysfunction in gestational diabetes. *Placenta,* 32(2), S159–S164. https://doi.org/10.1016/j.placenta.2010.12.011.

Soininen, S. K., Repo, J. K., Karttunen, V., Auriola, S., Vähäkangas, K. H., & Ruponen, M. (2015). Human placental cell and tissue uptake of doxorubicin and its liposomal formulations. *Toxicol Lett. Dec,* 239(2), 108-14. https://doi.org/10.1016/j.toxlet.2015.09.011.

Tang, Z., Abrahams, V. M., Mor, G., Guller, S. (2011). Placental Hofbauer cells and complications of pregnancy. *Ann. N. Y. Acad. Sci.,* 1221, 103-108. https://doi.org/10.1111/j.1749-6632.2010.05932.x.

Tarrade, A., Lai Kuen, R., Malassiné, A., Tricottet, V., Blain, P., Vidaud, M., & Evain-Brion, D. (2001). Characterization of human villous and extravillous trophoblasts isolated from first trimester placenta. *Laboratory investigation; a journal of technical methods and pathology,* 81(9), 1199–1211. https://doi.org/10.1038/labinvest.3780334.

Tessier, D. R., Yockell-Lelievre, J., & Gruslin. A. (2015). Uterine spiral artery remodeling: the role of uterine natural killer cells and extravillous trophoblasts in normal and high-risk human pregnancies. *Am. J. Reprod. Immunol.,* 74(1), 1-11. https://doi.org/10.1111/aji.12345.

Turco, M. Y., Gardner, L., Kay, R. G., Hamilton, R. S., Prater, M., Hollinshead, M. S., McWhinnie, A., Esposito, L., Fernando, R., Skelton, H., Reimann, F., Gribble, F. M., Sharkey, A., Marsh, S. G. E., O'Rahilly, S., Hemberger, M., Burton, G. J., & Moffett, A. (2018). Trophoblast organoids as a model for maternal-fetal interactions during human placentation. *Nature,* 564(7735), 263–267. https://doi.org/10.1038/s41586-018-0753-3.

Tüzel-Kox, S. N., Patel, H. M., & Kox, W. J. (1995). Uptake of drug-carrier liposomes by placenta: transplacental delivery of drugs and nutrients. *J Pharmacol Exp Ther,* 274(1), 104-9.

Vähäkangas, K., & Myllynen, P. (2009). Drug transporters in the human blood-placental barrier. *British journal of pharmacology,* 158(3), 665–678. https://doi.org/10.1111/j.1476-5381.2009.00336.x.

Wang, Y., & Zhao, S. (2010). Cell Types of the Placenta, Vascular Biology of the Placenta. *Morgan & Claypool Life Sciences.* San Rafael (CA) https://doi.org/10.4199/C00016ED1V01Y201008ISP009.

Watson, E. D., & Cross, J. C. (2005). Development of structures and transport functions in the mouse placenta. *Physiology (Bethesda),* 20, 180-93. https://doi.org/10.1152/physiol.00001.2005.

Wong, M. K., Shawky, S. A., Aryasomayajula, A., Green, M. A., Ewart, T., Selvaganapathy, P. R., & Raha, S. (2018). Extracellular matrix surface regulates self-assembly of three-dimensional placental trophoblast spheroids. *PloS one,* 13(6), e0199632. https://doi.org/10.1371/journal.pone.0199632.

Zhu, Y., Yin, F., Wang, H., Wang, L., Yuan, J., & Qin, J. (2018). Placental barrier-on-a-chip: modeling placental inflammatory responses to bacterial infection. *ACS Biomater. Sci. Eng,* 4(9), 3356-3363. https://doi.org/10.1021/acsbiomaterials.8b00653.

Chapter 7

The Blood-Nerve Barrier

Muzaffer Başak Tunalı*
Department of Histology and Embryology, Faculty of Veterinary Medicine, Istanbul University-Cerrahpasa, Istanbul, Turkiye

Abstract

This chapter presents an analysis of the blood-nerve barrier (BNB), a specialized structure that serves to protect the peripheral nervous system (PNS). The BNB plays a pivotal role in maintaining the homeostasis of the PNS. It acts as a barrier, preventing the passage of harmful substances, including toxins and pathogens, into nervous tissue. This allows the selective passage of nutrients and the removal of waste materials.

The BNB is a dynamic structure comprising not only endothelial cells but also a variety of other cells, including perineurial cells, pericytes, Schwann cells, basement membrane and axons. Recent research has facilitated a more comprehensive understanding of the structure and function of the BNB, as well as the elucidation of the pathogenesis of various peripheral nervous system disorders, such as peripheral neuropathies, autoimmune diseases and injuries.

Keywords: peripheral nerve, perineurium, endoneurium, Schwann cell, blood nerve barrier

---

* Corresponding Author's Email: basaktunali@iuc.edu.tr

In: A Histological Approach to Human Body Barriers
Editor: İlknur Keskin
ISBN: 979-8-89530-738-0

Introduction

Peripheral nerves and nerve roots transfer the signals between the central nervous system (CNS), comprising the brain and spinal cord and other parts of the body (including the gastrointestinal tract, skin, heart, secretory organs, and muscles) to regulate physiological processes and maintain homeostasis (Ubogu, 2020). Cranial and spinal nerves and associated nerve roots and ganglions are the main components of PNS. The peripheral nerve fibers are enclosed by a unique, selectively permeable structure called the blood-nerve barrier (BNB), a dedicated safeguard securing the well-being of peripheral nerves. It restricts the passage of potentially harmful bloodborne substances such as toxins, pathogens, and inflammatory molecules while favoring essential nutrients and oxygen (Gregor, 2017). The BNB is a functionally dynamic multicellular unit, consisting not only of highly specialized elaborated endoneurial endothelial cells but also interactive perineurial cells, pericytes, Schwann cells, basement membrane, and axons, providing the homeostasis of the PNS and correct repair of the peripheral nerve fibers (Mizisin & Weerasuriya, 2011).

Recent research has made a tremendous contribution to the understanding of peripheral nerve disorders with the development of in vitro cell culture models due to highly advanced novel technologies. The continuity of further research on these complex dynamic molecular principles of the BNB is of great significance in elucidating this vast scale of peripheral nerve disorders, including peripheral neuropathies, autoimmune disorders, and injuries (Lopes, 2022).

Peripheral Nerve Anatomy

A peripheral nerve is a bundle of nerve fibers held together by connective tissue. The peripheral nervous system (PNS) nerves are composed of a multitude of fibers, enabling the transmission of both sensory and motor (effector) information between the brain and spinal cord and the body's tissues and organs. The term "nerve fiber" refers to the axon in conjunction with the surrounding myelin and Schwann cells, or it can refer to the axon alone (Pawlina & Ross, 2015). Schwann cells are the glial cells of the peripheral nervous system and are found along the length of the axon. A Schwann cell not only provides myelin and a basal lamina to guide axons but also supports the maintenance of its neighboring axon as a source of trophic and growth factors.

Connective tissue plays a crucial role in maintaining peripheral nerve structural integrity (Franco, 2012). This connective tissue enveloping the peripheral nerves and nerve roots has three distinct components:

1) The outer epineurium consists of longitudinal strands of collagen fibers that are important for maintaining the nerve's structural integrity
2) The inner perineurium consists of concentric layers of specialized cells
3) The innermost endoneurium consists of a looser network of collagen fibers.

A nerve fascicle is a bundle of nerves composed of the endoneurium and the surrounding perineurium (Gregor, 2017) (Figure 1).

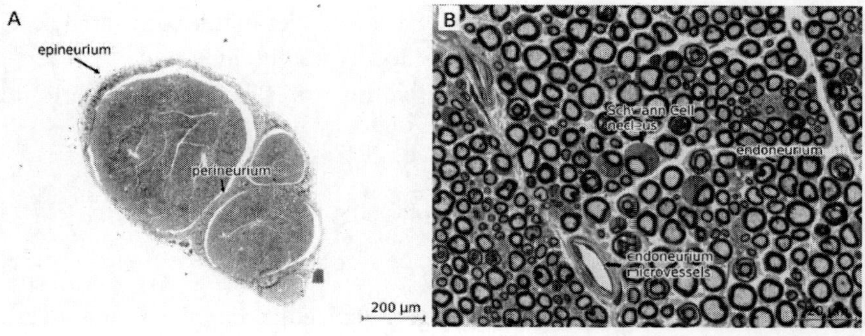

Figure 1. A plastic-embedded semi-thin sciatic nerve section of a rat, toluidine blue stain. (A) Epineurium surrounding the whole structure and perineural connective tissue within the nerve fascicles x10. (B) Endoneurium encircling the myelinated axons, endoneurial micro vessel and Schwann cell nucleus.

Epineurium

The epineurium consists of irregularly arranged collagen fibers, scattered fibroblasts, and occasional clusters of adipocytes (Weerasuriya & Mizisin 2010). The epineurium extends inwards, separating the fascicles (interfascicular epineurium). The layer between the epineurium and the surrounding tissue is called the paraneurium (Gregor, 2017).

Perineurium

Oblique, circular, and longitudinal collagen fibrils are located between perineurial cells. The outer lamellae of the perineurium contain endocytotic vesicles enabling the transfer of molecular components. Tight junctions between adjacent perineurial cells constitute the inner lamellae, restraining the intercellular transport of macromolecules and, thus, contributing significantly to the blood-nerve barrier's integrity. A disruption to the perineurium can impact the functionality of the axons it encircles. Furthermore, the perineurium is the nerve's primary source of tensile strength and carries the blood vessels (Gregor, 2017). An electron microscopic examination of the mouse sciatic nerve's perineural cells reveals the presence of many caveolae and filaments with opaque regions similar to those observed in smooth muscle. However, no myofilament-like structures or electron-opaque regions are observed in the plasma membrane. Aggregated filaments and numerous endoplasmic reticula, free ribosomes, and pinocytotic vesicles within their opaque regions indicate a cell with smooth muscle and fibrocyte characteristics. In this regard, these cells resemble peritubular contractile cells observed in the testes of rats and mice. Moreover, perineural cells generate nerve contraction and serve as a selective diffusion barrier (Ross & Reith, 1969; Weerasuriya & Mizisin, 2010).

Endoneurium

The endoneurium comprises fine longitudinal collagen fibrils and tightly connected microvessels, functioning as a blood-nerve barrier. Endoneurial homeostasis depends upon these microvessels, which regulate ions, solutes, water, nutrients, macromolecules, and leukocyte influx and outflow between the bloodstream and the endoneurium. Furthermore, the innermost layers of the perineurium regulate the flow of interstitial fluid components between the freely permeable epineurium and the endoneurium (Ubogu, 2020).

Structure of the Blood-Nerve Barrier (BNB)

The blood-nerve barrier (BNB) is recognized as a highly specialized and critical structure serving the homeostasis of the peripheral nervous system

(Ubogu, E. E. (2020). BNB prevents the influx of potentially harmful substances in the bloodstream from entering peripheral nerves. Furthermore, it was demonstrated to express transporter proteins for transporting nutrients, including glucose and amino acids, and removing waste products, functioning as an interface for maintaining the microenvironment in peripheral nerves. The blood-brain barrier (BBB) and BNB exhibit structural similarities. The basement membrane of both the blood-brain barrier (BBB) and the blood-nerve barrier (BNB) is composed of a complex mixture of extracellular matrix proteins, including collagen IV and laminin. Laminin is a trimeric molecule comprising α-, β- and γ-subunits, expressed explicitly in the central and peripheral nervous systems (Cardoso et al., 2010). Laminin α4 was observed to be rarely expressed in BNB compared to BBB. In contrast, α5, β1, β2, and γ1 were found to be widely expressed in BBB and BNB. On the other hand, the BBB primarily comprises brain microvascular endothelial cells, pericytes, astrocytes, and two distinct basement membranes (Takeshita Y et al., 2017). However, the BNB lacks astrocytes, which was previously assumed to have resulted in a less permeable barrier. Nevertheless, numerous studies have indicated that the BNB exhibits a similar barrier function to the BBB (Abe M et al., 2012).

The Vascularisation of Peripheral Nerves

The microcirculation of peripheral nerves is achieved by vasa nervorum, which primarily occurs along the longitudinal axis of the nerve. The radicular arteries supply the vasa nervorum that branches deeply into the epineurium as small arteries and arterioles, as well as precapillary arterioles running along the outer surface of the perineurium. Subsequently, these vessels diagonally cross the concentric multilayered perineurium and penetrate the endoneurium, giving rise to branches ultimately forming capillaries. The capillaries, merging with the venules that emerge from the perineurium, drain into the larger postcapillary venules within the endoneurium. Venules and small veins run longitudinally within the epineurium, eventually merging and draining into nearby vessels (Ubogu EE 2013).

Ultrastructurally, electron-dense intercellular tight junctions (TJs) and small intracellular pinocytic vesicles of 50 to 100 nm between the endothelial cells are the characteristics of the vasculature of the human peripheral nerve. The endothelial cells have no fenestration in the endoneurium. In contrast, epineurium and perineurium are characterized by a prevalence of endothelial cells with numerous fenestrations and the absence of TJs. These endothelial cells exhibit similarities to the restrictive blood-brain (BBB) and blood-testis barriers. Furthermore, TJs have been demonstrated to occur within the perineurium, particularly between perineurial myofibroblast cells within the inner concentric layers. In brief, the data indicates the occurrence of specialized interfaces with restrictive barrier properties within peripheral nerves (Reina MA et al., 2003).

Claudin family members, specifically claudin-5, are essential components of TJs, along with occludin, apart from cytoplasmic adapter molecules belonging to the ZO family, specifically ZO-1 and ZO-2. Claudin-5 and ZO-1 were detected within the human endoneurial microvascular tissue (Ubogu EE 2020). Occludin, claudin-1, claudin-3, claudin-19, tricellulin, and ZO-1 are expressed within the perineurium. ZO-1 is a critical scaffolding protein that binds junctional molecules such as claudin and occludin to the actin cytoskeleton by its PDZ domain, sealing tight junctions. Moreover, cadherins, catenins, and junctional adhesion molecules (JAMs) are responsible for forming adherens junctions. The JAM family comprises three members: JAM-A, eB, and eC. They belong to the immunoglobulin superfamily. JAMs interact with scaffolding molecules, such as ZO-1, through their intracellular C-terminal type II PDZ binding motif, responsible for binding to the actin skeleton. JAM-C, a member of the JAM family, has been predominantly identified in vascular and epithelial cells. In the PNS, it is located in the junctional regions of Schwann cells, facilitating myelinated peripheral neuron integrity (Reinhold AK et al., 2019). Recent data has pointed out the significance of the intercellular junctional complex, comprising tight and gap junctions and their respective adaptor proteins, and cytoskeletal components, for sustaining optimal endothelial and epithelial cell functionality (Ubogu EE 2020).

According to the data, of 133 intercellular junction complex molecules, 22 molecules are involved in tight junctions or junction-associated molecules, 45 in adherens junctions or junction-associated molecules, and 52 in cell junctions or adaptor molecules. Moreover, indirect fluorescence immunohistochemistry revealed the *in situ* expressions of α1-catenin (CTNNA1), cadherin-5 (CHD5), cadherin-6 (CDH6), claudin-4 (CLDN4), claudin-5 (CLDN5), crumps cell polarity component lin-7 homolog A (LIN7A), gap junction protein A1 (GJA1), multiple PDZ domain crumbs cell polarity component (MPDZ), protocadherin-1 (PCDH1), vezatin, Zonula Occludens-1 (ZO-1), and zyxin (ZYX), confirming the roles of these molecules in cell-cell adhesions. In particular, CLDN4 is an essential component of BNB tight junctions and CDH5 for adherens junctions. CTNNA1 links cell membranes to the cytoskeleton for structural integrity and the F-actin cytoskeleton to adherens junctions (Ubogu EE 2020).

Endoneurial endothelial cells' expression of specific mitogen receptors such as glial-derived neurotrophic factor (GDNF; GFRα1), vascular endothelial growth factor (VEGF; VEGFR2), basic fibroblast growth factor (bFGF; FGFR1), transforming growth factor-β (TGF-β; TGFRI/II) and glucocorticoids (GR) by autocrine or paracrine signaling has also been *in vitro* and *in situ* demonstrated. These molecules also secreted by Schwann cells, pericytes, mast cells, or endoneurial fibroblasts are known to maintain the BNB structural integrity. Schwann cells secrete GDNF *in vitro* and *in vivo*, and low nanomolar concentrations of GDNF have a dose-dependent effect on restrictive human BNB properties *in vitro* via RET tyrosine kinase-mitogen-activated protein kinase (MAPK) signaling, which implicates GDNF as an essential paracrine regulator of BNBs formation (Ubogu EE 2020).

Regulation of the Endoneurial Microenvironment

The endoneurium provides a specialized microenvironment within the peripheral nerves. Interactions between Schwann cells, axons, macrophages, and mast cells through cell-cell and cell-matrix signaling regulate the BNB permeability, enabling neural homeostasis (Mizisin AP &.Weerasuriya A 2011).

The endoneurium lacks lymphatic circulation, and microcirculation is sustained under positive hydrostatic pressure. However, the absence of lymphatic drainage is a hindrance to the removal of macromolecules such as albumin. Two pathways have been suggested for the removal of macromolecules from the endoneurium: metabolic degradation pathways to supply amino acids to axons and glia and proximo-distal convective flow of endoneurial fluid driven by hydrostatic pressure gradients, contributing to homeostasis of the nerve's microenvironment. Pathophysiological changes result from disturbances in endoneurial homeostasis and imbalances in this specialized area (Mizisin AP &.Weerasuriya A 2011).

The endoneurial fluid content of the sciatic nerve of the adult rat is approximately 70%, and the fluid is distributed between the intracellular and the extracellular compartments. The extracellular space within a nerve fascicle is approximately 20-25% of the total endoneurial volume. The water is either freely distributed or as a part of a hydrated gel-like ground substance. Even though electrolyte levels in these compartments are known to be more isotonic than in sera, initial studies have suggested that endoneurium sodium, chloride, and potassium are hypertonic compared to their serum counterparts. The immunoblotting method revealed that eluded endoneurial fluid contains 3.6% of total endoneurial protein, with albumin being the predominant protein (Mizisin AP & Weerasuriya A 2011).

The endoneurial extracellular matrix plays a crucial role in maintaining homeostasis and regulating nerve function. Glycosaminoglycans, particularly hyaluronan, create a hydrated microenvironment that supports ion balance and pH regulation essential for nerve impulse transmission (Melrose et al., 2021). The blood-nerve barrier, composed of endoneurial microvessels and the perineurium, regulates the exchange of materials between the endoneurium and surrounding tissues (Weerasuriya & Mizisin, 2011). This barrier is crucial for maintaining the optimal microenvironment for axons and Schwann cells (Ubogu, 2013). The extracellular matrix also provides guidance cues for neural development and repair. Proteoglycans and their glycosaminoglycan chains play diverse roles in nervous system function and pathology. Understanding the complex interactions between cells and the extracellular matrix is essential for developing therapeutic strategies for peripheral nerve disorders and central nervous system repair (Melrose et al., 2021).

BNB Dysfunction and Peripheral Nervous System Disorders

Advanced cell line technologies and *in vitro* models rendered the manipulation of BNB to search the pathophysiology of peripheral nervous system disorders such as peripheral neuropathy, potentially leading to the development of novel therapeutic strategies (Takeshita et al., 2020; Ubogu, 2020; Weerasuriya A & Mizisin AP 2011).

In the pathophysiology of peripheral neuropathy, the BNB is exposed to the invasion of leukocytes and the diffusion of potentially neurotoxic mediators like pain-inducing cytokines, with a reduction in the scaffolding protein ZO-1. JAM-C downregulation was noted after a sciatic crush injury, followed by convalescence in the subsequent course, compatible with neuron remyelination (Reinhold AK et al., 2019). Disruption of the endoneurial homeostasis was shown to be the cause of neuropathies as in the cases of experimental allergic neuritis, diabetic neuropathy, and lead neuropathy (Mizisin AP &.Weerasuriya A 2011).

BNB disorders exhibit distinct histopathological patterns, and these diverse histopathological changes observed in BNB-associated diseases may aid in diagnosing and understanding disease mechanisms. For instance, perivascular infiltration of T lymphocytes and monocytes is observed, with neuronal apoptosis in acute and chronic stages of Behçet's disease (Borhani-Haghighi A et al., 2019).

Endothelial cell damage of the BNB during inflammatory responses contributes to the development of peripheral neuropathy. This damage is characterized by the disruption of tight junctions, increased permeability and basement membrane hypertrophy. Vascular endothelial growth factors and advanced glycation end products are also involved in the breakdown of BNB (Takeshita Y et al, 2020). Therefore, understanding the underlying pathology is crucial for developing targeted therapies for neuropathies.

Diabetic neuropathy is a common complication of diabetes, and BNB dysfunction is also implicated in the development of diabetic neuropathy. Oxidative stress is a common pathway for several metabolic imbalances. In autoimmune neuropathies, there is a strong association between oxidative stress and the severity of BNB dysfunction. Oxidative stress is linked with oxidative stress activating inflammatory pathways and vice versa (Pang L et al, 2020). Demyelination in chronic inflammatory demyelinating polyradiculoneuropathy (CIDP) is associated with the severity of BNB impairment, manifested by clinical disability (Shimizu F et al., 2014).

Matrix metalloproteinases (MMPs) play an essential role in the degradation of tight junction proteins in the BNB and BBB, leading to increased permeability of the barriers with potential neurological complications. MMP-2 and MMP-9 are mainly involved in the degradation of tight junction proteins such as occludin, claudin-5, and ZO-1, facilitating the infiltration of immune cells into the central nervous system. Disruption of tight junctions by MMPs contributes to vasogenic edema and altered nerve function (Feng et al, 2011). Activated MMPs are also noted in diabetes, ischemia, and neuroinflammation.

Conclusion

In summary, neurophysiological homeostasis is linked with the structural integrity of the blood-nerve barrier (BNB), which protects neural tissues from external factors. Recent advances in understanding BNB biology have elicited potential therapeutic targets for peripheral neuroinflammation. Schwann cells have also emerged as a therapeutic target for the research of neuropathies. Identification of the underlying processes that comprise the BNB integrity, such as oxidative stress and inflammatory responses, is critical for the design of targeted therapeutic interventions, which may include the modulation of BNB permeability, regulation of adhesion molecule expression, and control of leukocyte trafficking, ultimately improving clinical outcomes of patients with neuropathic disorders. Future research should continue to focus on these molecular dynamics to improve the efficacy of current treatment options for such conditions.

References

Abe, M., Sano, Y., Maeda, T., Shimizu, F., Kashiwamura, Y., Haruki, H., ... & Kanda, T. (2012). Establishment and characterization of human peripheral nerve microvascular endothelial cell lines: a new in vitro blood-nerve barrier (BNB) model. *Cell structure and function,* 37(2), 89-100. doi: 10.1247/csf.11042.

Borhani-Haghighi, A., Kardeh, B., Banerjee, S., Yadollahikhales, G., Safari, A., Sahraian, M. A., & Shapiro, L. (2020). Neuro-Behcet's disease: an update on diagnosis, differential diagnoses, and treatment. *Multiple sclerosis and related disorders,* 39,101906. doi: 10.1016/j.msard.2019.101906.

Cardoso, F. L., Brites, D., & Brito, M. A. (2010). Looking at the blood–brain barrier: molecular anatomy and possible investigation approaches. *Brain research reviews,* 64(2), 328-363. doi: 10.1016/j.brainresrev.2010.05.003.

Feng, S., Cen, J., Huang, Y., Shen, H., Yao, L., Wang, Y., & Chen, Z. (2011). Matrix metalloproteinase-2 and-9 secreted by leukemic cells increase the permeability of blood-brain barrier by disrupting tight junction proteins. *PloS one,* 6(8), e20599. doi: 10.1371/journal.pone.0020599.

Franco, C. D. (2012). Connective tissues associated with peripheral nerves. *Regional Anesthesia and Pain Medicine,* 37(4), 363-365. doi: 10.1097/AAP.0b013 e31825a9485.

Gregor, Antoniadis. (2017). The Peripheral Nerve: Neuroanatomical Principles Before and After Injury. 1-10. doi: 10.1007/978-3-319-52319-4_1 doi:10.1007/978-3-319-52319-4_1.

Lopes B, Sousa P, Alvites R, Branquinho M, Sousa AC, Mendonça C, Atayde LM, Luís AL, Varejão, ASP, Maurício AC. (2022). Peripheral nerve injury treatments and advances: one health perspective. *International journal of molecular sciences,* 23(2), 918. doi:10.3390/ijms23020918.

Melrose, J., Hayes, A., & Bix, G. (2021). The CNS/PNS extracellular matrix provides instructive guidance cues to neural cells and neuroregulatory proteins in neural development and repair. *International Journal of Molecular Sciences,* 22. https://doi.org/10.3390/ijms22115583.

Mizisin, A. P., & Weerasuriya, A. (2011). Homeostatic regulation of the endoneurial microenvironment during development, aging and in response to trauma, disease and toxic insult. *Acta neuropathologica,* 121, 291-312. doi: 10.1007/s00401-010-0783-x.

Pang, L., Lian, X., Liu, H., Zhang, Y., Li, Q., Cai, Y., Ma, H., Yu, X. (2020). Understanding diabetic neuropathy: focus on oxidative stress. *Oxidative Medicine and Cellular Longevity,* 2020(1), 9524635. doi: 10.1155/2020/9524635.

Pawlina, W., & Ross, M. H. (2015). Histology: a text and atlas: with correlated cell and molecular biology. Lippincott Williams & Wilkins. ISBN 978-0-7817-7200-6.

Reina, M. A., López, A., Villanueva, M. C., De Andres, J. A., & Machés, F. (2003). The blood-nerve barrier in peripheral nerves. *Revista espanola de anestesiologia y reanimacion,* 50(2), 80-86.

Reinhold, A. K., Yang, S., Chen, J. T. C., Hu, L., Sauer, R. S., Krug, S. M., ... & Rittner, H. L. (2019). Tissue plasminogen activator and neuropathy open the blood-nerve barrier with upregulation of microRNA-155-5p in male rats. *Biochimica Et Biophysica Acta (BBA)-Molecular Basis of Disease,* 1865(6), 1160-1169. doi: 10.1016/j.bbadis.2019.01.008.

Ross, M. H., & Reith, E. J. (1969). Perineurium: Evidence for Contractile Elements. *Science,* 165(3893), 604–605. doi:10.1126/science.165.3893.604.

Shimizu, F., Sawai, S., Sano, Y., Beppu, M., Misawa, S., Nishihara, H., ... & Kanda, T. (2014). Severity and patterns of blood-nerve barrier breakdown in patients with chronic inflammatory demyelinating polyradiculoneuropathy: correlations with clinical subtypes. *PloS one,* 9(8), e104205. doi: 10.1371/journal.pone.0104205.

Takeshita, Y., Omoto, M., Fujikawa, S., & Kanda, T. (2017) Immunohistochemical analysis of laminin components in the blood–nerve barrier and blood–brain barrier. *Clinical and Experimental Neuroimmunology,* 8(1), 49-53. doi: 10.1016/j.expneurol.2020.113385.

Takeshita, Y., Sato, R., & Kanda, T. (2020). Blood–nerve barrier (BNB) pathology in diabetic peripheral neuropathy and in vitro human BNB model. *International Journal of Molecular Sciences,* 22(1), 62. doi: 10.3390/ijms2201006.

Ubogu, E. E. (2013). The molecular and biophysical characterization of the human blood-nerve barrier: current concepts. *Journal of vascular research,* 50(4), 289-303. doi: 10.1159/000353293.

Ubogu, E. E. (2020). Biology of the human blood-nerve barrier in health and disease. *Experimental neurology,* 328, 113272. doi: 10.1016/j.expneurol.2020.113272.

Weerasuriya, A., & Mizisin, A. P. (2010). The Blood-Nerve Barrier: Structure and Functional Significance. *The Blood-Brain and Other Neural Barriers,* 149–173. doi:10.1007/978-1-60761-938-3_6.

Chapter 8

The Blood-Brain Barrier

Işınsu Alkan*, PhD
Department of Basic Science, Faculty of Dentistry, Nevşehir Hacı Bektaş Veli University, Nevşehir, Türkiye

Abstract

The blood-brain barrier is a cellular barrier that tightly controls the microenvironment for the correct functioning of the nervous system and the creation of the appropriate neuronal environment. The blood-brain barrier comprises three cell types: endothelium, pericyte, and astrocyte. The connections between these cells are essential for the permeability of this barrier. In addition, it plays a significant role in the permeability of the BBB in the basement membrane on which the cells are located. The blood-brain barrier is a significant barrier in protecting the central nervous system. The permeability of this barrier regulates the microenvironment of the brain. For this reason, the permeability of the barrier is critical. Substance migration varies depending on its solubility in lipids, molecular weight, and number of bonds. While molecules dissolved in lipids and weighing less than 40Da enter the cell by passive diffusion, molecules with higher properties pass through transcytosis. This structure, which prevents the passage of matter, varies depending on different factors. This chapter will discuss the structure, solubility, and factors affecting the blood-brain barrier's solubility.

Keywords: astrocyte, pericyte, basement membrane, endothelium, tight junction

* Corresponding Author's Email: isinsuaydin@gmail.com, isinsu.alkan@nevsehir.edu.tr

In: A Histological Approach to Human Body Barriers
Editor: İlknur Keskin
ISBN: 979-8-89530-738-0

Introduction

Organs and tissues need energy and oxygen to maintain their functions, and a vast network of blood vessels meets these needs. However, the pathway through which each molecule in the blood affects different types of tissues is different. This situation reveals the need to protect vital organs particularly well. The central nervous system is one of the most critical systems responsible for the functioning of the entire organism. Especially in centers controlling the entire body, such as the brain, the encounter of tissues with every molecule in the blood produces harmful results.

The body has barrier systems to prevent such situations and protect critical areas. There are three protective barriers in the brain: the blood-brain barrier, the brain-cerebrospinal barrier, and the arachnoid barrier (Nag and Begley, 2005; Kadry et al., 2020). The blood-brain barrier is a membrane selectively permeable to substances that will pass from the blood to the brain to regulate the brain's microenvironment and control metabolic activity (Wu et al., 2023; Kadry et al., 2020). This membrane combines different cell types and their basement membranes with tight junction complexes (Abbott et al., 2010; Daneman and Prat, 2015; Kadry et al., 2020). The complements that make up the blood-brain barrier are capillary endothelial cells, astrocytes, and pericytes, and the capillaries here are continuous capillaries. Another barrier in the brain, the cerebrospinal barrier, consists of tight junctions between fenestrated capillaries and epidermal cells of the choroid plexus. Another barrier is the arachnoid barrier, which consists of arachnoid cells and a pial membrane.

One of these three barriers, the blood-brain barrier (BBB), plays a critical role in protecting the brain. This chapter summarizes the structure of the blood-brain barrier, substance passage, and factors affecting its function.

Blood-Brain Barrier Elements

Blood-Brain Barrier Cells

The blood-brain barrier consists of different cell types that are associated with each other and with plasma membranes through tight junctions. Endothelial cells of capillaries, pericytes, and astrocytes are the cells that form the BBB (Figure 1).

Endothelial Cells

Endothelial cells are single-layered squamous epithelial cells surrounding capillaries. They are histologically structured according to their area. Endothelial cells in the BBB have different morphological features from peripheral endothelial cells. The most important difference between them is that they form a continuous membrane, and the absence of fenestra spaces on them achieves this (Alhadidi et al., 2017). These continuous endothelial cells are the main component of the BBB. These cells have luminal and abluminal surfaces because they have both tight and adherens type connections. The luminal surface contains structures specialized for ion transport. Another structure that distinguishes the endothelial cells in the BBB from other endothelial cells is the large number of mitochondria. The abundance of mitochondria indicates that the need for energy is high. The endothelial cells in this area allow the passage of molecules with a molecular weight of less than 400 Da and fewer than eight hydrogen bonds (Pardridge, 2015; Kadry et al., 2020). Endothelial cells have two types of primary transporters for ion transitions (Daneman and Prat, 2015). While the first of these allows the diffusion of the lipophilic molecule on the lumenal surface, the other is high-specific nutrient transporters. These special transporters enable the passage of specific molecules from the blood to the brain while also allowing the passage of metabolic waste from the brain to the blood (Daneman and Prat, 2015). Endothelial cells can regulate molecules that pass through the barrier and reach the brain in three ways (Wu et al., 2023). The first of these is that cells repel negatively charged molecules because they are negatively charged. This situation ensures that the number of leukocytes is low in the environment. Another one is special substrates that control the inflow and outflow. The third pathway is that the cells have high transendothelial electrical resistance. This resistance limits the number of transcellular vesicles (Wu et al., 2023).

Pericyte

Pericytes are cells of neural crest origin that are located in the abluminal area of the capillary wall and share the same basal membrane with endothelial cells (Ballabh et al., 2004; Daneman and Prat, 2015; Wu et al., 2023). These cells can contract similarly to smooth muscle cells and regulate capillary diameter and cerebral blood flow (Ballabh et al., 2004; Daneman and Prat, 2015; Galea, 2021). However, pericytes have many cellular extensions, each connecting with several endothelial cells (Daneman and Prat, 2015). Between endothelial cells and pericytes, there are peg and socket junctions, as well as tight and gap junctions, mediated by these connection plates and cadherins. Pericytes also regulate the amount of tight junctions in endothelial cells (Wu et al., 2023). Another function of pericytes is the regulation of cerebral autoregulation through vascular mediators. These mediators, catecholamines, angiotensin, vasoactive intestinal peptides, endothelin-1, and vasopressin, are essential for regulation (Wu et al., 2023). In addition to all these, it is known that endothelial cells associated with pericytes are more resistant to apoptosis (Ballabh et al., 2004; Daneman and Prat, 2015; Wu et al., 2023). Although it is not fully understood whether multifunctional pericytes are managed by a single cell or have different subtypes, the vascular diameter is undoubtedly regulated by preventing transcytosis, which is the entry of solutes with two main functions (Galea, 2021).

Astrocyte

While astrocytes are glial cells that regulate neuronal processes, they extend legs that line blood vessels. It plays an essential role in forming and functioning the blood-brain barrier through these legs (Daneman and Prat, 2015). Astrocytes and pericytes surround blood vessels, creating an interface between neurons and endothelial cells (Wu et al., 2023). These cells also produce signals to regulate blood flow and thus regulate neuronal activity. Thus, it plays a role in regulating the contraction and relaxation of pericytes (Wu et al., 2023).

There are two types of astrocytes in the central nervous system. The first is protoplasmic astrocytes located in the vascular-rich gray matter, and the second is fibrous astrocytes located in the white matter with fewer vessels (Wu et al., 2023). The proteoglycan agrin connects the feet of astrocytes and the basal membrane. This junctional complex includes proteins such as aquaporin-4, dystroglycan, and dystropin (Wu et al., 2023). Aquaporim-4, located in this complex, regulates water flow across the BBB and plays a role in edema in neurodegenerative diseases (Galea, 2021).

The role of astrocytes in the BBB is controversial. While some studies say that astrocytes play a direct role in the formation of the barrier, other studies say that astrocyte development, in which the barrier is formed beforehand, occurs later (Bhasiin et al., 2023; Wu et al., 2023; Ballabh et al., 2004). Although different results are seen in studies, the relationship between the endothelium and astrocytes in the formation of the BBB is specific. The presence of astrocytes causes tightening of endothelial cells (Bhasiin et al., 2023).

Basement Membrane

The basal membrane is a specialized 50–100 nm thick extracellular matrix structure that supports endothelial cells (Xu et al., 2018). Its structure contains extracellular matrix elements such as collagen IV, laminin, nidogen, and perlecan (Thomsen et al., 2017). The basement membrane is divided into endothelial BM and parenchymal, which are separated by pericytes, and these two BM layers are indistinguishable from each other and appear as a single layer in areas where pericytes are absent (Figure 1) (Xu et al., 2018; Thomsen et al., 2017). Inner endothelial BM is also called vascular BM and is 20-200 nm thick. It contains integrins and transmembrane proteins on the vascular layer (Thomsen et al., 2017). External parenchymal BM is secreted primarily by astrocytic processes extending into the vascular system (Daneman and Prat, 2015). Together, both membranes regulate the permeability of the barrier. The three cells that form the basal membrane are kept in this membrane. This ensures that it remains fixed in the adhesion cells, and its localization is determined.

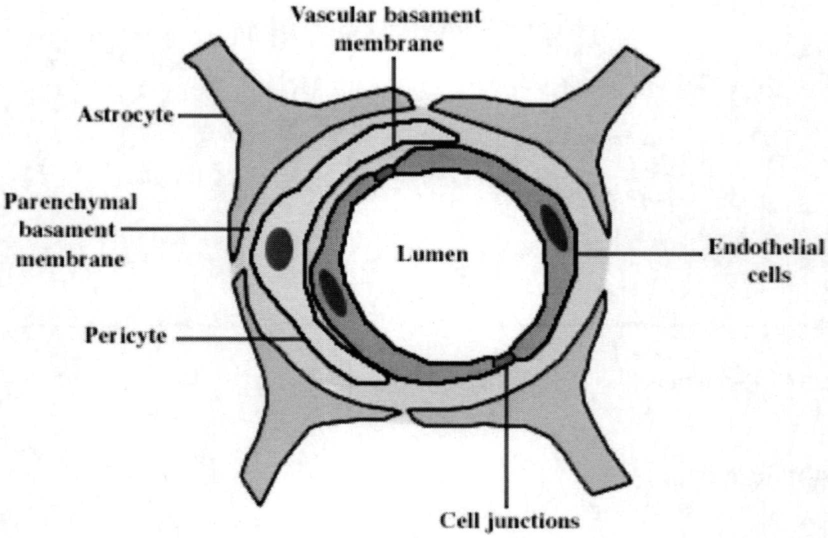

Figure 1. Schematic illustration of the blood–brain barrier.

Cell Connections

The most critical factor in the permeability of the blood-brain barrier is the connections between cells. Tight and adherent connections between the cells make up the Blood-Brain barrier (Figure 2). These two types of connections regulate the polarization and significantly limit the entry of matter.

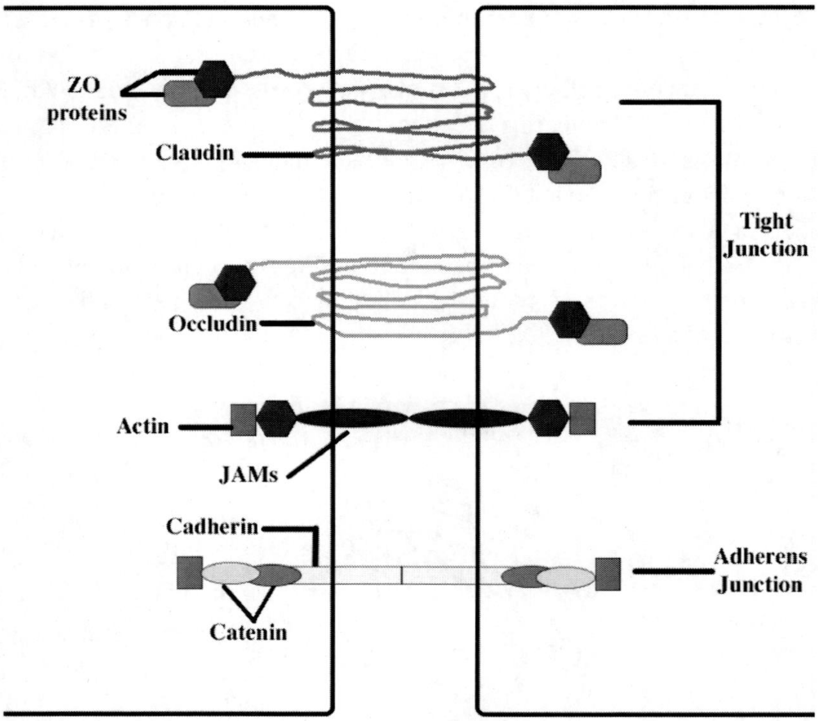

Figure 2. Schematic illustration of the cell junctions.

Tight Junction

In tight junction-type connections, the space between the cells is quite small, and the membranes of both cells appear to be fused. With this connection, the proteins on the apical surface cannot move to the side surfaces, and the apical surface always adheres to the same content. In addition, since these bindings prevent side-to-side transitions, they enable molecules to pass directly into the cell rather than between cells with paracellular pathways. Homotypic or heterotypic interactions can be observed at tight junctions. Even though tight junctions are tightly connected, they have pores smaller than 4nm and can allow the passage of molecules smaller than this size (Sugiyama et al., 2023; Daneman and Prat, 2015; Luissint et al., 2012). This permeability varies depending on the tissue. Tight junctions contain transmembrane proteins such as claudin, occludin, and junctional adhesion molecules (JAMs) (Sandoval and Witt, 2008).

Claudin is the essential protein of tight junctions and plays a role in paracellular barrier formation (Figure 2). Claudin consists of 4 membrane loops, and the protein residue on the first loop determines the width and ion charge of the pores (Kadry et al., 2020; Daneman and Prat, 2015). Claudins show homotypic interaction and are also associated with cytoplasmic proteins (Kadry et al., 2020; Luissint et al., 2012). Claudin 1 and 5 are primarily found in the central nervous system. While claudin 5 plays a role in the regulation of claudin 1, it regulates the size-selectivity of the barrier (Daneman and Prat, 2015). In recent studies, claudin 11, which has a function similar to claudin 5, has been identified (Kadry et al., 2020). Claudin 11 plays a role in paracellular tightness through oligomerization (Kadry et al., 2020).

Occludin is a transmembrane protein that is larger than claudin and does not have protein domains (Figure 2). Although it is highly expressed in endothelial cells in the central nervous system, it is reported in the literature that it is not found in the newborn brain (Ballabh et al., 2004). The cytoplasmic domains of occludin are directly associated with ZO proteins (Daneman and Prat, 2015). The homotypic interactions in the paracellular area are significant in the resistance of the BBB (Sugiyama et al., 2023; Sandoval and Witt, 2008). Studies show that occludin regulates calcium flux, and its density affects the integrity of the BBB (Sugiyama et al., 2023; Daneman and Prat, 2015).

JAMs are immunoglobulins that make homotypic connections with a single transmembrane domain (Figure 2). JAMs play a role in leukocyte extravasation and paracellular permeability. In particular, JAM1, JAM3, and JAM4 are located in the central nervous system (Kadry et al., 2020; Daneman and Prat, 2015).

Adherens Junctions

The type of connection connects cells to each other through actin filaments and cadherins. These connections create spatially, chemically, and mechanically separate microdomains in the paracellular space. Like tight junctions, adherence-type junctions connect to the cytoskeleton and are transmembrane proteins (Kadry et al., 2020). In these connections, while cadherins bind to actin filaments in the cytoplasm, they make connections with calcium-dependent cadherins between cells (Figure 2) (Ballabh et al., 2004). These links are essential to the integrity of the BBB.

Substance Transition through the Blood-Brain Barrier

The brain, which is the control center of the whole body, must be protected from toxins and pathological agents, and the balance of the microenvironment must be maintained. For this reason, the blood-brain barrier ensures the controlled passage of ions and substances from the blood to the brain and vice versa, as well as the controlled passage of metabolic wastes. The connections between the cells that make up the blood-brain barrier limit the passage of substances and do not allow the passage of molecules of a specific size. Substance passage through the blood-brain barrier is provided by passive diffusion, active affect, carrier-mediated transport and receptor-mediated transport (Kadry et al., 2020; Fu, 2018). The pathway through which the transition is achieved varies depending on the size of the substance, its lipid solubility, its ability to bind to specific carriers, and its electrical charge.

Two different transporters are used for substance passage in the BBB. The first of these, efflux transporters, are carriers that use ATP during the passage of substances and are mainly located on the lumenal surface. It plays a role in transferring substances from brain tissue to the blood (Daneman and Prat, 2015). Another transporter in the brain is the nutrition transporter. This transporter regulates the movement of specific nutrients from the blood to the brain down concentration gradients. These transporters are concentrated in neuronal, endothelial cells (Daneman and Prat, 2015).

Lipid-soluble molecules smaller than 40Da pass through passive diffusion from the blood into the brain. Lipid-soluble molecules cross the BBB through the transient formation of pores within the phospholipid bilayer (Wu et al., 2023). Likewise, molecules with fewer than eight hydrogen bonds cross the BBB by lipid-mediated diffusion (Daneman and Prat, 2015; Fu, 2018). Water-soluble substrates are transported by efflux transporters that allow bidirectional passage (Wu et al., 2023; Daneman and Prat, 2015; Fu, 2018). The BBB limits the diffusion of many essential polar nutrients, including glucose and amino acids essential for metabolism. Therefore, essential nutrients are transported by carrier-mediated transporters to reach the brain.

Therefore, essential nutrients are transported by carrier-mediated transporters to reach the brain. These transporters can also be located on both the luminal and abluminal sides of the membrane and provide bidirectional transport. Localizing tarnsporters may result in preferential transport of substrates (Kadry et al., 2020. Receptor-mediated transporters-mediated transcytosis is used for large peptides and proteins to cross the BBB (Kadry et al., 2020; Daneman and Prat, 2015). In transcytosis, macromolecular cell It comes together by binding to receptors specific to the ligands on their surface, and the ligand-receptor complex is taken into the cell and separated during this transition and exocytosis (Kadry et al., 2020; Daneman and Prat, 2015).

Factors of the Affecting Blood Brain Barrier Permeability

The permeability of the blood-brain barrier varies with many factors, such as chemical agents, age, temperature, etc. These factors change the permeability, and the changing permeability also changes the neural effects.

Inflammation markers are the primary factors that change permeability. The effect of inflammation markers such as Bradykinin, Endothelin 1, histamine, and substance P on BBB permeability has been shown in many studies (Zhao et al., 2022; Nokkari et al., 2018; Reijerkerk et al., 2013). It has been observed that bradykinin, a blood-brain barrier regulatory peptide, affects the BBB's permeability due to the downregulation of claudin-5 I. In addition, substance P, another neuropeptide secreted from cells such as macrophages, dendritic cells, and leukocytes, also affects the permeability of the BBB through cytokines (Zhao et al., 2022; Nokkari et al., 2018; O'Connor et al., 2004). Likewise, histamine binds to the H2 receptor and increases BBB permeability by increasing cAMP (Abbott, 2000). Endothelin-1 increases the permeability of monocytes through the BBB through endothelin-binding receptor signaling located on endothelial cells (Reijerkerk et al., 2013). In addition, the release of many cytokines such as interleukin-1 (IL-1), TNF-α, and eicosanoids, which play a role in the inflammation process, affects the integrity of the BBB. IL-1 changes BBB activity through TNF-α occludin expression (Zhao et al., 2022). VEGF, which plays an essential role in vascular angiogenesis in the development of the BBB, also plays a vital role in the permeability of the BBB (Shen et al., 2018; Morin-Brureau et al., 2011; Zhang et al., 2000). The effect of VEGF occurs through claudin-5 and occludin. VEGF disrupts claudin-5 and occludin, causing the tight junctions between endothelial cells to break down. This disruption increases the permeability of the BBB (Matsuno et al., 2022).

In addition to these chemical changes, agents such as age, gender, temperature, and physical activity also change the permeability of the BBB. It is known that aging causes many physiological disorders in the body. It is a known fact that aging disrupts physiological functions in the brain. Inflammatory mediators such as IL-1β, IFNγ, and TNF-α increase with age. As cellular inflammation increases, the expression of claudin, occludin, and ZO proteins, which form tight junctions between cells, decreases and becomes impaired. This causes the tight junctions to break down and the permeability of the BBB to increase (Zhao et al., 2022). It is also effective in changing the permeability of the BBB in the increasing degeneration of pericytes and astrocytes with age (Costea et al., 2019). In addition to aging, gender is essential in the permeability of the BBB. Gender-related hormonal changes regulate the permeability of the BBB. It has been observed that the hormones estrogen secreted in females and testosterone secreted in males ensure the stability of tight junctions. Both hormones have been shown to protect against tight junction degenerations caused by damage (Atallah et al., 2017; Maggioli et al., 2016).

Recent studies show that temperature plays a role in BBB permeability. Hyperthermia (38-42°C) causes increased fluid in the brain and cellular abnormalities, which increases BBB permeability. Hypothermia (32-34°C) has a protective effect on BBB integrity. However, under low-temperature conditions (15 °C), the localization of claudin-5 shifts to the cytoplasm, resulting in decreased resistance (Zhao et al., 2022).

In addition to all these, excessive physical activity increases inflammation and causes changes in the brain. It also increases oxidative stress and causes the formation of free oxygen radicals in cells. These changes are thought to arise from differences in serotonin levels through S100 levels and 5-HT2 receptors (Roh et al., 2017; Bailey et al., 2011).

Development of the Blood-Brain Barrier

Although the development of the BBB differs in timing due to the differences in each species, the formation steps are similar. Developmental stages are best studied and reported in rodents. According to these studies, the first blood vessels are observed around the neural tube. 10-11th day of embryonic life. (different time intervals are observed in different species) (Saili et al., 2017;

Engelhardt, 2003). Developing vessels anastomose to form a plexus in the ventricular region. While the capillaries in the neural tube are in the shape of sinusoids in the initial period, they lose their fenestration over time. The connecting strands of capillary endothelial cells are short and uncomplicated in early fetal capillaries. Later in development, endothelial connections become more extensive and interconnected (Saili et al., 2017; Engelhardt, 2003). Thus, BBB formation does not occur all at once but gradually, starting from some brain areas. During this gradual transition, differences begin to occur in the morphology of endothelial cells. Differentiation is achieved by vascular endothelial growth factor (VEGF). VEGF is highly expressed in the ventricular layer of the developing neuroectoderm. Cells that change with the help of the signal trigger the differentiation of other cells (Saili et al., 2017; Engelhardt, 2003).

Conclusion

The blood-brain barrier is a barrier that regulates the passage of substances between blood and the brain. This barrier consists of astrocytes, pericytes, endothelial cells, and the basal lamina of these cells. It is essential for substance permeability and the tight connections between endothelial cells. This regulation in the BBB protects the brain from toxic and pathogenic factors. Different physiological processes ensure the passage of substances across the BBB. While molecules under 40Da are allowed to pass through the pores in the BBB, transporters are used to pass molecules that are insoluble in fat and have more than eight hydrogen bonds. Different factors can achieve this selective permeability of the BBB. Many of these factors disrupt the regulation of tight junctions and increase the permeability of the BBB. This increase in permeability causes different neurodegenerative disorders. Although there are many studies in the literature on the structure and permeability of the BBB, the pathways by which the permeability of the BBB is regulated have yet to be fully explained. Defining this process is essential in the treatment of neurological disorders.

References

Abbott, N. J., Patabendige, A. A., Dolman, D. E., Yusof, S. R., Begley, D. J. (2010). Structure and function of the blood–brain barrier. *Neurobiol Dis*, 37(1),13–25.

Abbott, N. J. (2000). Inflammatory mediators and modulation of blood–brain barrier permeability. *Cell Mol Neurobiol* 20, 131–147.

Alhadidi, Q., Bin Sayeed, M. S., Shah, Z. A. (2017). The interplay between cofilin and phospho-cofilin: Its role in maintaining blood brain barrier integrity. *CNS Neurol. Disord. -Drug Targets* 16, 279–290 (2017).

Atallah A, Mhaouty-Kodja S, Grange-Messent V. Chronic depletion of gonadal testosterone leads to blood–brain barrier dysfunction and inflammation in male mice. *Journal of Cerebral Blood Flow & Metabolism*, 37(9),3161-3175.

Bailey, D. M., Evans, K. A., McEneny, J., Young, I. S., Hullin, D. A., James, P. E., Ogoh, S., Ainslie, P. N., Lucchesi, C., Rockenbauer, A., Culcasi, M., Pietri, S. (2011). Exercise-induced oxidative-nitrosative stress is associated with impaired dynamic cerebral autoregulation and blood-brain barrier leakage. *Exp Physiol,* 96(11), 1196-207.

Ballabh, P., Braun, A., Nedergaard, M. (2004). The blood-brain barrier: an overview: structure, regulation, and clinical implications. *Neurobiol Dis,* 16(1), 1-13. doi: 10.1016/j.nbd.2003.12.016.

Bhasiin, K., Heintz, O., Colodner, K. J. (2023). Optimization and technical considerations for the dye-exclusion protocol used to assess blood-brain barrier integrity in adult drosophila melanogaster. *Int. J. Mol. Sci.* 24, 1886.

Costea, L., Mészáros, Á., Bauer, H., Bauer, H. C., Traweger, A., Wilhelm, I., Farkas, A. E., Krizbai, I. A. (2019). The Blood–Brain Barrier and Its Intercellular Junctions in Age-Related Brain Disorders. *International Journal of Molecular Sciences*. 20(21), 5472.

Daneman, R., Prat, A. (2015). The blood-brain barrier. *Cold Spring Harb Perspect Biol*. 7(1), a020412. doi: 10.1101/cshperspect.a020412.

Engelhardt, B. (2003). Development of the blood-brain barrier. *Cell Tissue Res*. 314(1), 119-29. doi: 10.1007/s00441-003-0751-z.

Fu, B. M. (2018). Transport Across the Blood-Brain Barrier. *Adv Exp Med Biol*. 1097, 235-259.

Galea, I. (2021). The blood–brain barrier in systemic infection and inflammation. *Cell Mol Immunol* 18, 2489–2501.https://doi.org/10.1038/s41423-021-00757-x.

Kadry, H., Noorani, B., Cucullo, L. (2020). A blood–brain barrier overview on structure, function, impairment, and biomarkers of integrity. *Fluids Barriers CNS* 17, 69. https://doi.org/10.1186/s12987-020-00230-3.

Luissint, A. C., Artus, C., Glacial, F. *et al.* (2012). Tight junctions at the blood brain barrier: physiological architecture and disease-associated dysregulation. *Fluids Barriers CNS* 9, 23. https://doi.org/10.1186/2045-8118-9-23.

Maggioli, E., McArthur, S., Mauro, C., Kieswich, J., Kusters, D. H. M., Reutelingsperger, C. P. M., Yaqoob, M., Solito, E. (2016). Estrogen protects the blood-brain barrier from inflammation-induced disruption and increased lymphocyte trafficking. *Brain Behav Immun*. 51, 212-222.

Matsuno, H., Tsuchimine, S., O'Hashi, K. *et al.* (2022). Association between vascular endothelial growth factor-mediated blood–brain barrier dysfunction and stress-induced depression. *Mol Psychiatry* 27, 3822–3832.

Morin-Brureau, M., Lebrun, A., Rousset, M. C., Fagni, L., Bockaert, J., de Bock, F., Lerner-Natoli, M. (2011). Epileptiform activity induces vascular remodeling and zonula occludens 1 downregulation in organotypic hippocampal cultures: role of VEGF signaling pathways. *J Neurosci.* 31(29), 10677-88.

Nag, S., Begley, D. (2005). Blood–brain barrier, exchange of metabolites and gases. In: Pathology and genetics cerebrovascular diseases. *Basel: ISN Neuropath Press*; pp. 22–9.

Nokkari, A., Abou-El-Hassan, H., Mechref, Y., Mondello, S., Kindy, M. S., Jaffa, A. A., Kobeissy, F. (2018). Implication of the Kallikrein-Kinin system in neurological disorders: Quest for potential biomarkers and mechanisms. *Prog Neurobiol.* 165-167, 26-50.

O'Connor, T. M., O'Connell, J., O'Brien, D. I., Goode, T., Bredin, C. P., Shanahan, F. (2004). The role of substance P in inflammatory disease. *J Cell Physiol.* 201(2), 167-80. doi: 10.1002/jcp.20061. PMID: 15334652.

Pardridge, W. M. (2015). Blood–brain barrier endogenous transporters as therapeutic targets: a new model for small molecule CNS drug discovery. *Expert Opin Ther Targets.* 19(8), 1059–72.

Reijerkerk, A., Lopez-Ramirez, M. A., van Het Hof, B., Drexhage, J. A., Kamphuis, W. W., Kooij, G., Vos, J. B., van der Pouw Kraan, T. C., van Zonneveld, A. J., Horrevoets, A. J., Prat, A., Romero, I. A., de Vries, H. E. (2013). MicroRNAs regulate human brain endothelial cell-barrier function in inflammation: implications for multiple sclerosis. *J Neurosci.* 33(16), 6857-63.

Roh, H. T., Cho, S. Y., Yoon, H. G., So, W. Y. (2017). Effect of exercise intensity on neurotrophic factors and blood–brain barrier permeability induced by oxidative–nitrosative stress in male college students. *International journal of sport nutrition and exercise metabolism*, *27*(3), 239-246.

Saili, K. S., Zurlinden, T. J., Schwab, A. J., Silvin, A., Baker, N. C., Hunter, E. S. 3rd., Ginhoux, F., Knudsen, T. B. (2017). Blood-brain barrier development: Systems modeling and predictive toxicology. *Birth Defects Res.*109(20), 1680-1710. doi: 10.1002/bdr2.1180.

Sandoval, K. E., Witt, K. A. (2008). Blood-brain barrier tight junction permeability and ischemic stroke. *Neurobiol Dis.* 32(2), 200-19.

Shen, Y., Gu, J., Liu, Z., Xu, C., Qian, S., Zhang, X., Zhou, B., Guan, Q., Sun, Y., Wang, Y., Jin, X. (2018). Inhibition of HIF-1α Reduced Blood Brain Barrier Damage by Regulating MMP-2 and VEGF During Acute Cerebral Ischemia. *Front Cell Neurosci.* 12, 288.

Sugiyama, S., Sasaki, T., Tanaka, H. *et al.* (2023). The tight junction protein occludin modulates blood–brain barrier integrity and neurological function after ischemic stroke in mice. *Sci Rep* 13, 2892.

Thomsen, M. S., Routhe, L. J., Moos, T. (2017). The vascular basement membrane in the healthy and pathological brain. *J Cereb Blood Flow Metab.* 37(10), 3300-3317. doi: 10.1177/0271678X17722436.

Wu, D., Chen, Q., Chen, X. *et al.* (2023) The blood–brain barrier: structure, regulation, and drug delivery. *Sig Transduct Target Ther* 8, 217. doi: 10.1038/s41392-023-01481-w.

Xu, L., Nirwane, A., Yao, Y. (2018). Basement membrane and blood-brain barrier. *Stroke Vasc Neurol.* 4(2), 78-82. doi: 10.1136/svn-2018-000198.

Zhang, Z. G., Zhang, L., Jiang, Q., Zhang, R., Davies, K., Powers, C., Bruggen, Nv., Chopp, M. (2000). VEGF enhances angiogenesis and promotes blood-brain barrier leakage in the ischemic brain. *J Clin Invest*. 106(7), 829-38. doi: 10.1172/JCI9369.

Zhao, Y., Gan, L., Ren, L., Lin, Y., Ma, C., Lin, X. (2022). Factors influencing the blood-brain barrier permeability. *Brain Res*. 1788, 147937. doi: 10.1016/j.brainres.2022.147937.

Chapter 9

The Blood-Cerebrospinal Fluid Barrier

Tuba Demirci*, MD
Department of Histology and Embrology, Ataturk University, Erzurum, Turkiye

Abstract

There are many defense mechanisms to protect the human body against external and/or internal factors. Barriers in many organs such as the lungs, kidneys, brain, testicles, thymus, and eyes form an important part of defense mechanisms. The barrier systems in the body are responsible for preventing foreign substance penetration and maintaining normal cell signaling. Protecting the central nervous system (CNS) from blood-borne microorganisms, waste products, toxins, proteins, and other molecules is crucial for the maintenance of normal function of the CNS. The blood-cerebrospinal fluid (CSF) barrier, an important part of the central nervous system, is one of these barriers and acts as a protective barrier surrounding the cerebrospinal fluid. The blood-CSF barrier and the blood-brain barrier work together to protect the CNS and ensure its homeostasis. The blood-cerebrospinal fluid barrier specifically regulates the composition of cerebrospinal fluid (CSF), while the blood-brain barrier controls the passage between blood and brain tissue. These two barriers help keep the microenvironment in different parts of the CNS stable and maintain the functionality of the CNS. The complex interaction of endothelial cells and ependymal cells forms the blood-CSF barrier. The structure, functions, and disorders of this barrier are important for understanding neurological diseases and developing treatment approaches. In this section, the structure, functions, disorders, and effects on the health of the blood-CSF barrier will be examined in detail.

* Corresponding Author's Email: drtubademirci@gmail.com

In: A Histological Approach to Human Body Barriers
Editor: İlknur Keskin
ISBN: 979-8-89530-738-0

Keywords: blood-CSF barrier, choroid plexus, choroid plexus epithelial cells

Introduction

The blood-CSF barrier is a selectively permeable barrier settled in the brain and spinal cord. It has an essential role in regulating the chemical and biological composition of the CSF by controlling the exchange of molecules between the CSF and the blood. The barrier, formed by the choroid plexus (CP) epithelium, protects the CNS from harmful substances in the external environment and regulates the homeostasis of the cerebrospinal fluid, besides the formation of cerebrospinal fluid (Abbott, 2004; Saunders et al., 2015).

The blood-CSF barrier consists of epithelial cells of the CP located in the brain ventricles, fenestrated capillary vessels, and basal laminas of these two epithelia, with the stroma accompanying these structures. The inner surface of the ventricle cavities is lined with the ependymal cells in the brain (Figure 9.1). Tight junctions between the CP epithelial cells role as one of the most important parts of the barrier by preventing the free passage of molecules (C. Johanson et al., 2011). Thus, the central nervous system is protected from the harmful effects of foreign molecules such as cells, toxins, microorganisms, and pathogens. This barrier protects the brain by not allowing harmful substances, toxins, and pathogens to pass into the cerebrospinal fluid, and keeps the CNS healthy.

In addition, it plays a critical role in cerebral functioning by allowing the passage of various neurotransmitters, ions, and nutrients into the cerebrospinal fluid (Fong et al., 2024; Saunders et al., 2015). The barrier layer controls blood-brain ionic traffic through ion transporters and channels and maintains an optimal ionic environment in the cerebral interstitial fluid (ISF) and CSF (Abbott, 2004). It performs this function thanks to its selective permeability. The barrier blocks the passage of small molecules that can be harmful to the brain. In addition to harmful substances and microorganisms, it also prevents the passage of large molecules. For example, glucose and certain amino acids can pass through the barrier, while large proteins and some drugs cannot (C. Johanson et al., 2011). Thus, it is ensured that homeostasis in the brain and therefore the neurons maintain their optimal function (Abbott, 2004; Abbott et al., 2010). Another function of the blood-CSF barrier is its contribution to the protection of neurological health by clearing metabolic wastes and by-products in the brain and spinal fluid (Vendel et al., 2019). The epithelium of the CP, an important part of the blood-CSF barrier, controls CSF production through secretion promoted by apical Na, K, and ATPase. This process regulates the production rate and composition of CSF.

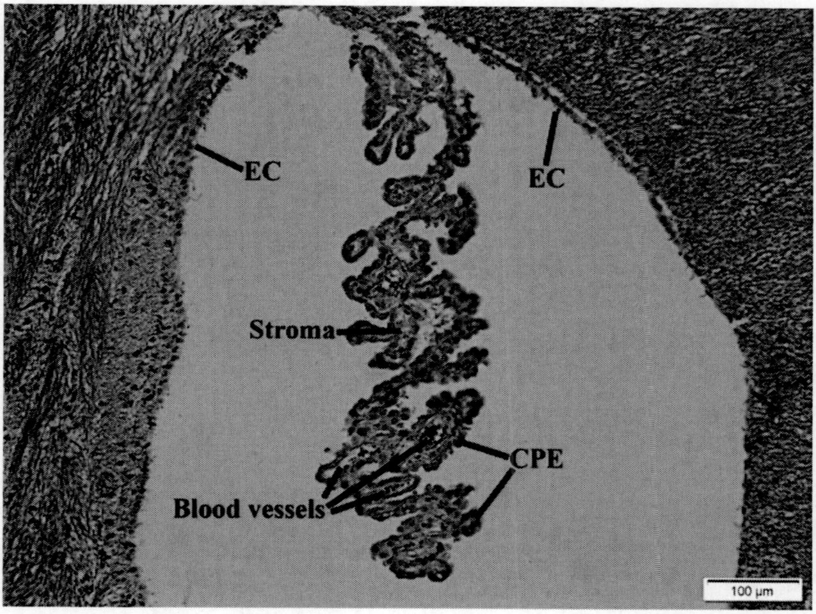

Figure 9.1. Rat choroid plexus in the ventricle. CPE, choroid plexus epithelium, EC, ependymal cells lining the inner surface of the ventricle.

The Significance of the Blood-CSF Barrier in the CNS Health

The healthy functioning of the blood-CSF barrier is extremely important for the protection of CNS health. A small disruption in this barrier structure may contribute to the development of various neurological and neuroinflammatory diseases by affecting its functions. Therefore, understanding and maintaining the functionality of the blood-CSF barrier is important for diagnosing and treating neurological diseases (Saunders et al., 2015).

Any disruption that occurs in the blood-CSF barrier leads to CNS disorders and especially plays a crucial role in the pathophysiology of many neurological diseases, such as meningitis and multiple sclerosis. During these diseases, the functionality of this barrier is disrupted, and the normal components of CSF may be altered. Even the permeability of the blood-CSF barrier may be affected, and the CNS may be more vulnerable (Zlokovic, 2008).

The blood-CSF barrier plays a role in the control of brain edema. As a result of damage or impaired function of the barrier, cerebral edema can occur (Abbott, 2004). Cerebral edema is swelling that occurs with fluid accumulation in and around brain tissue. This condition increases intracranial pressure (ICP) by increasing the volume of the brain and can severely affect brain functions (Simard et al., 2007).

The blood-CSF barrier has an important responsibility in the transfer of drugs into in the CNS taken into the body and regulates drug concentrations and distribution in the cerebral interstitial fluid. The fact that many drugs cannot pass through this barrier brings difficulties in the treatment of CNS diseases. Therefore, the investigation of the ability of drugs to cross the blood-CSF barrier is an important research topic to improve the effectiveness of neurological therapies (Zlokovic, 2008).

Cerebrospinal Fluid (CSF)

Cerebrospinal fluid is a transparent and colorless fluid secreted by the CP and found in the cerebral ventricles, the subarachnoid space around the brain and spinal cord, and the canalis centralis of the spinal cord. It coordinates various functions, such as aiding in the transport of nutrients and their waste products, and regulates the chemical environment of the brain and spinal cord. Also, it protects the CNS from numerous harmful conditions and impacts (Spector et al., 2015). In addition, CSF found in and around the brain reduces the net weight of the brain within the cranial cavity. CSF prevents brain injuries by slowing down the fluctuations of the brain, especially during sudden head movements. However, this effect does not protect against significant injuries (Rea, 2015).

Its basic components include water, glucose, proteins, electrolytes, vitamins, and a minimum amount of cellular components (Spector et al., 2015). CSF has a higher concentration of sodium and chloride but less protein, glucose, potassium, and calcium than blood (Rea, 2015). The contents of CSF and serum are compared in Table 9.1. (Gartner, 2017).

Table 9.1. The content of cerebrospinal fluid and serum (Gartner, 2017)

	Cerebrospinal Fluid	Serum
White blood cells (cells/mL)	0–5	0
Protein (g/L)	Insignificant	60–80
Glucose (mmol/L)	2.1–4.0	4.0–5.5
Na^+ (mmol/L)	135–150	135–150
K^+ (mmol/L)	2.8–3.2	4.0–5.1
Cl^- (mmol/L)	115–130	100–105
Ca^{2+} (mmol/L)	1.0–1.4	2.1–2.5
Mg^{2+} (mmol/L)	0.8–1.3	0.7–1.0
pH	7.3	7.4

Secretion, Circulation, and Absorption of CSF

The CP produces CSF from blood, which is transported through the ventricles to other areas of the CNS. Ependymal cells found in the CP produce approximately two-thirds of the circulating CSF. The ventricular surfaces and the lining of the subarachnoid space produce the remainder of the CSF. CSF secretion is a complex process, and it is regulated by both physiological and biochemical mechanisms (Damkier et al., 2013; Rea, 2015). Approximately 500-600 ml CSF is produced each day. CSF circulates within the brain ventricles, canalis centralis, and around the brain and spinal cord. CSF flows into the subarachnoid space, passing from the lateral ventricles to the third and fourth ventricles. In the subarachnoid space, CSF circulates around the brain and spinal cord. Since absorption also occurs during this circulation, the volume at any given time is approximately 100–150 ml. In other words, the CSF in the body is renewed 3-4 times a day. (Rea, 2015). CSF absorption is mainly carried out by arachnoid villi on the brain's surface, and CSF returns to the venous circulation. CSF is constantly replenished in this absorption process and waste products are removed (Brinker et al., 2014). To understand the formation and secretion of CSF let's look at the structure of the CP.

Choroid Plexus

The choroid plexus (CP) is located in the area covering the surface of the brain ventricles, and is a secretory epithelial tissue comprising the CP epithelial cells, stroma, and fenestrated blood vessels (Figure 9.2 and Figure 9.3) (Neman & Chen, 2015). During the embryonic stage, the choroid plexus is derived from ependymal cells lining the inner surfaces of the lateral, third, and fourth ventricles, as well as the vascular mesoderm of the meninges. By the proliferation of ventricular ependymal cells and vascular mesenchymal cells found just beneath them, sac-like invaginations occur towards the ventricles. These projections form the choroid plexus (Sadler, 2018).

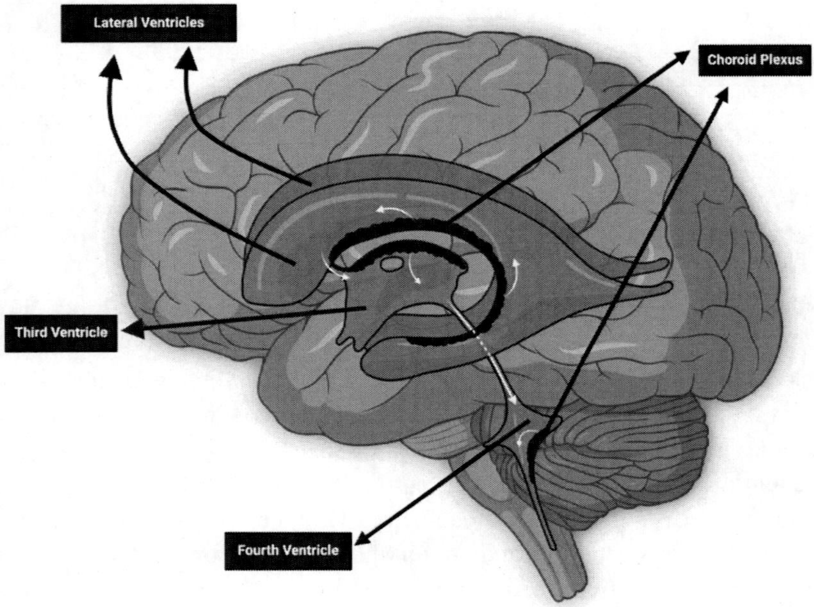

Figure 9.2. Lateral view of the choroid plexus and ventricles. The white arrows indicate the direction of the CSF flow (*Biorender*, n.d.).

Although it is known that the primary function of the CP is to produce and secrete CSF, interestingly, it also plays a role in nourishing the brain parenchyma and helps to clear metabolic byproducts from the nervous system (Bitanihirwe et al., 2022). Although it is known that the primary function of the CP is to produce and secrete CSF, interestingly, it also plays a role in nourishing the brain parenchyma and helps to clear metabolic byproducts from the nervous system (Bitanihirwe et al., 2022). It also helps to transport other molecules, including hormones, to the brain. It does this by regulating the movement of CSF within and around the brain ventricles (Spector et al., 2015). The CP, consisting of a cuboidal epithelium, is a highly vascularized tissue quite delicate. The apical surfaces of the cells are in contact with the CSF in the ventricles, while their basal surfaces are on the basement membrane

(Figure 9.4) (Bitanihirwe et al., 2022). These structures, via a series of CP components, selectively regulate and control the movement of materials between blood and brain tissue (Liddelow, 2015). CP produces various biological factors, including growth factors of several types, neurotrophins, cytokines, and other hormones. These factors are carried through the cerebral fluid (CSF) to different brain regions, where they promote nerve repair by up-regulating neurogenesis and angiogenesis. So, it ensures the healthy function of the neurons and glial cells. Thus, if the cues that CP gives to the brain for the occurrence of new neurons are damaged, then this situation may lead to various pathological conditions (Redzic, 2011). The blood vessels within the stroma of CP are permeable to circulating inflammatory cells, and CSF may contain inflammatory cells, such as T cells, macrophages, and dendritic cells, in healthy as well as diseased conditions (Engelhardt & Ransohoff, 2012; Ransohoff & Engelhardt, 2012; Shechter et al., 2013).

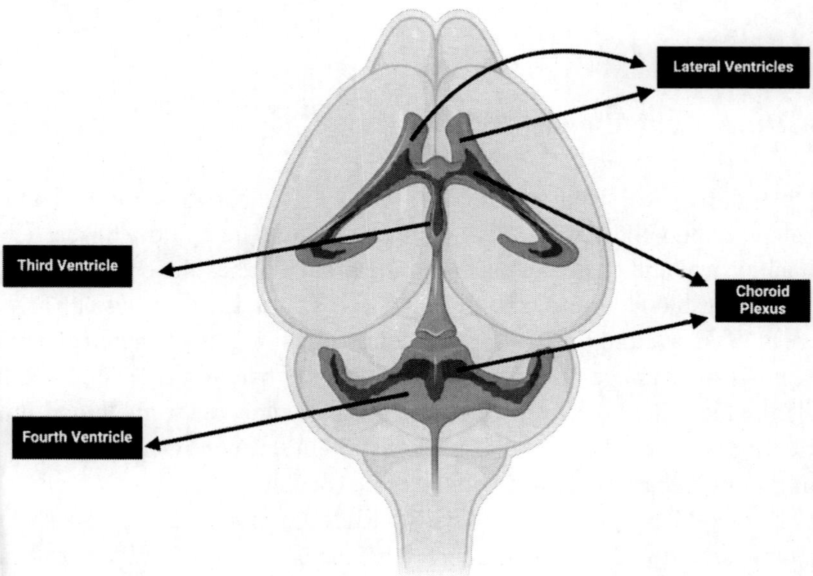

Figure 9.3. Dorsal view of the choroid plexus and ventricles (*Biorender*, n.d.).

Different pathological conditions result from imbalances in the production and functions of CP. This can result in conditions such as hydrocephalus when too much is produced or not enough is absorbed. This also may increase intracranial pressure (Bateman & Siddique, 2014; Spector et al., 2015). Similarly, the interaction of hormones such as atrial natriuretic peptide (ANP) and arginine vasopressin (AVP) with the choroid plexus has also been reported. It is also remarkable that ANP has an inherent relationship to the intracranial pressure and AVP controls body liquid and CSF amount (C. E. Johanson et al., 2008).

Aging can cause some changes in the structure of the CP. As a result of aging, intellectual abilities may be decreased or even lost. Because of this structural and functional deterioration in CP, the structure of CSF is affected, and this leads to both biochemical and immunological changes (Spector et al., 2015).

The apical surface of the ependymal cells on the inner surface of the ventricles contains cilia, as will be discussed in more detail later. These cilia, with ependymal ciliary activity, provide the transport of CSF within the ventricles by undulating motion. Any structural and functional deterioration that may occur in CP will both cause conditions such as hydrocephalus, as described above, and will adversely affect brain functions (Sawamoto et al., 2006).

Structure of the Blood-CSF Barrier

The blood–CSF barrier is situated between the lumen of choroidal blood vessels and the CSF (Zheng & Chodobski, 2005). The blood-CSF barrier is both a physical and chemical barrier in the brain that has the crucial function of separating blood from CSF. In other words, it acts as a physical barrier between the blood and the CSF, while at the same time, it is a chemical barrier that allows the passage of drugs and biomolecules between the blood and the CSF. The blood-CSF barrier is more permeable compared to the blood-brain barrier and allows the passage of plasma protein through pinocytosis. It acts as an important barrier to access to the brain (Sadler, 2018).

The blood CSF barrier, which will fulfill this important task, has a special structure formed in three parts: choroid plexus epithelium (CPE) cells, basal laminas of CPE and fenestrated endothelial cells, and fenestrated endothelial cells (Figure 9.4). (Zheng & Chodobski, 2005). The structure formed by the choroid plexus epithelial cells, which are connected by tight connections, forms the main component of the blood-CSF barrier. Endothelial cells with stroma and fenestra, located just below this structure, act as supporting components of the barrier and affect the movement of substances between the blood and the CSF. This triple structure, by working together, forms a barrier system that regulates the passage of molecules into the CSF.

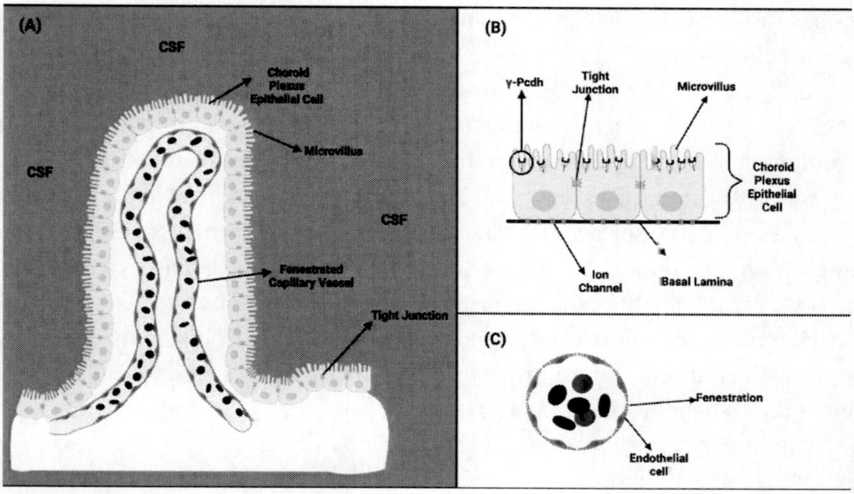

Figure 9.4. A. Cross-section of choroid plexus. B. Choroid plexus epithelial cells C. Cross section of the fenestrated capillary vessel (Biorender, n.d.).

Ependymal Cells

The ependymal cells originate from neural ectoderm (McMillan & Harris, 2018) and are arranged as one cell layer and form a simple epithelium lining the inner surfaces of the ventricles in the brain and the canalis centralis in the spinal cord (Groh et al., 2024). The ependymal cells lining the inner surface of the ventricles form an inner limiting membrane, while those located below the pia mater form an outer limiting membrane. Both structures are formed by finely fused pedicels (Gartner, 2017). Ependymal cells form an epithelium-like lining on the inner surface of the ventricles (Figure 9.1). Ependymal cells are mostly cuboidal in shape. Also, they may be flattened or low columnar. They have a centrally located round nucleus and have microvilli or motile cilia on their apical surfaces. Microvilli are responsible for the absorption of the CSF. Ciliated ependymal cells found in some regions are responsible for sustaining the local flow and distribution of the CSF (Lechtreck et al., 2008). Furthermore, ependymal cells are tightly bound to each other via junctional complexes such as zonula adherens and zonulae occludentes (Gartner, 2017; Groh et al., 2024; Lechtreck et al., 2008; Ross & Pawlina, 2016). The tight junctions between the cells control the movement of molecules and force them to follow a transcellular pathway. Therefore, CSF production depends on facilitated and active transport through the ependymal cells. As a result, this causes differences between CSF and plasma content (Gartner, 2017). Plenty of mitochondria and intermediate filaments are found in their cytoplasm (Gartner, 2017). The cytoskeleton of ependymal cells contains intermediate filaments such as vimentin and cytokeratin, which play an important role in maintaining cell shape and stabilizing junctional proteins (Groh et al., 2024).

Some specialized ependymal cells lining the third ventricle are named tanycytes. The free surfaces of these cells are in contact with the CSF but have no cilia on their apical surfaces (Ross & Pawlina, 2016). The extensions of tanycytes reach the hypothalamus and terminate there. These cells, which are closely related to blood vessels and neurosecretory cells, contact the CSF, and it is considered that they transport CSF to these neurosecretory cells. These cells may respond to changes in hormone levels in the CSF, and they may play a role in important processes in the body, such as controlling body weight and energy balance (Bolborea & Dale, 2013; Gartner, 2017).

Choroid Plexus Epithelial Cells

Some special ependymal cells in the ventricles participate in the structure of the choroidal plexus (Gartner, 2017). These cells are specialized cells synthesizing of CSF, which is responsible for washing and protecting the brain. (McMillan & Harris, 2018; Neman & Chen, 2015). As mentioned above, the CP is located within the brain ventricles and consists of modified ependymal cells and adjacent capillary vessels (Ross & Pawlina, 2016). The choroid plexus epithelium consists of specialized ependymal cells and a continuous basal membrane just beneath the cells. The choroidal epithelial cells in direct contact with the ventricular CSF have numerous cytoplasmic projections or microvilli on the apical surface, and complex basolateral foldings and interdigitations are present in the basal part of the cells (Figure 9.4A and 9.4B). (MacAulay et al., 2022; Neman & Chen, 2015). There are tight junctions between cells and also where adhesive contacts are formed from the interactions between cadherin and catenin proteins (Neman & Chen, 2015). These tight junctions are involved in the formation of the blood-CSF barrier. It acts as a protective barrier by limiting the substances that can pass into the CSF. Furthermore, the presence of γ-Pcdh cell adhesion molecules is observed on the apical surfaces of cells. There are many ion channels in the basement membrane, and these ion channels are critical for maintaining fluid balance and the functionality of CPE (Figure 9.4B). (Liu et al., 2022).

Stroma, the Basal Lamina of the CPE, and the Basal Lamina of the Fenestrated Capillaries

The choroid plexuses, which form an interface between the blood and CSF, consist of a ciliated cubic epithelium surrounding a loose connective tissue stroma. The blood vessels found in this stroma form large fenestrated capillaries adjacent to the tight epithelium that form the blood-CSF barrier (Ghersi-Egea et al., 2018). The stromal space is bounded on one side by the basal lamina of endothelial cells of the fenestrated capillaries and on the other side by the basal lamina of the CPE. The endothelial basal lamina surrounding the fenestrated capillaries forms the inner lamina of the stromal space, and the subepithelial basal lamina of CPE forms the outer lamina. Both basal laminae continue uninterruptedly (Figure 9.4A, 9.4B and 9.4B) (Liu et al., 2022) (Zheng & Chodobski, 2005).

The stroma consists of loose connective tissue and contains many connective tissue cells, such as immune cells, microglia, fibroblasts, and macrophages, and structural components, with the distance between cells being large. This loose connective tissue structure also includes collagen fibers, reticular fibers, and a small amount of elastic fibers. This structure gives flexibility to the stroma and allows the movement of fluids and molecules during CSF production; moreover, it supports the functionality of the blood-CSF barrier and contributes to CSF production. The stromal cells and CPE cells are sensitive to physiological changes in the brain and damage, such as inflammation. In these cases, it usually responds with a rapid secretion of chemokines (Ghersi-Egea et al., 2018). Plenty of macrophages, T cells, and bone marrow-origin dendritic cells passing through the fenestra capillaries are found in the choroidal stroma (Baruch et al., 2013; Nathanson & Chun, 1989; Serot et al., 1997). These cells function immunologically to protect the brain in various pathological conditions.

Fenestrated Capillaries

CPE provides a balance between blood and CSF, and to maintain this balance, a thin layer of connective tissue and fenestrated capillaries are found in CP (Liu et al., 2022). The vessels in the choroid plexus, which participate in the blood-CSF barrier structure, are fenestrated and form a nonrestrictive barrier (Figure 9.4A and 9.4C) (MacAulay et al., 2022; Neman & Chen, 2015;

Saunders et al., 2008). The choroidal endothelium, which forms the first cellular layer between blood and CSF, is permeable, allowing macromolecules to pass through into the surrounding stroma (Ghersi-Egea et al., 2018; Neman & Chen, 2015). The formation and maintenance of fenestra and their diaphragms in capillary vessels are under the control of the plasmalemma vesicle-associated protein (Plvap) gene and vascular endothelial growth factor (VEGF) (Maharaj et al., 2008; Stan et al., 2012).

The peripheral blood, and therefore the inflammatory cells in it, come to the stroma of the choroid plexus through these vessels. By the expression of various receptors and adhesion molecules on the CPE cells, the cells that will pass to CSF are controlled and determined (Neman & Chen, 2015).

Consequences of Disorders in the Blood-CSF Barrier and Their Relationship with Diseases

The deterioration of the blood-CSF barrier, about which we have given information about its properties, structure, and functions above, leads to several neurological diseases. Any disorder that may occur in the structure or functions of the blood-CSF barrier, mainly in CPE, causes the brain tissue to be exposed to harmful substances or even systemic inflammatory events, and this triggers neurodegenerative and neuroinflammatory diseases (Liu et al., 2022). Various bacteria and viruses cause deterioration in the epithelium, cell death, deterioration of barrier function and increased barrier permeability while crossing the blood-CSF barrier. These disruptions can contribute to the progression of the disease by triggering inflammatory responses during CNS infections (Schwerk et al., 2015).

If the CSF is constantly produced, absorption decreases or any blockage occurs during the flow of the CSF in the brain ventricles or subarachnoid area, swelling of brain tissue occurs, and then this leads to the head expanding in the fetus or neonates. This condition results in hydrocephalus, which is clinically characterized by impaired mental and muscle function and, if left untreated, results in death (Gartner, 2017; Sadler, 2018).

Neurodegenerative and neuroinflammatory diseases such as Alzheimer's disease, multiple sclerosis and Parkinson's disease, and brain injury accompanied by acute inflammation such as stroke also have deterioration in the blood-CSF barrier. Let's briefly look at these diseases under separate headings:

Alzheimer's Disease

Alzheimer's disease (AD) is the most common neurodegenerative disease in the central nervous system in the elderly. In addition to cognitive impairment, dementia, synaptic loss, and speech disorders are also seen in patients. Delaying the occurrence of this incurable disease is the most important treatment method. In the pathophysiology of Alzheimer's disease, there are amyloid plaques occur due to the overproduction and accumulation of β-amyloid in the brain tissue. Fibrillar tangles formed due to the accumulation of tau protein in neurons also accompany these plaques. As the disease progresses, β-amyloid accumulation increases (Bolos et al., 2013; Liu et al., 2022). Studies have shown the presence of β-amyloid accumulation in CPE cells in Alzheimer's disease. This affects the CSF secretion of CPE cells and contributes to the progression of the disease (Bolos et al., 2013; Raha-Chowdhury et al., 2019). The presence of β-amyloid in CPE causes capillary damage and interstitial fibrosis, following an increase in IgG by activating immune system responses (Prineas et al., 2016). Aging and β-amyloid accumulation in CPE lead to a decrease in tight junctions, CSF secretion, and the ability to clean waste products. In the early stages of the disease, β-amyloid accumulation increases the secretion of proinflammatory cytokines and matrix metalloproteinases (MMP-3), resulting in downregulation of tight junction proteins such as ZO-1, Claudin-1, Claudin-5, and occludin. Moreover, the decrease in tight junctions of the CPE increases the permeability of the blood-CSF barrier, allowing inflammatory cells to enter the brain, which leads to an increase in neuroinflammation (Brkic et al., 2015). In Alzheimer's disease, the Atrophy of CPE cells due to accumulation of lipofuscin vacuoles, stromal fibrosis, and thickening of basement membranes (capillary walls and CPE) are other disorders of the blood-CSF barrier. These disorders, by affecting the integrity of the blood-CSF barrier, lead to changes in the composition of the CSF, and this situation plays an important role in the pathology of the disease (Solár et al., 2020). In conclusion, the functionality of CPE plays a critical role in the development of Alzheimer's disease, which is further complicated by the abnormalities that CPE presents with aging.

Multiple Sclerosis

Multiple sclerosis (MS), an autoimmune demyelinating disease, is more common in women than in men. It leads to many negative consequences such as vision problems, sensory disturbances, and muscle weakness in patients. It has been emphasized that this disease, the etiology of which is not clearly understood, occurs as a result of the destruction of the immune system and the demyelination of nerve cells with the entry of inflammatory cells such as T and B lymphocytes and macrophages into the brain. In the brains of multiple sclerosis patients, the decrease in the expression of claudin-3, a tight junction protein, in CPE cells increases the permeability of the blood-CSF barrier to inflammatory cells. This creates an important pathway for the infiltration of inflammatory cells, especially lymphocytes, into the brain. Lymphocytes that leak into the brain are found both in the vessels and in the stroma (Baecher-Allan et al., 2018; Liu et al., 2022; Solár et al., 2020). Furthermore, in the brains of patients with multiple sclerosis, in the CPE cells, it has been determined that there is more hypoxia than in normal individuals. In other words, it can be said that this condition impairs the secretory function of CPE in MS patients to a substantial extent (Rodríguez-Lorenzo et al., 2020). As a result, a structural change in the blood CSF barrier, especially in CPE, increases barrier permeability and causes neurodegeneration and neuroinflammation following the entry of inflammatory cells into the brain.

Parkinson's Disease

Parkinson's disease is characterized by resting tremors, muscle rigidity, and slow movement. Although the cause of the disease, a common neurodegenerative disease, is not known exactly, it is thought that more than one genetic factor and aging play a role in the pathogenesis (Elbaz et al., 2016). Decreased dopamine synthesis leads to a decrease in striatal dopamine content. This decrease leads to the appearance of several symptoms, such as resting tremors and slow movement (Fernández-Sotos et al., 2019). It is noted that in Parkinson's disease, feroxidase ceruloplasmin is oxidized and deaminated by pathological CSF. Oxidized and deaminated ceruloplasmin in CPE cells has also been reported to impair the function of CPE cells and prevent cell proliferation (Barbariga et al., 2020). In another study, the Parkinson 's-associated gene Parkin co-regulated gene (PACRG) was shown to be expressed in the choroidal plexus of the lateral ventricle, third ventricle, and fourth ventricle in mouse brains. The presence of PACRG in CPE cells shows that Parkinson's disease may be related to the blood-CSF barrier (Liu et al., 2022; Wilson et al., 2009) Alpha-synuclein is an important protein involved in the pathology of Parkinson's disease. Studies have shown that

Alpha-synuclein is expressed in CPE cells and that the choroidal plexus may play a role in the transport of this protein between the blood and CSF (Bates et al., 2015; Solár et al., 2020). In conclusion, although studies are showing that there may be a relationship between Parkinson's disease and the blood-CSF barrier, there is no definitive information on this issue and there is a need for many studies to be done.

Stroke

Stroke is a common disease in which brain tissue is damaged due to sudden occlusion or rupture of blood vessels in the brain. In stroke, brain cells die in a short time, leaving irreversible damage to the brain tissue. This damage manifests clinically in the form of deterioration in neurological functions and disability (Hornung & Sievert, 2021).

Since CPE cells do not come into contact with blood, the changes in the CPE are not directly related to stroke. But, there are cellular abnormalities in CPE in hypertension, which is an important cause of stroke. In addition, CPE plays an important role in the mechanisms of cell damage and death that occurs in the brain after stroke (Liu et al., 2022). Studies have shown that the cause of cellular damage to the brain after a stroke is neuroinflammation as well as ischemia. During neuroinflammation, inflammatory cells attack brain cells. It is noted that CPE cells play an important role in this process. In fact, some studies show that T cells accumulate in CPE after a stroke and migrate from there to brain tissue (Liu et al., 2022; Llovera et al., 2017). In conclusion, a better understanding of the role of CPE in both hypertension and post-stroke neuroinflammation will be one of the therapeutic goals to reduce post-stroke brain injury.

Conclusion

The blood-CSF barrier is a critical structure with essential functions in the central nervous system. In addition to functions such as CSF secretion and regulation of its content, this barrier, which protects the CNS from harmful substances and allows the passage of necessary molecules, acts both structurally and functionally. The permeability of the blood-CSF barrier is an important factor in the pathogenesis of diseases associated with neuroinflammation and neurodegeneration. A good understanding of the role of this barrier in the development of neuroinflammation and diseases may pave the way for new approaches in the treatment of neurological diseases.

References

Abbott, N. J. (2004). Evidence for bulk flow of brain interstitial fluid: significance for physiology and pathology. *Neurochemistry International*, *45*(4), 545–552. https://doi.org/10.1016/J.NEUINT.2003.11.006.

Abbott, N. J., Patabendige, A. A. K., Dolman, D. E. M., Yusof, S. R., & Begley, D. J. (2010). Structure and function of the blood–brain barrier. *Neurobiology of Disease*, *37*(1), 13–25. https://doi.org/10.1016/J.NBD.2009.07.030.

Baecher-Allan, C., Kaskow, B. J., & Weiner, H. L. (2018). Multiple Sclerosis: Mechanisms and Immunotherapy. *Neuron*, *97*(4), 742–768. https://doi.org/10.1016/J.NEURON.2018.01.021.

Barbariga, M., Zanardi, A., Curnis, F., Conti, A., Boselli, D., Di Terlizzi, S., & Alessio, M. (2020). Ceruloplasmin oxidized and deamidated by Parkinson's disease cerebrospinal fluid induces epithelial cells proliferation arrest and apoptosis. *Scientific Reports 2020 10:1*, *10*(1), 1–10. https://doi.org/10.1038/s41598-020-72447-z.

Baruch, K., Ron-Harel, N., Gal, H., Deczkowska, A., Shifrut, E., Ndifon, W., Mirlas-Neisberg, N., Cardon, M., Vaknin, I., Cahalon, L., Berkutzki, T., Mattson, M. P., Gomez-Pinilla, F., Friedman, N., & Schwartz, M. (2013). CNS-specific immunity at the choroid plexus shifts toward destructive Th2 inflammation in brain aging. *Proceedings of the National Academy of Sciences of the United States of America*, *110*(6), 2264–2269. https://doi.org/10.1073/PNAS.1211270110/-/DCSUPPLEMENTAL/PNAS.201211270SI.PDF.

Bateman, G. A., & Siddique, S. H. (2014). Cerebrospinal fluid absorption block at the vertex in chronic hydrocephalus: Obstructed arachnoid granulations or elevated venous pressure? *Fluids and Barriers of the CNS*, *11*(1), 1–10. https://doi.org/10.1186/2045-8118-11-11/FIGURES/1.

Bates, C. A., Fu, S., Ysselstein, D., Rochet, J. C., & Zheng, W. (2015). Expression and Transport of a-Synuclein at the Blood-Cerebrospinal Fluid Barrier and Effects of Manganese Exposure. *ADMET and DMPK*, *3*(1), 15–33. https://doi.org/10.5599/ADMET.3.1.159.

Biorender. (n.d.). Retrieved November 18, 2024, from https://app.biorender.com/gallery.

Bitanihirwe, B. K. Y., Lizano, P., & Woo, T.-U. W. (n.d.). *Perspective Deconstructing the functional neuroanatomy of the choroid plexus: an ontogenetic perspective for studying neurodevelopmental and neuropsychiatric disorders*. https://doi.org/10.1038/s41380-022-01623-6.

Bolborea, M., & Dale, N. (2013). Hypothalamic tanycytes: potential roles in the control of feeding and energy balance. *Trends in Neurosciences*, *36*(2), 91. https://doi.org/10.1016/J.TINS.2012.12.008.

Bolos, M., Spuch, C., Ordoñez-Gutierrez, L., Wandosell, F., Ferrer, I., & Carro, E. (2013). Neurogenic effects of β-amyloid in the choroid plexus epithelial cells in Alzheimer's disease. *Cellular and Molecular Life Sciences: CMLS*, *70*(15), 2787. https://doi.org/10.1007/S00018-013-1300-X.

Brinker, T., Stopa, E., Morrison, J., & Klinge, P. (2014). A new look at cerebrospinal fluid circulation. *Fluids and Barriers of the CNS*, *11*(1), 10. https://doi.org/10.1186/2045-8118-11-10.

Brkic, M., Balusu, S., Van Wonterghem, E., Gorlé, N., Benilova, I., Kremer, A., Van Hove, I., Moons, L., De Strooper, B., Kanazir, S., Libert, C., & Vandenbroucke, R. E. (2015). Amyloid β Oligomers Disrupt Blood-CSF Barrier Integrity by Activating Matrix Metalloproteinases. *The Journal of Neuroscience : The Official Journal of the Society for Neuroscience*, *35*(37), 12766–12778. https://doi.org/10.1523/JNEUROSCI.0006-15.2015.

Damkier, H. H., Brown, P. D., & Praetorius, J. (2013). Cerebrospinal fluid secretion by the choroid plexus. *Physiological Reviews*, *93*(4), 1847–1892. https://doi.org/10.1152/PHYSREV.00004.2013/ASSET/IMAGES/LARGE/Z9J0041326730014.JPEG.

Elbaz, A., Carcaillon, L., Kab, S., & Moisan, F. (2016). Epidemiology of Parkinson's disease. *Revue Neurologique*, *172*(1), 14–26. https://doi.org/10.1016/J.NEUROL.2015.09.012.

Engelhardt, B., & Ransohoff, R. M. (2012). Capture, crawl, cross: the T cell code to breach the blood–brain barriers. *Trends in Immunology*, *33*(12), 579–589. https://doi.org/10.1016/J.IT.2012.07.004.

Fernández-Sotos, P., López-Arcas Calleja, P., Lozano-Vicario, L., García-Tercero, E., Jesús Del Yerro-Álvarez, M., & López-álvarez, J. (2019). [Posterior reversible leukoencephalopathy syndrome in a patient with Parkinson's disease and initial psychiatric symptoms: a complex clinical presentation]. *Revista de Neurologia*, *68*(10), 426–430. https://doi.org/10.33588/RN.6810.2018435.

Fong, H. , Zhou, B. , Feng, H. , Luo, C. , Bai, B. , Zhang, J. , Wang, Y., Fong, H., Zhou, B., Feng, H., Luo, C., Bai, B., Zhang, J., & Wang, Y. (2024). Recapitulation of Structure–Function–Regulation of Blood–Brain Barrier under (Patho)Physiological Conditions. *Cells 2024, Vol. 13, Page 260*, *13*(3), 260. https://doi.org/10.3390/CELLS13030260.

Gartner, L. P. (2017). Textbook of Histology (4th Ed). In *Academic Medicine* (Vol. 9, Issue 6). Elsevier.

Ghersi-Egea, J. F., Strazielle, N., Catala, M., Silva-Vargas, V., Doetsch, F., & Engelhardt, B. (2018). Molecular anatomy and functions of the choroidal blood-cerebrospinal fluid barrier in health and disease. *Acta Neuropathologica 2018 135:3*, *135*(3), 337–361. https://doi.org/10.1007/S00401-018-1807-1.

Groh, A. M. R., Song, Y. L., Tea, F., Lu, B., Huynh, S., Afanasiev, E., Bigotte, M., Del Bigio, M. R., & Stratton, J. J. A. (2024). Multiciliated ependymal cells: an update on biology and pathology in the adult brain. *Acta Neuropathologica 2024 148:1*, *148*(1), 1–23. https://doi.org/10.1007/S00401-024-02784-0.

Hornung, M., & Sievert, H. (2021). It Is Time to Fight Ischemic Stroke the Best Possible Way. *JACC: Cardiovascular Interventions*, *14*(7), 793–795. https://doi.org/10.1016/J.JCIN.2021.02.017.

Johanson, C. E., Duncan, J. A., Klinge, P. M., Brinker, T., Stopa, E. G , & Silverberg, G. D. (2008). Multiplicity of cerebrospinal fluid functions: New challenges in health and disease. *Cerebrospinal Fluid Research*, *5*. https://doi.org/10.1186/1743-8454-5-10.

Johanson, C., Stopa, E., Mcmillan, P., Roth, D., Funk, J., & Krinke, G. (2011). The Distributional Nexus of Choroid Plexus to Cerebrospinal Fluid, Ependyma and Brain:Toxicologic/Pathologic Phenomena, Periventricular Destabilization, and Lesion Spread. *Toxicologic Pathology*, *39*(1), 186–212. https://doi.org/10.1177/0192623310394214/ASSET/IMAGES/LARGE/10.1177_0192623310394214-FIG12.JPEG.

Lechtreck, K. F., Delmotte, P., Robinson, M. L., Sanderson, M. J., & Witman, G. B. (2008). Mutations in Hydin impair ciliary motility in mice. *Journal of Cell Biology*, *180*(3), 633–643. https://doi.org/10.1083/JCB.200710162/VIDEO-6.

Liddelow, S. A. (2015). Development of the choroid plexus and blood-CSF barrier. *Frontiers in Neuroscience*, *9*(MAR), 123479. https://doi.org/10.3389/FNINS.2015.00032/BIBTEX.

Liu, R., Zhang, Z., Chen, Y., Liao, J., Wang, Y., Liu, J., Lin, Z., & Xiao, G. (2022). Choroid plexus epithelium and its role in neurological diseases. *Frontiers in Molecular Neuroscience*, *15*, 949231. https://doi.org/10.3389/FNMOL.2022.949231/BIBTEX.

Llovera, G., Benakis, C., Enzmann, G., Cai, R., Arzberger, T., Ghasemigharagoz, A., Mao, X., Malik, R., Lazarevic, I., Liebscher, S., Ertürk, A., Meissner, L., Vivien, D., Haffner, C., Plesnila, N., Montaner, J., Engelhardt, B., & Liesz, A. (2017). The choroid plexus is a key cerebral invasion route for T cells after stroke. *Acta Neuropathologica*, *134*(6), 851–868. https://doi.org/10.1007/S00401-017-1758-Y/FIGURES/6.

MacAulay, N., Keep, R. F., & Zeuthen, T. (2022). Cerebrospinal fluid production by the choroid plexus: a century of barrier research revisited. *Fluids and Barriers of the CNS*, *19*(1). https://doi.org/10.1186/S12987-022-00323-1.

Maharaj, A. S. R., Walshe, T. E., Saint-Geniez, M., Venkatesha, S., Maldonado, A. E., Himes, N. C., Matharu, K. S., Ananth Karumanchi, S., & D'Amore, P. A. (2008). VEGF and TGF-β are required for the maintenance of the choroid plexus and ependyma. *The Journal of Experimental Medicine*, *205*(2), 491. https://doi.org/10.1084/JEM.20072041.

McMillan, D. B., & Harris, R. J. (2018). An Atlas of Comparative Vertebrate Histology. *An Atlas of Comparative Vertebrate Histology*, 1–604. https://doi.org/10.1016/C2012-0-06909-8.

Nathanson, J. A., & Chun, L. L. Y. (1989). Immunological function of the blood-cerebrospinal fluid barrier. *Proceedings of the National Academy of Sciences of the United States of America*, *86*(5), 1684–1688. https://doi.org/10.1073/PNAS.86.5.1684.

Neman, J., & Chen, T. C. (2015). The Choroid Plexus and Cerebrospinal Fluid: Emerging Roles in CNS Development, Maintenance, and Disease Progression. In *The Choroid Plexus and Cerebrospinal Fluid: Emerging Roles in CNS Development, Maintenance, and Disease Progression*. Elsevier Inc. https://doi.org/10.1016/C2014-0-00275-4.

Prineas, J. W., Parratt, J. D. E., & Kirwan, P. D. (2016). Fibrosis of the Choroid Plexus Filtration Membrane. *Journal of Neuropathology & Experimental Neurology*, *75*(9), 855–867. https://doi.org/10.1093/JNEN/NLW061.

Raha-Chowdhury, R., Henderson, J. W., Raha, A. A., Vuono, R., Bickerton, A., Jones, E., Fincham, R., Allinson, K., Holland, A., & Zaman, S. H. (2019). Choroid Plexus Acts as Gatekeeper for TREM2, Abnormal Accumulation of ApoE, and Fibrillary Tau in

Alzheimer's Disease and in Down Syndrome Dementia. *Journal of Alzheimer's Disease: JAD*, *69*(1), 91–109. https://doi.org/10.3233/JAD-181179.

Ransohoff, R. M., & Engelhardt, B. (2012). The anatomical and cellular basis of immune surveillance in the central nervous system. *Nature Reviews Immunology 2012 12:9*, *12*(9), 623–635. https://doi.org/10.1038/nri3265.

Rea, P. (2015). Chapter 10 – Brainstem Tracts. In *Essential Clinical Anatomy of the Nervous System* (Issue 4). http://www.sciencedirect.com:5070/book/9780128020302/essential-clinical-anatomy-of-the-nervous-system.

Redzic, Z. (2011). Molecular biology of the blood-brain and the blood-cerebrospinal fluid barriers: similarities and differences. *Fluids and Barriers of the CNS 2011 8:1*, *8*(1), 1–25. https://doi.org/10.1186/2045-8118-8-3.

Rodríguez-Lorenzo, S., Ferreira Francisco, D. M., Vos, R., Van Het Hof, B., Rijnsburger, M., Schroten, H., Ishikawa, H., Beaino, W., Bruggmann, R., Kooij, G., & De Vries, H. E. (2020). Altered secretory and neuroprotective function of the choroid plexus in progressive multiple sclerosis. *Acta Neuropathologica Communications*, *8*(1), 1–13. https://doi.org/10.1186/S40478-020-00903-Y/FIGURES/4.

Ross, M. H., & Pawlina, W. (2016). *Histology: a text and atlas: with correlated cell and molecular biology* (Seventh edition). Wolters Kluwer Health.

Sadler, T. W. (2018). Langman's medical embryology. In *Lippincott Williams & Wilkins, 2018.ippincott Williams & Wilkins, 2018.* (Vol. 5, Issue 4). Lippincott Williams & Wilkins. https://doi.org/10.1016/0890-6238(91)90102-l.

Saunders, N. R., Dziegielewska, K. M., Møllgård, K., & Habgood, M. D. (2015). Markers for blood-brain barrier integrity: how appropriate is Evans blue in the twenty-first century and what are the alternatives? *Frontiers in Neuroscience*, *9*(OCT), 385. https://doi.org/10.3389/FNINS.2015.00385.

Saunders, N. R., Ek, C. J., Habgood, M. D., & Dziegielewska, K. M. (2008). Barriers in the brain: a renaissance? *Trends in Neurosciences*, *31*(6), 279–286. https://doi.org/10.1016/J.TINS.2008.03.003.

Sawamoto, K., Wichterle, H., Gonzalez-Perez, O., Cholfin, J. A., Yamada, M., Spassky, N., Murcia, N. S., Garcia-Verdugo, J. M., Marin, O., Rubenstein, J. L. R., Tessier-Lavigne, M., Okano, H., & Alvarez-Buylla, A. (2006). New neurons follow the flow of cerebrospinal fluid in the adult brain. *Science*, *311*(5761), 629–632. https://doi.org/10.1126/SCIENCE.1119133/SUPPL_FILE/SAWAMOTO.SOM.PDF.

Schwerk, C., Tenenbaum, T., Kim, K. S., & Schroten, H. (2015). The choroid plexus-a multi-role player during infectious diseases of the CNS. *Frontiers in Cellular Neuroscience*, *9*. https://doi.org/10.3389/FNCEL.2015.00080.

Serot, J.-M., Foliguet, B., Béné, M.-C., & Faure, G.-C. (1997). Ultrastructural and immunohistological evidence for dendritic-like cells within human choroid plexus epithelium. *Neuroimmunology*.

Shechter, R., Miller, O., Yovel, G., Rosenzweig, N., London, A., Ruckh, J., Kim, K. W., Klein, E., Kalchenko, V., Bendel, P., Lira, S. A., Jung, S., & Schwartz, M. (2013). Recruitment of Beneficial M2 Macrophages to Injured Spinal Cord Is Orchestrated by Remote Brain Choroid Plexus. *Immunity*, *38*(3), 555–569. https://doi.org/10.1016/J.IMMUNI.2013.02.012.

Simard, J. M., Kent, T. A., Chen, M., Tarasov, K. V., & Gerzanich, V. (2007). Brain oedema in focal ischaemia: molecular pathophysiology and theoretical implications. *Lancet Neurology*, *6*(3), 258. https://doi.org/10.1016/S1474-4422(07)70055-8.

Solár, P., Zamani, A., Kubíčková, L., Dubový, P., & Joukal, M. (2020). Choroid plexus and the blood–cerebrospinal fluid barrier in disease. *Fluids and Barriers of the CNS 2020 17:1*, *17*(1), 1–29. https://doi.org/10.1186/S12987-020-00196-2.

Spector, R., Robert Snodgrass, S., & Johanson, C. E. (2015). A balanced view of the cerebrospinal fluid composition and functions: Focus on adult humans. *Experimental Neurology*, *273*, 57–68. https://doi.org/10.1016/J.EXPNEUROL.2015.07.027.

Stan, R. V., Tse, D., Deharvengt, S. J., Smits, N. C., Xu, Y., Luciano, M. R., McGarry, C. L., Buitendijk, M., Nemani, K. V., Elgueta, R., Kobayashi, T., Shipman, S. L., Moodie, K. L., Daghlian, C. P., Ernst, P. A., Lee, H. K., Suriawinata, A. A., Schned, A. R., Longnecker, D. S., … Carrière, C. (2012). The diaphragms of fenestrated endothelia – gatekeepers of vascular permeability and blood composition. *Developmental Cell*, *23*(6), 1203. https://doi.org/10.1016/J.DEVCEL.2012.11.003.

Vendel, E., Rottschäfer, V., & De Lange, E. C. M. (2019). The need for mathematical modelling of spatial drug distribution within the brain. *Fluids and Barriers of the CNS*, *16*(1). https://doi.org/10.1186/S12987-019-0133-X.

Wilson, G. R., Tan, J. T., Brody, K. M., Taylor, J. M., Delatycki, M. B., & Lockhart, P. J. (2009). Expression and localization of the Parkin co-regulated gene in mouse CNS suggests a role in ependymal cilia function. *Neuroscience Letters*, *460*(1), 97–101. https://doi.org/10.1016/J.NEULET.2009.05.043.

Zheng, W., & Chodobski, A. (2005). The blood-cerebrospinal fluid barrier. In *CRC Press*. CRC Press.

Zlokovic, B. V. (2008). The blood-brain barrier in health and chronic neurodegenerative disorders. *Neuron*, *57*(2), 178–201. https://doi.org/10.1016/J.NEURON.2008.01.003.

Chapter 10

The Blood-Retina Barrier: Histological Structure and Functions

Gul Ipek Gundogan*, PhD
Department of Histology and Embryology, Faculty of Medicine, Biruni University, Istanbul, Turkey

Abstract

This chapter comprehensively examines the histological structure and functions of the blood-retina barrier (BRB), as well as the embryonic development and histology of the retina. The BRB is a critical structure that separates retinal tissue from the blood circulation, ensuring the protection and maintenance of retinal cells and their functions. The BRB consists of two main components: the inner retina barrier (iBRB) and the outer retina barrier (oBRB). The inner retina barrier is formed by tight junctions between retinal capillary endothelial cells, providing selective permeability to the retinal tissue. The outer retina barrier is composed of retinal pigment epithelial (RPE) cells, which offer physical and biochemical protection to the outer part of the retina. These two structures play a central role in maintaining the homeostasis and health of the retinal tissue. The BRB protects the internal environment of the eye from toxins, pathogens, and inflammatory cells, thus preserving the health of retinal cells. Disruption of the BRB can lead to the development of various retinal diseases.

The process of retinal embryonic development, the formation of retinal layers, and retinal histology are also addressed in this chapter. The retina is a complex structure in which photoreceptor cells and other neuronal cells are formed and organized in a specific arrangement. This process is

---

* Corresponding Author's Email: gulipekgundogan@gmail.com

In: A Histological Approach to Human Body Barriers
Editor: İlknur Keskin
ISBN: 979-8-89530-738-0

regulated by various genetic factors and molecular mechanisms. The retinal histology section provides a detailed description of the retinal layers and the cell types within these layers. Photoreceptor cells are divided into cones and rods, which play a crucial role in transmitting visual information to the brain.
This information contributes to the development of new strategies for maintaining retinal health and treating retinal diseases. Current literature places significant emphasis on research concerning the anatomical structure, physiological functions, and disease associations of the BRB. In this context, the histological and physiological properties of the BRB and its role in pathophysiological processes are examined in detail.

Keywords: Blood-Retina Barrier (BRB), retinal embryonic development, retinal histology, photoreceptor cells, Retinal Pigment Epithelium (RPE)

Introduction

The retina is a complex and delicate structure at the center of visual function, composed of photoreceptor cells and supporting cells. The retina perceives visual information through photoreceptors, which are light-sensitive cells, and converts this information into signals transmitted to the brain. Retinal embryonic development begins with the formation of the eyelids and capillary layers and progresses through the interaction of various genetic, cellular, and molecular mechanisms. During this process, retinal layers form in a specific sequence, and each layer acquires distinct functional properties.

The blood-retina barrier (BRB) is a critical barrier that protects retinal tissue and regulates the passage of substances between the bloodstream and the retina. The BRB consists of two main components: the inner retina barrier (iBRB) and the outer retina barrier (oBRB). The inner retina barrier is formed by tight junctions between retinal capillary endothelial cells, providing selective permeability to the retinal tissue. The outer retina barrier is composed of retinal pigment epithelial (RPE) cells, which offer physical and biochemical protection to the outer part of the retina. These two structures play a central role in maintaining the homeostasis and health of the retinal tissue.

The histological structure of the Blood-Retina Barrier (BRB) is of great importance in maintaining retinal health and sustaining visual function (Cunha-Vaz, 2017). The BRB controls the passage of substances between the retina and systemic circulation, protecting retinal cells from toxins, pathogens, and inflammatory cells. Through these functions, it ensures the homeostasis and integrity of retinal tissue. Disruption of the BRB can lead to the development of various retinal diseases, such as diabetic retinopathy and age-related macular degeneration. Current literature places significant emphasis on research concerning the anatomical structure, physiological functions, and disease associations of the BRB. In this context, the histological and physiological features of the BRB and its role in pathophysiological processes are being thoroughly examined.

In this chapter, the embryonic development of the retina, retinal histology, and the histological structure and functions of the blood-retina barrier will be detailed. Additionally, the molecular mechanisms of the BRB and the roles of genetic factors in retinal development will be discussed. This information will contribute to the development of new strategies for preserving retinal health and treating retinal diseases.

Embryonic Development of the Retina

The embryonic development of the retina is a complex process that encompasses the formation of the retina and other eye structures during an organism's developmental stages. This process spans from the embryonic period to the prenatal stage, involving various genetic, cellular, and molecular mechanisms. The retina, a structure composed of light-sensitive cells that transmit visual information to the brain, is formed through this intricate developmental sequence.

Stages of Retinal Development

Formation of Outer and Inner Vascular Layers

Retinal embryonic development typically begins with the development of the eyelids and the formation of the vascular layers. During this stage, communication between the retinal pigment epithelium (RPE) and the retinal layers lays the foundation for retinal formation. The optic vesicle, a fundamental structure in brain and eye development during the embryonic stage, undergoes a series of morphogenetic changes to form the anterior and posterior segments of the eye (Raeisossadati et al., 2021). The Retinal Pigment Epithelium (RPE) plays a critical role in retinal development and assists in the formation of photoreceptor cells (Grigoryan, 2022).

Formation of Retinal Layer

The retina is composed of various layers, which form in a specific sequence during embryonic development (Grigoryan, 2022).The development of the retina includes the orderly formation of the inner and outer layers. These layers contain different functional properties and structures across the retina. The organization of photoreceptor cells and other retinal cell types plays a role in the formation of these retinal layers (Grigoryan, 2022).

Formation of Synaptic Connections

During the development of the retina, synaptic connections are established, facilitating cellular communication within the retina (Kolb, 1995). Synaptic plasticity during retinal development enhances the functionality of the retina through developmental changes, a process known as synaptic plasticity (Raeisossadati et al., 2021). This comprehensive overview not only sheds light on the developmental intricacies of the retina but also highlights the critical stages that ensure proper retinal function and structure, pivotal for visual perception.

Molecular Mechanisms and Genetic Factors

Genetic Factors

Several key genes play crucial roles in retinal development, including RHO, CRX, Pax6, and Six3 (Grigoryan, 2022; Johnsen et al., 2018):

- *RHO and CRX Genes:* These genes are critical for the development and function of photoreceptor cells and play significant roles in retinal development.
- *Pax6 and Six3 Genes:* These genes are influential in retinal formation and morphogenesis, holding fundamental functions in eye development.

Molecular Pathways

The molecular pathways involved in retinal development include:

- *Notch and Wnt Pathways:* These are instrumental in the formation of retinal layers and cellular differentiation processes (Raeisossadati et al., 2021).
- *SHH and BMP Pathways:* These serve as fundamental signaling pathways in retinal development (Grigoryan, 2022).

Current research focuses on understanding embryonic retinal development to advance in areas such as treatment of genetic diseases and repair of retinal damage. Advanced research techniques and model organisms are being utilized to gather more insights into retinal development and potential treatment methods (Drag et al., 2023; Takita & Seko, 2024).

Retinal Histology and Function

The retina consists of two main parts: the neural retina (retina proper) and the pigment epithelium (Burns et al., 2019). The neural retina contains the photoreceptors, while the retinal pigment epithelium is tightly connected to the choroidal choroid capillaries through Bruch's membrane (Kevany & Palczewski, 2010).

The neural retina is functionally divided into two parts. The non-photosensitive part extends between the inner side of the ciliary body and the posterior surface of the iris (Kolb, 1995). The photosensitive part (optical part) is located on the inner surface of the eye behind the ora serrata (Sterling, 1988).

The region where the optic nerve connects to the retina is called the optic papilla or optic disc. Since no photoreceptors are present at the optic disc, this region is a blind spot in the visual field (Curcio & Allen, 1990). About 2.5 mm lateral to the optic disc is the fovea centralis, a slight depression where visual acuity is highest. The fovea is surrounded by the macula lutea, a yellowish area, and represents the region of the retina with the highest concentration of visual elements (Yuodelis & Hendrickson, 1986).

The histological structure of the retina is complex, with numerous cell types whose bodies and extensions are organized for contact and communication. It is known that there are at least 15 types of neurons making 38 different types of synapses in the retina (R. H. Masland, 2001).

There are four types of cells in the retina: photoreceptors, transmitting neurons, interconnecting neurons, and supportive cells. Photoreceptors consist of cone and rod cells (Kolb, 1995). Transmitting neurons include bipolar and ganglion cells (Richard H. Masland, 2012). Interconnecting neurons, or other neurons, include horizontal, centrifugal, and amacrine cells (R. H. Masland, 2001). Among the supportive cells are Müller cells, microglia, and astrocytes (Reichenbach & Bringmann, 2010).

This cellular organization creates ten different layers in the retina from outer to inner (Berson, 2008):

1) Retinal pigment epithelium
2) Cone and rod layer
3) Outer limiting membrane
4) Outer nuclear layer (granular)
5) Outer plexiform layer (stratum reticulare)
6) Inner nuclear layer (granular)
7) Inner plexiform layer (stratum reticulare)
8) Ganglion cell layer
9) Layer of optic nerve fibers
10) Inner limiting membrane

Retinal Pigment Epithelium (RPE)

The retinal pigment epithelium (RPE) is a single layer of cuboidal cells that rests against the Bruch's membrane of the choroid (Strauss, 2005). In the fovea region, the tall pigment cells make this area appear darker (Kolb, 1995). The cells are interconnected by zonula occludens and gap junctions; these connection complexes form the blood-retina barrier (Cunha-Vaz, 2009).

The apical surfaces of RPE cells feature microvilli that associate with the photoreceptor extensions of cone and rod cells (Marmorstein et al., 2009). The nuclei in the basal area are indented, and the cytoplasm contains extensive granular endoplasmic reticulum and a prominent supranuclear Golgi complex (Strauss, 2005). Surrounding the melanin granules in the cytoplasm, phagosomes or residual bodies containing lamellar materials phagocytosed from the extensions of photoreceptors are seen (Feeney-Burns, 1980).

The RPE absorbs light, preventing reflection and glare, thus enhancing visual acuity (Takita & Seko, 2024). It is also a crucial component of the blood-retina barrier and provides photosensitivity to the visual pigments that decompose in response to light (Marmorstein et al., 2009). RPE cells have the ability to synthesize visual pigments and eliminate worn-out membranous disks from retinal photoreceptor cells by phagocytosis (Strauss, 2005).

Photoreceptor Cells: Cone and Rod Layer

The cone and rod layer is a layer of photoreceptor cells that extends from the outer part of the neural retina to the pigment epithelium. These cells function as visual receptors, and their nuclei form the outer nuclear layer of the retina (Kolb, 1995). The retina contains approximately 120 million rods and 7 million cones. Rods are functionally more sensitive to light (Chen et al., 2024).

Both cell types have a non-nucleated basal part that consists of three sections:

- *Outer Segment:* This segment, considered in the naming of photoreceptor cells, is cylindrical or conical (for cone or rod cells). Closely associated with microvilli extending from the underlying pigment epithelium, this part contains numerous horizontal disks regularly spaced in the cytoplasm (Campbell & Humphries, 2013). These structures result from the folding of the plasma membrane. In rods, these disks are continuously produced throughout life, while in cones, disk production is not as regular (Young, 1967). Rods lose the connection with the membranes from which the disks originate, whereas in cones, this connection continues (Strauss, 2005).
- *Connecting Cilium:* Arising from the basal body, this modified cilium consists of nine peripheral microtubule doublets. It forms a narrow transition zone between the inner and outer segments. A thin and tapering extension, known as the calycal process, emerges from the distal part of the inner segment and encircles the proximal part of the outer segment (Besharse & Horst, 1990).
- *Inner Segment:* The inner segment comprises two parts: the outer ellipsoid area, rich in mitochondria, and the inner myoid area, containing a prominent Golgi apparatus, extensive granular endoplasmic reticulum, and numerous free ribosomes. The nuclei of cones are generally located close to the limiting membrane, while the nuclei of rods are located in the middle of the inner segment (Kolb, 1995).
- *Photoreceptor Pigments:* Rod cells contain rhodopsin, and cone cells contain iodopsin. Rhodopsin is situated on the outer, cytoplasmic face of the membranous disks' lipid layer and initiates the visual process upon light absorption (Palczewski, 2006). Rod cells facilitate twilight or night vision. Cone cells, containing iodopsin, are specialized to

respond maximally to red, green, and blue light, providing better visual acuity under high light conditions (Nathans, 1989).

- *Disk Structures and Renewal:* Rhodopsin and iodopsin consist of two units: opsin and chromophore. Rod opsins are scotopsins, while cone opsins are photopsins. The chromophore in rods is retinal, a carotenoid derived from vitamin A, and deficiency in vitamin A can lead to night blindness (Wald, 1968). In rods, newly synthesized visual pigment is incorporated into disks at the base of the outer segment, and it takes days to reach the apex. In cones, retinal pigment is continuously produced, and the pigment can join disks at any part of the outer segment. Disks are normally shed, and the shed parts are phagocytosed by pigment epithelial cells for elimination. Lost disks are replaced by newly synthesized disks (Young, 1967).
    - *Outer Limiting Membrane:* This is not a true membrane. In this area, zonula adherens type connection complexes are found, linking the apical ends of Müller cells to each other and to cone/rod cells. Müller cells terminate at the base of the receptors' inner segments and create a barrier that prevents large molecules from passing deeper into the retina (Bringmann et al., 2006).
    - *Outer Nuclear Layer:* Consists of the nuclei of cone and rod cells. The nuclei of rod cells are surrounded by a thin ring of cytoplasm, while the nuclei of cone cells are enveloped in a broad swath of cytoplasm (Kolb, 1995).
    - *Outer Plexiform Layer:* This layer contains no nuclei and is composed of the extensions of cone and rod cells, as well as horizontal, interplexiform, amacrine, and bipolar neurons. These extensions are found in this layer and facilitate the synaptic connections between photoreceptors and interneurons. The outer plexiform layer is the first synaptic layer of the retina (R. H. Masland, 2001).
    - *Inner Nuclear Layer:* Includes bipolar neurons, horizontal cells, interplexiform cells, amacrine cells, and Müller cells. The nuclei of horizontal cells are located in the outer part, the nuclei of bipolar cells in the middle, and the nuclei of amacrine cells on the inner side. The basal part of Müller cells forms the inner limiting membrane, and the apical part forms the outer limiting membrane (Bringmann et al., 2006).
    - *Inner Plexiform Layer:* This is the synaptic area between the axons of bipolar neurons and the dendrites of ganglion cells. The

parallel arrangement of cell extensions in this layer gives it a horizontally striped appearance (Kolb, 1995).

- *Ganglion Cell Layer:* Contains large multipolar neurons with vesicular nuclei and prominent nucleoli. These cells' cytoplasm contains numerous Nissl bodies. The axons emerging from the cell bodies cross the nerve fiber layer and enter the optic nerve (Selhorst & Chen, 2009).
- *Nerve Fiber Layer:* Comprised of the axons of ganglion cells. The nerve fibers are thin and unmyelinated. Glial cells are found among the parallel-running fibers, and retinal blood vessels are located in this layer (Kolb, 1995).
- *Inner Limiting Membrane:* Constitutes the boundary of the vitreous body with a basal membrane structure. It is formed by the retinal and iris capillary endothelia and the ciliary and retinal epithelia (Strauss, 2005).

Histological Structure of the Blood-Retina Barrier (BRB)

The retina is protected by the aqueous-blood barrier and the blood-retina barrier (BRB). The aqueous-blood barrier includes the ciliary epithelium and iris capillaries, while the BRB consists of tight junction complexes in the retinal pigment epithelium and the uninterrupted capillaries of the retina, preventing the entry of large molecules from the choroidal layer (Cunha-Vaz, 2009).

Structures and Cells of the Blood-Retina Barrier

The retina is a complex neural tissue that converts light into electrochemical signals transmitted to the brain via the optic nerve. It comprises two layers: the inner neural layer adjacent to the vitreous and the outer layer strengthened by the retinal pigment epithelium (RPE). The retina maintains homeostasis through the BRB, which regulates the exchange of molecules and fluids between the retinal parenchyma and vascular components (Cunha-Vaz, 2009).

Structure of the Blood-Retina Barrier

The BRB is divided into the inner BRB (iBRB) and outer BRB (oBRB):

- *Inner BRB (iBRB)* consists of vascular endothelial cells, pericytes, glial cells, and neurons, forming a complex structure that fine-tunes tissue viability.
- *Outer BRB (oBRB)* is managed by the RPE and regulates nutrient flow between the choriocapillaris and the photoreceptor layer (Campbell & Humphries, 2013).

The BRB is crucial for maintaining a specific retinal environment necessary for proper visual function.

Components of the Blood-Retina Barrier

- *Inner Blood-Retinal Barrier (iBRB):* Composed of retinal capillary endothelial cells, pericytes, astrocytes, and Müller cells. The endothelial cells of the retina are the primary component of the iBRB and are linked by tight junctions, which prevent the uncontrolled passage of substances and help protect the retinal tissue (Campbell & Humphries, 2013). Pericytes surrounding the endothelial cells provide capillary stability and control permeability (Santos et al., 2018), while glial cells like astrocytes and Müller cells offer structural support to the endothelial cells, contributing to the barrier function (Strauss, 2005).
- *Outer Blood-Retinal Barrier (oBRB):* Composed of retinal pigment epithelium (RPE) cells and structural components like the Bruch's membrane. RPE cells, located between the photoreceptor cells and Bruch's membrane, form the oBRB. They are connected by tight junctions which allow selective permeability (Klaassen et al., 2013). The Bruch's membrane, located at the base of RPE cells, regulates the exchange of substances between the retina and choroid (Campbell & Humphries, 2013). The barrier created by RPE cells facilitates the passage of nutrients necessary for photoreceptors while regulating the removal of waste products. The tight junctions between RPE cells control the passage of substances, preserving the homeostasis and integrity of the retinal tissue.

Cells Involved in the Blood-Retina Barrier

1) *Endothelial Cells:* These cells form the iBRB by creating tight junctions that restrict substance passage from the blood to the retina, supported by the tips of surrounding Müller glial cells, playing a crucial role in maintaining BRB integrity and regulating retinal homeostasis (Simons et al., 2016).
2) *Retinal Pigment Epithelium (RPE) Cells:* These cells form the oBRB, regulating the exchange of nutrients and waste between the retina and choroid and protecting the retina from potential harmful substances in the blood flow(Strauss, 2005).
3) *Müller Glial Cells:* These glial cells extend from the inner to the outer retina, providing structural support and preserving the stability of the BRB. They also help metabolize neurotransmitters and protect neurons from oxidative stress (Bringmann et al., 2006).
4) *Pericytes:* Embedded in the basal membrane of retinal capillaries, pericytes help maintain capillary stability and regulate blood flow within the retina (Armulik et al., 2011).

Functions of the Blood-Retina Barrier

The BRB undertakes various critical functions to preserve retinal health and sustain cellular activities. It provides selective permeability, allowing the passage of nutrients and oxygen to the retinal tissue while blocking toxins and pathogens (Cunha-Vaz, 2017). It also facilitates the removal of metabolic wastes by RPE cells (Strauss, 2005), maintains ion balance and fluid regulation necessary for retinal cell functions, and establishes an immune defense mechanism by limiting the entry of pathogens and inflammatory cells, thus preventing inflammation and cellular damage (Klaassen et al., 2013). These functions are vital for keeping the retinal tissue healthy and functional.

Molecular Structures in Cell-Cell Connections

The functionality of the Blood-Retina Barrier (BRB) is maintained through tight junctions (TJs) and adherens junctions among its constituent cells. Tight junctions form a physical barrier between endothelial and epithelial cells, controlling paracellular (between cells) permeability. Key components of these junctions include claudins, occludin, and zonula occludens (ZO) proteins (Niessen, 2007).

Tight Junctions

Tight junctions are fundamental components of the BRB and consist of over 40 different transmembrane and intracellular scaffolding proteins. These include claudins, occludin, junctional adhesion molecules (JAMs), and ZO proteins. ZO proteins balance the connection between transmembrane TJ proteins and the actin cytoskeleton, ensuring structural integrity (Campbell & Humphries, 2013). Tight junctions seal the intercellular spaces, regulating the passage of ions and other molecules. They are comprised of transmembrane proteins like claudins and occludin, which are linked to the cellular skeleton by ZO proteins. Claudins, particularly claudin-5, play a crucial role in the BRB by providing selective permeability (Wolburg & Lippoldt, 2002).

Extracellular Vesicles (EVs) and Intracellular Communication

Extracellular vesicles (EVs) are small membrane-bound particles that regulate and facilitate intercellular communication. EVs contain proteins, lipids, and RNA molecules and transport these molecules to target cells, affecting cellular functions. In the BRB, EVs play a role in maintaining intercellular communication and homeostasis (Tkach & Théry, 2016). Once released by cells, EVs are directed to target cells via surface molecules and receptors and bind to these cells. Integrins and tetraspanins on the surface of EVs play significant roles in the binding and uptake processes by target cells. This interaction allows EVs to transmit molecular information to target cells, facilitating intercellular communication and functional regulation. This process is especially critical in the functionality of the BRB and intercellular coordination (Raposo & Stoorvogel, 2013).

Eye Angiogenesis and Formation of the Blood-Retina Barrier

Eye angiogenesis and the formation of the Blood-Retina Barrier (BRB) are two essential processes in the embryonic development of the eye. Angiogenesis, the formation of new blood vessels, is vital for the development and health of various tissues, including the retina (Gariano & Gardner, 2005). The BRB protects the retina's delicate microscopic environment and provides selective permeability (Campbell & Humphries, 2013).

Basic Mechanisms of Angiogenesis

Eye angiogenesis is important not only in pathological conditions such as preeclampsia and retinopathy but also in normal physiological processes (Eilken & Adams, 2010). Angiogenesis occurs through the sprouting of new vessels from existing blood vessels, requiring the coordination of a series of cellular and molecular events.

- *Endothelial Cell Activation and Migration:* Growth factors like Vascular Endothelial Growth Factor (VEGF) activate endothelial cells, prompting their migration from existing vessel structures (Simons et al., 2016).
- *Cell Proliferation and Formation of Tubular Structures:* Under VEGF signaling, endothelial cells undergo proliferation and form new tubular structures. This process is also supported by other growth factors like basic Fibroblast Growth Factor (bFGF) (Carmeliet & Jain, 2011).

Features of Retinal Angiogenesis

The retina is a highly vascularized tissue with two main vascular systems: the inner and outer capillary layers. These systems distribute oxygen and nutrients throughout the retina.

- *Inner Capillary Layer:* Originates from the central retinal artery at the optic nerve head and spreads across the retinal surface (Gariano & Gardner, 2005).
- *Outer Capillary Layer:* Is nourished from the choroid and meets the high energy demands of photoreceptor cells (Saint-Geniez & D'Amore, 2004).

Retinal angiogenesis is a complex and multistage process tightly regulated by various molecular mechanisms. A detailed understanding of these mechanisms enables the development of new strategies for treating retinal diseases.

Molecular Mechanisms of Retinal Angiogenesis

Retinal angiogenesis is the process of new blood vessel formation within the retina and plays a crucial role in various conditions such as normal development, wound healing, and pathological states. Understanding the molecular mechanisms of retinal angiogenesis is vital for the treatment and prevention of retinal diseases (Gariano & Gardner, 2005). The understanding of cells and molecular mechanisms in the Blood-Retina Barrier (BRB) is critical for developing treatment strategies for retinal diseases characterized by BRB breakdown, such as diabetic retinopathy and age-related macular degeneration (Tomkins-Netzer et al., 2024).

Growth Factors and Receptors

Vascular Endothelial Growth Factor (VEGF) plays a role in angiogenesis and in increasing vascular permeability. VEGF is a principal growth factor in retinal angiogenesis, promoting endothelial cell proliferation, migration, and new vessel formation. The action of VEGF is mediated through VEGF receptors (VEGFR-1 and VEGFR-2), with VEGFR-2 having critical roles in mitogenic, chemotactic, and vascular permeability effects in endothelial cells (Ferrara, 2004). While essential for normal vascular development, overexpression of VEGF can lead to pathological conditions like diabetic retinopathy that disrupt BRB integrity.

Hypoxia and Hypoxia-Induced Factors

Hypoxia is a potent stimulator of retinal angiogenesis, initiating cellular responses via Hypoxia-Inducible Factor-1 (HIF-1). HIF-1 increases the expression of several angiogenic genes, including VEGF. This mechanism plays a crucial role especially in pathological conditions like retinal ischemia and diabetic retinopathy (Semenza, 2012).

Notch Signaling Pathway

The Notch signaling pathway is critical in regulating endothelial cell fate and vascular branching in angiogenesis. Notch signaling controls the differentiation of endothelial cells into tip cells or stalk cells. Tip cells lead new vessel growth with filopodia, while stalk cells follow and form the main structure of the vessel (Gridley, 2010).

Extracellular Matrix and MMPs

The extracellular matrix (ECM) provides the physical structure necessary for endothelial cell migration and vessel formation. Matrix metalloproteinases (MMPs) facilitate the remodeling of the ECM and enhance cell mobility. Regulation of MMPs is a critical stage in the control of the angiogenic process (Page-McCaw et al., 2007).

Cell-Cell Connections and Integrins

Tight Junction Proteins such as occludin, claudins, and junctional adhesion molecules (JAMs) form tight junctions among endothelial cells in the iBRB and RPE cells in the oBRB. These junctions are critical for the barrier function of the BRB and prevent the leakage of blood-borne substances into the retinal tissue.

Integrins are transmembrane receptors that facilitate the attachment and signaling of endothelial cells to the ECM. Integrin signals are important for cell migration, proliferation, and survival. Additionally, cell-cell connections play a significant role in maintaining vascular permeability and cellular integrity (Hynes, 2002).

Wnt/β-Catenin Signaling Pathway

The Wnt/β-catenin signaling pathway is crucial for the development and maintenance of the BRB. This pathway regulates the expression of tight junction proteins necessary for maintaining BRB integrity. During retinal development and in response to injury or disease, the Wnt/β-catenin pathway promotes the formation of a functional BRB. Dysregulation of this pathway is associated with retinal vascular diseases and is therefore considered a significant target for therapeutic interventions (Nguyen et al., 2022; Wang et al., 2019).

Carriers and Channels

Various carriers such as glucose transporters (e.g., GLUT1) and monocarboxylate transporters (MCTs) are expressed in BRB cells to facilitate the controlled movement of nutrients and metabolic waste products. These carriers are crucial for meeting the metabolic demands of the highly active retinal cells (Tomkins-Netzer et al., 2024).

Extracellular Vesicles and Cell Communication

Extracellular vesicles (EVs) are vital tools for intercellular communication. EVs carry growth factors, mRNA, miRNA, and other biomolecules, spreading angiogenic signals and facilitating intercellular coordination. This mechanism plays a significant role, especially in pathological angiogenesis (Raposo & Stoorvogel, 2013).

The interaction of EVs with cells and their specific roles in cellular processes form the basis for developing various clinical applications, diagnostics, and drug delivery systems. The ability to modulate cellular functions highlights the therapeutic potential of manipulating this process in disease contexts.

EVs' capabilities to modulate cellular processes are promising for therapeutic applications. They can be used to treat diseases by carrying specific molecular signals to target cells. Especially, EVs could be an important tool in developing treatment strategies against BRB dysfunction (Martins et al., 2024).

Cellular Communication and Disease Pathogenesis

EVs play a crucial role in cellular communication, affecting cellular functions and the pathogenesis of diseases. For example, in diabetes mellitus, the disruption of cellular communication through EVs has been shown to affect the dysfunction in the BRB. In diabetes, impaired signaling through EVs between vascular pericytes and endothelial cells adversely affects microvascular stabilization and remodeling, leading to increased BRB permeability and impaired retinal functions (Martins et al., 2024).

The role of EVs in the pathogenesis of retinal diseases is increasingly understood. In pathological conditions, EVs can affect the structure and function of the BRB, leading to barrier dysfunction. For instance, in conditions like diabetic retinopathy, EVs have been suggested to disrupt intercellular communication, potentially increasing BRB permeability (Martins et al., 2024).

The Blood-Retina Barrier (BRB)

The Blood-Retina Barrier (BRB) is a critical structure that surrounds the retina, part of the central nervous system, and separates it from systemic circulation. The primary function of the BRB is to maintain the homeostasis of the retina and protect it from potentially harmful substances. The BRB consists of two main components: the inner BRB (iBRB) and the outer BRB (oBRB) (Cunha-Vaz, 2009).

Inner BRB (iBRB)

The iBRB is formed by retinal capillary endothelial cells, which are interconnected by tight junctions. These junctions prevent the passage of substances between endothelial cells, thereby creating a barrier between the blood and the retina. Various molecular components and signaling pathways play critical roles in the formation and maintenance of the iBRB. Tight junction proteins are crucial for the structural integrity of the iBRB, including occludin, claudins, and zonula occludens-1 (ZO-1) (Campbell & Humphries, 2013).

Outer BRB (oBRB)

The oBRB is formed by retinal pigment epithelium (RPE) cells and is located between the photoreceptors and the choroid. RPE cells create the oBRB, providing a selective barrier between the retina and the choroid and regulating retinal metabolism (Strauss, 2005).

Molecular Components and Signaling Pathways of the BRB

Tight Junction Proteins

The functionality and integrity of the BRB are maintained by tight junction proteins, which create a physical barrier between cells and regulate substance passage. Key proteins include occludin, claudins, and ZO-1. Occludin is located in the cell membrane and stabilizes tight junctions (Niessen, 2007). Claudins strengthen intercellular connections and control permeability. ZO-1 is a scaffolding protein that organizes the connections of these proteins.

VEGF and Anti-VEGF Therapies

Vascular Endothelial Growth Factor (VEGF) is a crucial factor that increases the permeability of the BRB. VEGF is released in response to stress factors such as hypoxia and promotes the formation of new blood vessels. However, overexpression of VEGF can disrupt the integrity of the BRB and lead to pathological conditions (Ferrara, 2004). Anti-VEGF therapies block the effects of VEGF, helping to protect the BRB and reduce its permeability in pathological conditions. These treatments are particularly used in the management of diseases such as diabetic retinopathy and age-related macular degeneration (Avery et al., 2006).

Wnt/β-Catenin Signaling Pathway

The Wnt/β-catenin signaling pathway is critically important for the development and protection of the BRB. This pathway regulates the expression of tight junction proteins and promotes the formation of a functional BRB during retinal development and in response to injury or disease. Dysregulation of this pathway is associated with retinal vascular diseases and is a significant target for therapeutic interventions (Wang et al., 2019).

Notch Signaling Pathway

The Notch signaling pathway plays a significant role in regulating endothelial cell fate and vascular branching. Notch signaling controls the differentiation of endothelial cells into tip cells or stalk cells. Proper functioning of this pathway is necessary for maintaining healthy angiogenesis (Gridley, 2010).

The formation and function of the Blood-Retina Barrier (BRB) play a central role in preserving retinal health. The structural and functional components of the inner and outer BRB are regulated by tight junction proteins and various signaling pathways. Understanding the molecular mechanisms of the BRB allows for the development of new strategies to treat retinal diseases. Signaling pathways such as VEGF and Wnt/β-catenin are crucial targets for maintaining the function of the BRB and managing pathological conditions.

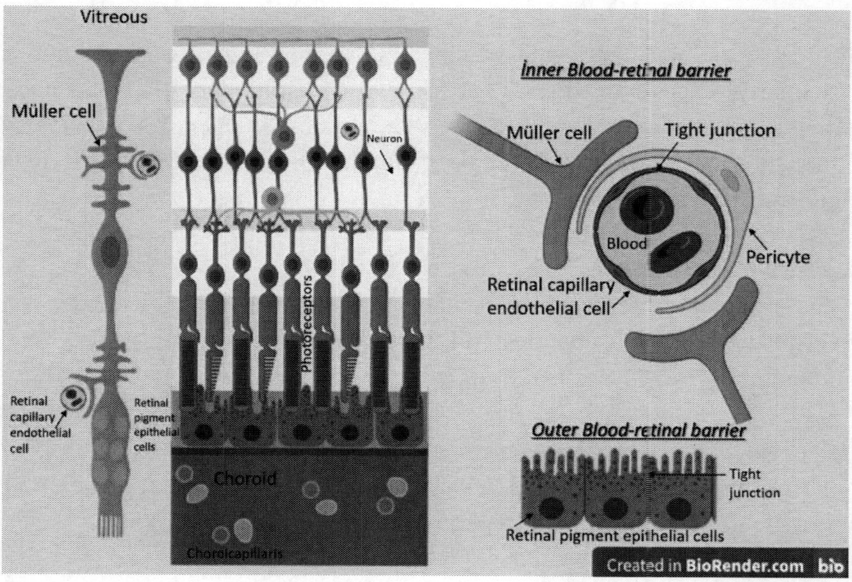

Figure 1. The inner and outer layers of the blood-retina barrier. (Created by the author).

Disruption of the Blood-Retina Barrier and Associated Diseases

The disruption of the Blood-Retina Barrier (BRB) plays a significant role in the development of various retinal diseases. For example, diabetic retinopathy is influenced by high blood sugar levels that damage capillary endothelial cells, leading to disruption of the inner Blood-Retina Barrier (iBRB) and causing edema and hemorrhages in the retinal tissue (Klaassen et al., 2013). Similarly, in Age-related Macular Degeneration (AMD), functional loss of Retinal Pigment Epithelium (RPE) cells and disruption of the outer Blood-Retina Barrier (oBRB) lead to degeneration of photoreceptor cells and consequent vision loss (Strauss, 2005). Genetic conditions like retinitis pigmentosa also disrupt the BRB due to mutations in photoreceptor and RPE cells, contributing to retinal degeneration (Cunha-Vaz, 2017).

Eye angiogenesis and BRB dysfunction can lead to various retinal diseases. Diseases such as diabetic retinopathy and AMD are characterized by abnormal regulation of these processes (Antonetti et al., 2021).

Retinal Angiogenesis Dysregulation and Its Association with Diseases

Disorders in retinal angiogenesis can lead to various pathological conditions. Particularly, excessive VEGF expression can disrupt the BRB and cause complications such as macular edema (Gariano & Gardner, 2005). Diabetic retinopathy and AMD are common examples of disorders resulting from angiogenesis dysregulation.

Diabetic Retinopathy

In this condition, hyperglycemia-induced increased VEGF production leads to abnormal new vessel formation and BRB disruption. This can result in edema and hemorrhages in the retina, leading to vision loss (Klaassen et al., 2013).

Age-Related Macular Degeneration (AMD)

In AMD, loss of function in RPE cells and subsequent disruption of the oBRB contribute to the degeneration of photoreceptor cells (Strauss, 2005).

Regenerative Medicine and Stem Cell Therapies

Regenerative medicine involves using stem cells and bioengineering methods to repair and regenerate damaged or diseased tissues. Stem cell-based therapies show promising results in treating retinal diseases associated with BRB disruption. Research on deriving RPE cells from stem cells and their transplantation is particularly noteworthy.

Current research has developed various innovative treatment approaches to maintain and repair the function of the BRB. Anti-VEGF therapies, particularly in diseases like diabetic retinopathy and AMD, aim to control abnormal vessel formation and barrier disruption by using vascular endothelial growth factor (VEGF) inhibitors. These treatments have proven effective in reducing vascular permeability and retinal edema (Jager et al., 2008).

Cell-based approaches such as RPE cell transplants and stem cell therapies are promising strategies for repairing the damaged retinal barrier. These methods involve direct transplantation of RPE cells and conversion of pluripotent stem cells into RPE cells, aiming to reconstitute retinal tissue (Uyama et al., 2021). Gene therapies aim to preserve or correct the function of the retinal barrier in genetic diseases like retinitis pigmentosa through targeted gene therapies. These therapeutic approaches are achieving significant advancements in repairing genetic mutations or enhancing BRB functions through gene therapies (Drag et al., 2023). These modern treatment strategies are leading to significant advancements in the preservation of the BRB and the management of various retinal diseases.

Embryonic Stem Cells (ESCs)

Embryonic stem cells (ESCs) are pluripotent, meaning they have the capability to differentiate into various cell types, including retinal pigment epithelium (RPE) cells. A study by Schwartz et al. (2012) demonstrated that RPE cells derived from human ESCs can be used to treat Age-related Macular Degeneration (AMD), significantly improving patients' visual abilities. This research highlights the potential of ESCs in regenerative medicine, especially for eye diseases where the loss of specific cell types, like RPE cells, leads to vision impairment (Schwartz et al., 2012).

Induced Pluripotent Stem Cells (iPSCs)

Induced pluripotent stem cells (iPSCs) are derived from a patient's own somatic cells and reprogrammed to a pluripotent state, allowing them to differentiate into RPE cells among others. A review by Uyama et al. (2021) discussed the efficacy of iPSC-derived RPE cells in treating retinal degenerative diseases. This approach reduces the risk of immunological incompatibility, enhancing the effectiveness of the treatment and offering a promising avenue for personalized medicine in regenerative therapies (Uyama et al., 2021).

Mesenchymal Stem Cells (MSCs)

Mesenchymal stem cells (MSCs) are known for their immunomodulatory properties and accessibility, making them a viable option for repairing the Blood-Retina Barrier (BRB). Research by Drag et al. (2023) has shown that MSCs can repair damaged BRB, reduce inflammation, and promote cellular regeneration. These cells can be sourced from various tissues such as bone marrow, adipose tissue, and dental pulp, offering diverse opportunities for clinical applications in regenerative medicine (Drag et al., 2023).

CRISPR-Cas9 Technology

Genetic engineering techniques play a crucial role in regenerative medicine. Technologies like CRISPR-Cas9 offer the capability to directly target and correct genetic mutations causing the disruption of the BRB. This precision editing tool can be used in conjunction with stem cell-based approaches to treat retinal diseases, providing a dual strategy that corrects the underlying genetic defects while replacing or repairing damaged tissues. This integrated approach could potentially lead to more effective and long-lasting treatments for retinal conditions (Bovi dos Santos et al., 2024).

These advancements in stem cell technology and genetic engineering are paving the way for innovative treatments for retinal diseases, offering hope for restoring vision and improving the quality of life for patients with currently incurable eye conditions. Each of these technologies has its own set of challenges and benefits, but together, they represent the forefront of efforts to combat blindness and other severe visual impairments.

Conclusion

Stem cell-based treatments hold great potential for repairing the BRB and treating retinal diseases. However, more research is needed for these therapies to transition into clinical practice. Studies continue on the long-term safety, efficacy, and immunological responses of stem cells. Advances in regenerative medicine and stem cell technologies are opening new horizons in the treatment of retinal diseases.

The Blood-Retina Barrier (BRB) plays a critical role in maintaining retinal health and visual function. The histological structure of the BRB is vital in protecting retinal tissue and defending against various diseases. Comprising two main components, the inner and outer BRB, it functions to provide selective permeability, waste removal, ion and fluid balance, and immune defense, preserving the homeostasis of retinal cells. Disruption of the BRB is a fundamental factor in the pathogenesis of various retinal diseases such as diabetic retinopathy, AMD, and retinitis pigmentosa (Cunha-Vaz, 2017; Klaassen et al., 2013; Santos et al., 2018; Strauss, 2005). In this context, ongoing research and treatment approaches aimed at protecting and repairing the retina barrier are making significant advances in the management of eye diseases. Modern strategies like anti-VEGF treatments, cell therapies, and gene therapies aim to preserve the function of the BRB and provide effective solutions in treating retinal diseases (Klaassen et al., 2013).

References

Antonetti, D. A., Silva, P. S., & Stitt, A. W. (2021). Current understanding of the molecular and cellular pathology of diabetic retinopathy. In *Nature Reviews Endocrinology* (Vol. 17, Issue 4, pp. 195–206). Nature Publishing Group. https://doi.org/10.1038/s41574-020-00451-4.

Armulik, A., Genové, G., & Betsholtz, C. (2011). Pericytes: Developmental, Physiological, and Pathological Perspectives, Problems, and Promises. In *Developmental Cell* (Vol. 21, Issue 2, pp. 193–215). Elsevier. https://doi.org/10.1016/j.devcel.2011.07.001.

Avery, R. L., Pieramici, D. J., Rabena, M. D., Castellarin, A. A., Nasir, M. A., & Giust, M. J. (2006). Intravitreal bevacizumab (Avastin) for neovascular age-related macular degeneration. *Ophthalmology*, *113*(3), 363-372.e5. https://doi.org/10.1016/j.ophtha.2005.11.019.

Berson, D. M. (2008). Retinal Ganglion Cell Types and Their Central Projections. In *The Senses: A Comprehensive Reference* (Vol. 1, pp. 491–519). Academic Press. https://doi.org/10.1016/B978-012370880-9.00280-2.

Besharse, J. C., & Horst, C. J. (1990). The Photoreceptor Connecting Cilium A Model for the Transition Zone. In *Ciliary and Flagellar Membranes* (pp. 389–417). Springer, Boston, MA. https://doi.org/10.1007/978-1-4613-0515-6_15.

Bovi dos Santos, G., de Lima-Vasconcellos, T. H., Móvio, M. I., Birbrair, A., Del Debbio, C. B., & Kihara, A. H. (2024). New Perspectives in Stem Cell Transplantation and Associated Therapies to Treat Retinal Diseases: From Gene Editing to 3D Bioprinting.

Stem Cell Reviews and Reports, *20*(3), 722–737. https://doi.org/10.1007/s12015-024-10689-4.

Bringmann, A., Pannicke, T., Grosche, J., Francke, M., Wiedemann, P., Skatchkov, S. N., Osborne, N. N., & Reichenbach, A. (2006). Müller cells in the healthy and diseased retina. In *Progress in Retinal and Eye Research* (Vol. 25, Issue 4, pp. 397–424). Pergamon. https://doi.org/10.1016/j.preteyeres.2006.05.003.

Burns, S. A., Elsner, A. E., Sapoznik, K. A., Warner, R. L., & Gast, T. J. (2019). Adaptive optics imaging of the human retina. In *Progress in Retinal and Eye Research* (Vol. 68, pp. 1–30). Pergamon. https://doi.org/10.1016/j.preteyeres.2018.08.002.

Campbell, M., & Humphries, P. (2013). The blood-retina barrier tight junctions and barrier modulation. *Advances in Experimental Medicine and Biology*, *763*, 70–84. https://doi.org/10.1007/978-1-4614-4711-5_3.

Carmeliet, P., & Jain, R. K. (2011). Molecular mechanisms and clinical applications of angiogenesis. In *Nature* (Vol. 473, Issue 7347, pp. 298–307). Nature Publishing Group. https://doi.org/10.1038/nature10144.

Chen, C., Adler, L., Milliken, C., Rahman, B., Kono, M., Perry, L. P., Gonzalez-Fernandez, F., & Koutalos, Y. (2024). The First Steps of the Visual Cycle in Human Rod and Cone Photoreceptors. *Investigative Ophthalmology & Visual Science*, *65*(8), 9. https://doi.org/10.1167/iovs.65.8.9.

Cunha-Vaz, J. (2009). The Blood–Retinal Barrier in Retinal Disease. *European Ophthalmic Review*, *03*(02), 105. https://doi.org/10.17925/eor.2009.03.02.105.

Cunha-Vaz, J. (2017). The Blood-Retinal Barrier in the Management of Retinal Disease: EURETINA Award Lecture. *Ophthalmologica*, *237*(1), 1–10. https://doi.org/10.1159/000455809.

Curcio, C. A., & Allen, K. A. (1990). Topography of ganglion cells in human retina. *Journal of Comparative Neurology*, *300*(1), 5–25. https://doi.org/10.1002/cne.903000103.

Drag, S., Dotiwala, F., & Upadhyay, A. K. (2023). Gene Therapy for Retinal Degenerative Diseases: Progress, Challenges, and Future Directions. In *Investigative ophthalmology & visual science* (Vol. 64, Issue 7, p. 39). The Association for Research in Vision and Ophthalmology. https://doi.org/10.1167/iovs.64.7.39.

Eilken, H. M., & Adams, R. H. (2010). Dynamics of endothelial cell behavior in sprouting angiogenesis. In *Current Opinion in Cell Biology* (Vol. 22, Issue 5, pp. 617–625). Elsevier Current Trends. https://doi.org/10.1016/j.ceb.2010.08.010.

Feeney-Burns, L. (1980). Lipofuscin of human retinal pigment epithelium. *American Journal of Ophthalmology*, *90*(6), 783–787. https://doi.org/10.1016/S0002-9394(14)75193-1.

Ferrara, N. (2004). Vascular endothelial growth factor: Basic science and clinical progress. In *Endocrine Reviews* (Vol. 25, Issue 4, pp. 581–611). https://doi.org/10.1210/er.2003-0027.

Gariano, R. F., & Gardner, T. W. (2005). Retinal angiogenesis in development and disease. In *Nature* (Vol. 438, Issue 7070, pp. 960–966). Nature Publishing Group. https://doi.org/10.1038/nature04482.

Gridley, T. (2010). Notch signaling in the vasculature. In *Current Topics in Developmental Biology* (Vol. 92, Issue C). Academic Press. https://doi.org/10.1016/S0070-2153(10)92009-7.

Grigoryan, E. N. (2022). Self-Organization of the Retina during Eye Development, Retinal Regeneration In Vivo, and in Retinal 3D Organoids In Vitro. In *Biomedicines* (Vol. 10, Issue 6). MDPI. https://doi.org/10.3390/biomedicines10061458.

Hynes, R. O. (2002). Integrins: Bidirectional, allosteric signaling machines. *Cell, 110*(6), 673–687. https://doi.org/10.1016/S0092-8674(02)00971-6.

Jager, R. D., Mieler, W. F., & Miller, J. W. (2008). Age-Related Macular Degeneration. *New England Journal of Medicine*, *358*(24), 2606–2617. https://doi.org/10.1056/NEJMRA0801537.

Johnsen, E. O., Frøen, R. C., Olstad, O. K., Nicolaissen, B., Petrovski, G., Moe, M. C., & Noer, A. (2018). Proliferative Cells Isolated from the Adult Human Peripheral Retina only Transiently Upregulate Key Retinal Markers upon Induced Differentiation. *Current Eye Research*, *43*(3), 340–349. https://doi.org/10.1080/02713683.2017.1403630.

Kevany, B. M., & Palczewski, K. (2010). Phagocytosis of retinal rod and cone photoreceptors. In *Physiology* (Vol. 25, Issue 1, pp. 8–15). https://doi.org/10.1152/physiol.00038.2009.

Klaassen, I., Van Noorden, C. J. F., & Schlingemann, R. O. (2013). Molecular basis of the inner blood-retinal barrier and its breakdown in diabetic macular edema and other pathological conditions. In *Progress in Retinal and Eye Research* (Vol. 34, pp. 19–48). Pergamon. https://doi.org/10.1016/j.preteyeres.2013.02.001.

Kolb, H. (1995). Simple Anatomy of the Retina. In *Webvision: The Organization of the Retina and Visual System*. http://europepmc.org/books/NBK11533.

Marmorstein, A. D., Cross, H. E., & Peachey, N. S. (2009). Functional roles of bestrophins in ocular epithelia. In *Progress in Retinal and Eye Research* (Vol. 28, Issue 3, pp. 206–226). Pergamon. https://doi.org/10.1016/j.preteyeres.2009.04.004.

Martins, B., Pires, M., Ambrósio, A. F., Girão, H., & Fernandes, R. (2024). Contribution of extracellular vesicles for the pathogenesis of retinal diseases: shedding light on blood-retinal barrier dysfunction. In *Journal of Biomedical Science* (Vol. 31, Issue 1, p. 48). https://doi.org/10.1186/s12929-024-01036-3.

Masland, R. H. (2001). Neuronal diversity in the retina. In *Current Opinion in Neurobiology* (Vol. 11, Issue 4, pp. 431–436). Elsevier Current Trends. https://doi.org/10.1016/S0959-4388(00)00230-0.

Masland, Richard H. (2012). The Neuronal Organization of the Retina. In *Neuron* (Vol. 76, Issue 2, pp. 266–280). Elsevier. https://doi.org/10.1016/j.neuron.2012.10.002.

Nathans, J. (1989). The genes for color vision. In *Scientific American* (Vol. 260, Issue 2, pp. 42–49). https://doi.org/10.1038/scientificamerican0289-42.

Nguyen, H., Lee, S. J., & Li, Y. (2022). Selective Activation of the Wnt-Signaling Pathway as a Novel Therapy for the Treatment of Diabetic Retinopathy and Other Retinal Vascular Diseases. In *Pharmaceutics* (Vol. 14, Issue 11). https://doi.org/10.3390/pharmaceutics14112476.

Niessen, C. M. (2007). Tight junctions/adherens junctions: Basic structure and function. In *Journal of Investigative Dermatology* (Vol. 127, Issue 11, pp. 2525–2532). Elsevier. https://doi.org/10.1038/sj.jid.5700865.

Page-McCaw, A., Ewald, A. J., & Werb, Z. (2007). Matrix metalloproteinases and the regulation of tissue remodelling. In *Nature Reviews Molecular Cell Biology* (Vol. 8, Issue 3, pp. 221–233). Nature Publishing Group. https://doi.org/10.1038/nrm2125.

Palczewski, K. (2006). G protein-coupled receptor rhodopsin. In *Annual Review of Biochemistry* (Vol. 75, Issue Volume 75, 2006, pp. 743–767). *Annual Reviews.* https://doi.org/10.1146/annurev.biochem.75.103004.142743.

Raeisossadati, R., Ferrari, M. F. R., Kihara, A. H., AlDiri, I., & Gross, J. M. (2021). Epigenetic regulation of retinal development. In *Epigenetics and Chromatin* (Vol. 14, Issue 1). https://doi.org/10.1186/s13072-021-00384-w.

Raposo, G., & Stoorvogel, W. (2013). Extracellular vesicles: Exosomes, microvesicles, and friends. In *Journal of Cell Biology* (Vol. 200, Issue 4, pp. 373–383). The Rockefeller University Press. https://doi.org/10.1083/jcb.201211138.

Reichenbach, A., & Bringmann, A. (2010). Müller cells in the healthy and diseased retina. In *Müller Cells in the Healthy and Diseased Retina*. https://doi.org/10.1007/978-1-4419-1672-3.

Saint-Geniez, M., & D'Amore, P. A. (2004). Development and pathology of the hyaloid, choroidal and retinal vasculature. In *International Journal of Developmental Biology* (Vol. 48, Issues 8–9, pp. 1045–1058). UPV/EHU Press. https://doi.org/10.1387/ijdb.041895ms.

Santos, G. S. P., Prazeres, P. H. D. M., Mintz, A., & Birbrair, A. (2018). Role of pericytes in the retina. In *Eye (Basingstoke)* (Vol. 32, Issue 3, pp. 483–486). https://doi.org/10.1038/eye.2017.220.

Schwartz, S. D., Hubschman, J. P., Heilwell, G., Franco-Cardenas, V., Pan, C. K., Ostrick, R. M., Mickunas, E., Gay, R., Klimanskaya, I., & Lanza, R. (2012). Embryonic stem cell trials for macular degeneration: A preliminary report. *The Lancet*, *379*(9817), 713–720. https://doi.org/10.1016/S0140-6736(12)60028-2.

Selhorst, J. B., & Chen, Y. (2009). The optic nerve. In *Seminars in Neurology* (Vol. 29, Issue 1, pp. 29–35). © Thieme Medical Publishers. https://doi.org/10.1055/s-0028-1124020.

Semenza, G. L. (2012). Hypoxia-inducible factors in physiology and medicine. In *Cell* (Vol. 148, Issue 3, pp. 399–408). Elsevier. https://doi.org/10.1016/j.cell.2012.01.021.

Simons, M., Gordon, E., & Claesson-Welsh, L. (2016). Mechanisms and regulation of endothelial VEGF receptor signalling. In *Nature Reviews Molecular Cell Biology* (Vol. 17, Issue 10, pp. 611–625). Nature Publishing Group. https://doi.org/10.1038/nrm.2016.87.

Sterling, P. (1988). The retina. An approachable part of the brain. *Cell*, *53*(2), 175–176. https://doi.org/10.1016/0092-8674(88)90378-9.

Strauss, O. (2005). The retinal pigment epithelium in visual function. In *Physiological Reviews* (Vol. 85, Issue 3, pp. 845–881). American Physiological Society. https://doi.org/10.1152/physrev.00021.2004.

Takita, S., & Seko, Y. (2024). Zebrafish as an experimental model for inherited retinal diseases. In *Zebrafish Research - An Ever-Expanding Experimental Model*. IntechOpen. https://doi.org/10.5772/intechopen.1004858.

Tkach, M., & Théry, C. (2016). Communication by Extracellular Vesicles: Where We Are and Where We Need to Go. In *Cell* (Vol. 164, Issue 6, pp. 1226–1232). Cell Press. https://doi.org/10.1016/j.cell.2016.01.043.

Tomkins-Netzer, O., Niederer, R., Greenwood, J., Fabian, I. D., Serlin, Y., Friedman, A., & Lightman, S. (2024). Mechanisms of blood-retinal barrier disruption related to intraocular inflammation and malignancy. In *Progress in Retinal and Eye Research* (Vol. 99, p. 101245). Pergamon. https://doi.org/10.1016/j.preteyeres.2024.101245.

Uyama, H., Mandai, M., & Takahashi, M. (2021). Stem-cell-based therapies for retinal degenerative diseases: Current challenges in the establishment of new treatment strategies. *Development Growth and Differentiation*, *63*(1), 59–71. https://doi.org/10.1111/dgd.12704.

Wald, G. (1968). Molecular basis of visual excitation. In *Science* (Vol. 162, Issue 3850, pp. 230–239). American Association for the Advancement of Science. https://doi.org/10.1126/science.162.3850.230.

Wang, Z., Liu, C. H., Huang, S., & Chen, J. (2019). Wnt Signaling in vascular eye diseases. In *Progress in Retinal and Eye Research* (Vol. 70, pp. 110–133). Pergamon. https://doi.org/10.1016/j.preteyeres.2018.11.008.

Wolburg, H., & Lippoldt, A. (2002). Tight junctions of the blood-brain barrier: Development, composition and regulation. *Vascular Pharmacology*, *38*(6), 323–337. https://doi.org/10.1016/S1537-1891(02)00200-8.

Young, R. W. (1967). The renewal of photoreceptor cell outer segments. *The Journal of Cell Biology*, *33*(1), 61–72. https://doi.org/10.1083/jcb.33.1.61.

Yuodelis, C., & Hendrickson, A. (1986). A qualitative and quantitative analysis of the human fovea during development. *Vision Research*, *26*(6), 847–855. https://doi.org/10.1016/0042-6989(86)90143-4.

Chapter 11

The Bone Marrow-Blood Barrier

Duygu Gürsoy Gürgen[1,2,*], PhD
[1]Department of Histology and Embryology, Ankara Medipol University, Istanbul, Turkey
[2]Research Institute for Health Sciences and Technologies (SABITA)
Istanbul Medipol University, Istanbul, Turkey

Abstract

Tissue barriers are among the structures that separate tissues from the circulatory system and play essential roles in the organism. Bone tissue surrounds the bone marrow, which is the center of hematopoietic cell production, forming a barrier that separates hematopoiesis from the circulatory system. Composed of calcified matrix and osteocytes, the bone is organized in a structure that begins with the periosteum. Bone tissue is organized in a regular pattern consisting of outer and inner circumferential lamellae, osteons, and interstitial lamellae. Bone marrow is a complex organ that provides a suitable microenvironment for hematopoiesis and, with this property, supports the production of hematopoietic cells. The bone marrow–blood barrier consists of endothelial cells, a basal lamina, and reticular connective tissue. This barrier plays a critical role in the regulation of the hematopoietic microenvironment and the control of vascular permeability. Hematopoietic cells mature, differentiate, and pass into the circulatory system within this microenvironment. Bone marrow provides a sterile environment for the production of blood cells, making it a structure of great importance in hematopoiesis. The challenges in studying the organizational structure of the bone marrow have hindered the full understanding of hematopoietic processes and mechanisms. This necessitates a more detailed examination of the hematopoietic

* Corresponding Author's Email: dgursoy@medipol.edu.tr

In: A Histological Approach to Human Body Barriers
Editor: İlknur Keskin
ISBN: 979-8-89530-738-0

microenvironment and the bone marrow–blood barrier. The barrier system that ensures the preservation of the hematopoietic process consists of the arterial endothelium, the basal lamina of the endothelium, the reticular connective tissue immediately preceding the bone marrow, and the calcified bone matrix. The heterogeneity and intrinsic homeostasis of the bone marrow are of considerable interest, particularly in toxicology studies. This section provides a detailed examination of the histology of the bone marrow, the structure of the bone marrow–blood barrier, the processes of hematopoiesis, and its embryological development. It explains the role of hematopoiesis in the organization by examining the structure and function of the bone marrow in detail.

Keywords: bone marrow, blood barrier, hematopoiesis, endothelium, basal membrane

Introduction

Tissue barriers are responsible for separating the tissue parenchyma from the circulatory system. In order to protect the productive component of the circulatory system—hematopoiesis—from the circulatory system itself, a tissue with a matrix as solid as rock is required: bone tissue. Bone tissue consists of bone marrow surrounded by lamellar systems formed by osteoblasts embedded in a calcified matrix. Bone marrow tissue is a vital center for the formation of blood cells in hematopoiesis. This complex microenvironment, situated between bone structures, possesses a unique vascular network that regulates the movement of cells between the bone marrow and the circulatory system. The onset of circulation—the hematopoietic process—must be preserved and remain sterile. Hematopoiesis is the production of blood cells (Ross Histology Text and Atlas 6th Txtbk (1), n.d.). According to Lucas, due to the difficulty in visualizing the bone marrow, the anatomy of hematopoiesis and how local spatial signaling is established have not been fully defined (Lucas, 2021). The bone marrow–blood barrier, composed of endothelial cells, basal lamina, and reticular connective tissue, plays a significant role in regulating the hematopoietic environment and controlling vascular permeabilization. This section discusses in detail the histology of bone marrow and the components involved in the bone marrow–blood barrier. In addition to addressing the hematopoietic process and its embryology, examples of bone marrow disorders are also provided.

Main Body

Bone Tissue Histology

As we move from the periphery of the bone toward the bone marrow, the first structure encountered is the membrane that surrounds the bone, the periosteum. Beneath the periosteum lie osteoblasts, which are immature bone cells that support the osteogenic process. As we move away from the membrane, mature osteocytes embedded in the calcified matrix adhere to each other through their canaliculi. The cytoplasmic extensions that osteocytes project toward each other within the calcified matrix are called canaliculi. These canaliculi form the lamellar systems. Due to their peripheral location, osteocytes are observed as outer circumferential lamellae, unlike the circular lamellae deeper in the tissue. The circular lamellae are formed by osteocytes surrounding central blood vessels within the tissue parenchyma. This structure, composed of concentric lamellae arranged in parallel and made up of osteocytes and their canaliculi, is referred to as the Haversian system (osteon). Because osteons have a round structure, the regions between them in the tissue parenchyma are lined with interstitial lamellae. Deeper in the tissue, osteocytes are arranged as non-circular inner circumferential lamellae. These lamellae also surround the bone marrow. At the center of the bone, bone marrow is observed.

In long bones, a nutrient artery and one or two nutrient veins enter the bone obliquely and reach the bone marrow cavity. After entering, the artery branches upward and downward in parallel with the bone and becomes wrapped around the central vein of the bone marrow (Travlos, 2006). In flat bones, this organization is replaced by a more extensive vascular network. In long bones, the entering artery divides upward and downward along the longitudinal axis and forms a spiral arrangement around the central longitudinal vein. This artery gives rise to small, thin-walled arterioles and capillaries extending outward toward the cortical bone. The capillary arteries forming the Haversian canals within the bone tissue return to the bone marrow and open into venous sinusoids. Near the bone, the arterioles open into venous sinusoids and form an anastomosing plexus. These venous sinusoids drain into the central longitudinal vein nourished by the nutrient vein through collector tubules that return to the central vein. Thus, a circulatory network is established that forms a circular path from the center of the bone marrow to the periphery and back to the center.

The bone marrow is the part where bone trabeculae are located along with connective tissue and the nutrient artery. The production of blood cells takes place here. This process is called hematopoiesis.

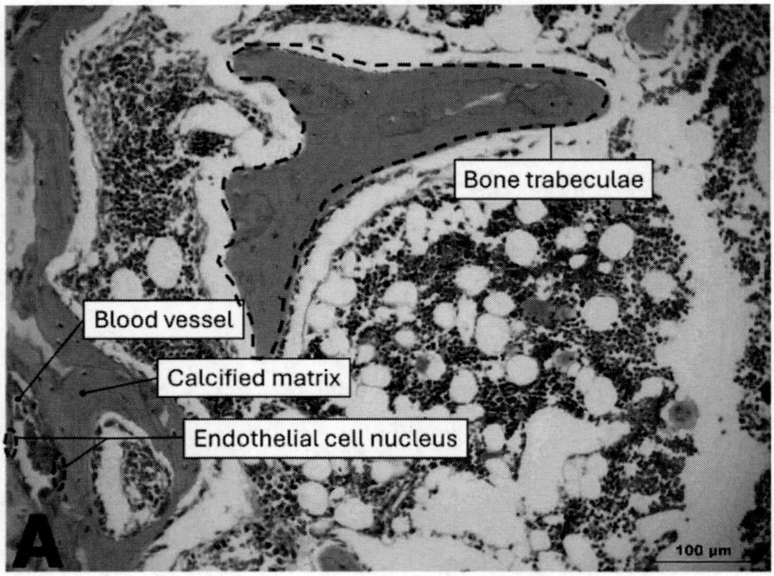

Figure 1. H&E-stained section showing concentric lamellae, osteocytes, and canaliculi in compact bone.

Hematopoiesis

The initiation of circulation—the hematopoietic process—must be protected and remain sterile. Hematopoiesis is the production of blood cells, and it takes place in the spaces between blood vessels, bone tissue, and reticular cells within the bone marrow (Lucas, 2021; Ross Histology Text and Atlas 6th Txtbk (1), n.d.). In general, three types of blood cells—erythrocytes, granulocytes, and agranulocytes—are produced in the bone marrow and released into circulation. Hematopoiesis is staged throughout the embryonic period, occurring first in the yolk sac, then in the liver and spleen, and finally in the bone marrow. The bone marrow phase begins in the second trimester of gestation and continues into adulthood. Blood cell life is maintained through continuous synthesis and degradation, and their lifespan is limited. The primary purpose of hematopoiesis is to maintain a stable number of different cell types in circulation. Erythrocytes and platelets spend their entire lifespan in circulation, whereas other blood cells enter the circulation and migrate to peripheral tissues, and their lifespans may vary. Thus, approximately 400 billion platelets, 10 billion granulocytes, and over 200 billion erythrocytes enter circulation daily, while an equivalent number exit (Mehdi Tavassoli, 1990). The level of cells in circulation is maintained in this way. Additionally, numerous lymphocytes (B and T cells) and monocytes are produced from totipotent progenitor cells. At any given time, one trillion cells are present in our bone marrow.

While the hematopoietic process exhibits spatial and regional differences within the bone marrow, this enables the regulation of different hematopoietic stem cells (HSCs) within the microenvironment (Lucas, 2021). This heterogeneity highlights the presence of specific sinusoidal and arteriolar niches. HSCs are located in different regions regulated by local signals derived from various microenvironments (Acar et al., 2015; Kokkaliaris et al., 2020; Kunisaki et al., 2013; Zhao et al., 2019). Studies indicate that HSCs are particularly localized in sinusoidal and arteriolar areas. Furthermore, due to the bulkiness of the sinusoids, HSCs are observed approximately 30 μm from the sinusoids, and each arteriolar or endosteal niche necessarily contains a sinusoid. The differences in cell populations in these areas and the balance between them serve as a guide for potential stem cell-based rejuvenation therapies (Pinho et al., 2018). This structural organization is critically important for HSC function and homeostasis. Megakaryocytes are significant cells that influence the localization and activity of HSCs. Studies show that HSCs around megakaryocytes are regulated by factors such as CXCL4 and TGFβ secreted by these cells (Bruns et al., 2014). It is also stated that HSCs located near megakaryocytes exhibit a tendency toward proliferation in the event of megakaryocyte loss (Pinho et al., 2018; Zhao et al., 2014). The endosteal region provides an essential niche for the localization and function of HSCs. Donor HSCs have been observed to accumulate in regions close to endosteal cells in recipient mice (Lo Celso et al., 2009). Furthermore, $CD48^-CD49b^-$ HSCs in this region are proposed to be resistant to chemotherapy and represent the reserve HSC (rHSC) population (Zhao et al., 2014). While multipotent progenitor cells are ranked below HSCs in the hematopoietic hierarchy, they play a significant role in blood cell production (Kwon et al., 2024). Studies using various imaging methods have proposed two opposing views on whether HSCs and multipotent progenitor cells share the same niches (Christodoulou et al., 2020; Cordeiro Gomes et al., 2016). Further research is needed to clarify this issue.

Myeloid cell production (myelopoiesis) is regulated by signals from microenvironmental components such as endothelial cells, perivascular cells, osteocytes, megakaryocytes, and neutrophils (Boettcher et al., 2014; Hérault et al., 2017; Hoyer et al., 2020; Nagareddy et al., 2013; Schürch et al., 2014; Shi et al., 2011). It has been shown that in emergencies, signals that trigger myeloid cell production create clusters of myeloid progenitors in specific areas (Boettcher et al., 2014; Cordeiro Gomes et al., 2016; Hérault et al., 2017). Lymphopoiesis, on the other hand, depends on signaling produced by perivascular stroma, endothelial cells, osteoblastic progenitors, osteoblasts, and osteocytes, and it has been reported that lymphoid progenitors accumulate in endosteal regions (Cordeiro Gomes et al., 2016; Ding & Morrison, 2013; Sato et al., 2013; Silberstein et al., 2016; Yu et al., 2015; Zhu et al., 2007).

Classically, erythropoiesis is a regional organization in which erythroblasts mature within a niche formed by macrophages located near the sinusoids (Bessis, 1958; Mohandas & Prenant, 1978). Since erythroid progenitors are regulated by the secretion of reticular stromal cells located in perisinusoidal regions, sinusoids are erythropoietic areas (Comazzetto et al., 2019; Lucas, 2021).

Studies reveal the balance of heterogeneity within the bone marrow microenvironment and highlight the critical role of cellular interactions in the hematopoietic process.

Embryology and Histology of the Bone Marrow

The embryological process of the bone marrow begins with the infiltration of blood vessels and mesenchymal cells into the cavities formed in the diaphysis, the central part of the long bones. Osteoblasts, which differentiate from these cells, begin to deposit bone tissue onto the cartilage matrix. As a result, bone trabeculae emerge, consisting of a core of calcified cartilage tissue and a surface of bone tissue. Bone marrow is formed in the spaces between the bone trabeculae and blood vessels through the settlement of reticular connective tissue and blood cells differentiated from mesenchymal cells. During these events, in the region between the epiphyses and the diaphysis of the cartilage model, chondrocytes continuously proliferate through mitosis, forming stacked groups. Thus, the length of the cartilage template increases continuously. The bone collar also continues to develop, thickening and extending toward the epiphyses, surrounding the region with chondrocytes from the outside. In this region, chondrocytes enlarge and begin to die. As in the primary ossification center, cartilage matrix first forms, followed by bone trabeculae in these areas. These trabeculae are a continuation of those formed earlier. While the bone tissue completely surrounds the bone marrow, creating a spatial boundary, it also extends trabecular projections toward the bone marrow, integrating into the bone marrow parenchyma (Lucas, 2021). The bone marrow cavity is lined by a dense network of fenestrated sinusoids formed by arterioles traversing through the bone. This vascular structure is in close association with perivascular reticular cells that extend throughout the bone marrow.

The vascularization of the bone marrow can be categorized into three stages: vasculogenesis, angiogenesis, and hematopoietic niche formation. Vasculogenesis is the process by which blood vessels form de novo. It is observed in synchrony with hematopoiesis. Therefore, endothelial cells and blood cells share a common progenitor cell origin. During early embryogenesis, vascular endothelial growth factor (VEGF) plays a critical role. Angiogenesis refers to the formation of new blood vessels from preexisting ones. This process is limited to the bone marrow and occurs through tissue-specific signaling. One of the primary roles of vascularization is the regulation of existing stem and progenitor cells, which governs the processes of osteogenesis and hematopoiesis. The formation of a microenvironment that houses hematopoietic stem cells is referred to as hematopoietic niche formation. This niche provides essential signals for the survival, quiescence, mobility, and differentiation of hematopoietic stem cells. Endothelial cells and the angiocrine factors they secrete play a vital role in maintaining hematopoietic stem cell homeostasis (Sivan et al., 2019).

In humans, bone marrow tissue constitutes approximately 3% of total body mass (Picker & Siegelman, 1999). The components of the bone marrow can be categorized under two main compartments (HISTOLOGY AND CELL BIOLOGY: An Introduction to Pathology, Fourth Edition, n.d.): the marrow stromal compartment and the hematopoietic cell compartment. The stromal compartment is composed of blood vessels, endothelial cells lining these vessels, the basal lamina of the endothelium, stromal (reticular) cells, fibroblasts, macrophages, and adipocytes. The hematopoietic cell compartment contains all immature blood cell types involved in the process of hematopoiesis. These include erythrocytes, granulocytes (neutrophils, eosinophils, basophils), and agranulocytes (monocytes, lymphocytes, platelets). Once they complete their maturation, they pass through the sinusoids and enter circulation. The sinusoids within the barrier are characterized by discontinuous endothelium and basal lamina. It has been reported that, rather than forming tight junctions, adjacent endothelial cells overlap and slide over one another, allowing vascular dilation (Branemark, 1959; Mehdi Tavassoli & Shaklai, 1979). According to Chamberlain and Lichtman, the pores that permit cellular passage are not pre-existing but appear during cell migration and close afterward (Chamberlain & Lichtman, n.d.). Otherwise, if closure did not occur, the endothelial cell would eventually destroy itself by forming an excessive number of pores. However, calculations have shown that the number of cells forming the sinusoidal wall does not change.

In the blood vessels of the bone marrow, particularly in the sinusoids, a receptor-dependent inhibition system exists to prevent the passage of immature cells. Only cells that express specific membrane proteins, such as aquaporin and glycophorin, on their surface are allowed to pass through the endothelium (Abraham L. Kierszenbaum, n.d.). Due to their suitability for blood cell migration, the sinusoids exhibit a variably thick adventitial layer.

In the 1970s, researchers questioned whether equilibrium or disequilibrium existed between the extravascular spaces and the circulation in the bone–blood interface (W. F. Neuman et al., 1979; William F. Neuman et al., 1982; Talmage et al., 1977). The characteristic features of vascular sinusoids, such as the known ability of granulocytes to migrate across the barrier due to their lobulated nuclei (Lichtman & Kearney, 1970), and the observation that, unlike in birds—where nucleated erythrocytes enter circulation due to intravascular erythropoiesis—in humans, erythrocytes migrate through the barrier by leaving their nucleus behind and passing only the cytoplasm (F. Campbell, 1967), have contributed to the definitive understanding of the existence of the marrow–blood barrier (MBB).

In a study using carbon particles, the particles were observed in the extravascular area of the bone marrow, but not in the junctional spaces between endothelial cells. In another study analyzing serial sections, it was reported that transmural passage in the bone marrow occurs via a transendothelial rather than an interendothelial route (Mehdi Tavassoli & Shaklai, 1979). This finding highlights the presence and selectivity of the barrier. Migrating cells contact the endothelial membrane, exert pressure, and undergo fusion with the endothelial membrane, followed by separation (fusion–fission) (Mehdi Tavassoli, 1979), thereby creating a passage into the lumen. Differences in membrane proteins between the luminal and tissue-facing surfaces of endothelial cells have also been reported, which may play a critical role in determining the direction of transport. Thus, the selectivity of the barrier is maintained.

In light of all these findings, the structures comprising the bone marrow–blood barrier can be listed, from the lumen toward the parenchyma, as follows: endothelial cell (/cell membrane), fenestrated basal membrane belonging to the endothelium, adventitial cells, reticular connective tissue, stromal cells (reticular cells and macrophages), and calcified matrix.

Endothelial cell: The fenestrated structure allows endothelial cells to communicate with the hematopoietic compartment while also enabling contraction, dilation, or closure of the cells (Lichtman et al., 2011). In transmission electron microscopy, endothelial cells appear as thin structures with reduced cytoplasm of varying sizes and are interrupted by fenestrations of different dimensions (Zhang et al., 2023). In scanning electron microscopy, two types of fenestrae are observed: large ones that allow the passage of blood cells and smaller pores composed of cribriform plaque-like aggregates.

Basal membrane: Although discontinuity of the basal membrane was reported as early as the 1970s, this could not be fully clarified due to preparation artifacts (F. R. Campbell, 1972a; Weiss, 1965, 1976). In electron microscopy studies, Inoue and Osmond reported that the basal membrane of the bone marrow has a distinct organization and composition (Inoue & Osmond, 2001). It mainly consists of laminin and a small amount of discontinuous type II collagen (Zhang et al., 2023). The low presence of heparan sulfate proteoglycan (HSPG) in the basal membrane renders it more prone to disruption and facilitates cellular migration. Due to the role of HSPG in connecting other components of a typical membrane structure, its scarcity prevents the formation of a mesh-like architecture. The abundant presence of chondroitin sulfate proteoglycan (CSPG) is thought to serve as a reservoir for the CD44 receptor, which is essential for hematopoiesis, and to play a critical role in the development and differentiation of hematopoietic cells (Kolset & Gallagher, 1990; Laurie, 1985; Spooncer et al., 1983; Verfaillie et al., 1994). The remodeling of the basal membrane that allows cellular passage is thought to be associated with adventitial cells. Since known laminin isoforms cannot self-assemble, an unorganized basal

Adventitial cells: These cells cover approximately two-thirds of the vascular endothelial surface (Zhang et al., 2023). They regulate the opening and closing of fenestrae by contracting their cell bodies, and by stretching the junctions of endothelial cells, they regulate blood volume and the flow of blood cells into the hematopoietic compartment (F. R. Campbell, 1972; Yamada, 1975). Their thin and elongated cytoplasmic extensions form a mesh-like structure in the tissue outside the vascular area (Valdez et al., 2012).

Reticular cells exhibit fibroblastic characteristics with reticulin fibers and are thought to be involved in protein synthesis and to be associated with preosteoblasts (N. Tavassoli & Friedenstein, 1983). Based on their positivity for alkaline phosphatase, it has been suggested that they are involved in granulopoietic areas of hematopoietic cords (Westen & Bainton, 1979).

Macrophages within the stromal compartment can be divided into two subgroups: those that form erythroblastic islands surrounded by developing erythroid cells, and perisinusoidal macrophages located adjacent to sinuses that penetrate the sinus wall to perform intravascular phagocytosis (Shaklai & Tavassoli, 1979; M. Tavassoli, 1974, 1977).

Calcified matrix: Collagen fibers produced by osteoblasts form a major component of the matrix, contributing to the structural integrity of bone marrow and shaping the bone (Ali Sahebekhtiari & Tavassoli, 1978; N. Tavassoli & Friedenstein, 1983). Reticular fibers associated with collagen occupy a large area within the matrix and play a role in protein synthesis via their connections with rough endoplasmic reticulum (RER) in the extensions of reticular cells (N. Tavassoli & Friedenstein, 1983).

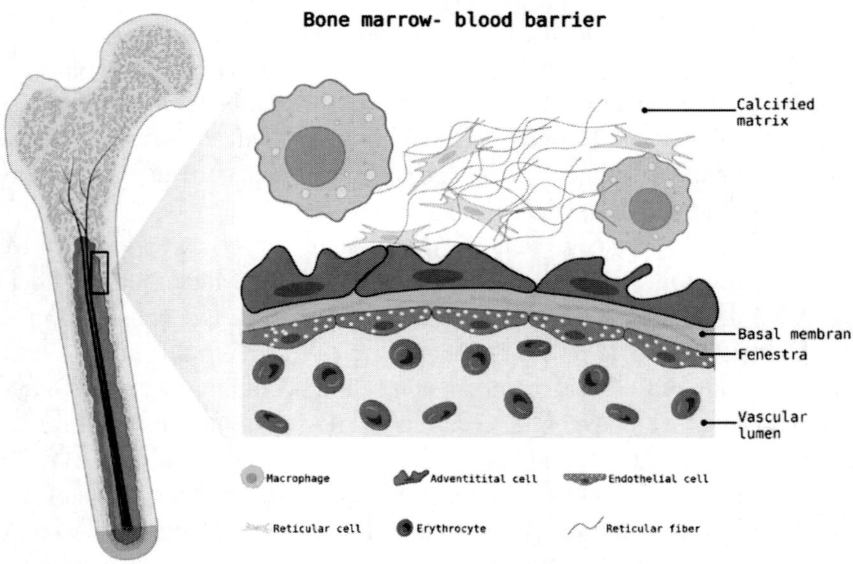

Figure 2. Schematic representation of the marrow–blood barrier and its components from lumen to bone matrix.

Conclusion

The barrier system that ensures the preservation of this process consists of the arterial endothelium, the basal lamina of the endothelium, the reticular connective tissue immediately preceding the bone marrow, and the calcified bone matrix. The selectivity of the barrier and its decisive role in cellular trafficking indicate its regulatory function within the bone marrow. The heterogeneity and intrinsic homeostasis of the bone marrow have attracted significant interest in various fields, particularly in toxicology studies. Imaging and evaluation performed in the bone marrow using appropriate methods are of great importance, as they can provide more information than a peripheral blood smear and may facilitate clinical intervention in any hematopoietic disorder.

References

Abraham L. Kierszhenbaum. (n.d.). Histology and Cellular Biology. In *Elsevier* (Fifth edition, Vol. 1).

Acar, M., Kocherlakota, K. S., Murphy, M. M., Peyer, J. G., Oguro, H., Inra, C. N., Jaiyeola, C., Zhao, Z., Luby-Phelps, K. & Morrison, S. J. (2015). Deep imaging of bone marrow shows non-dividing stem cells are mainly perisinusoidal. *Nature*, *526*(7571), 126–130. https://doi.org/10.1038/NATURE15250.

Ali Sahebekhtiari, H. & Tavassoli, M. (1978). Studies on bone marrow histogenesis: morphometric and autoradiographic studies of regeneration marrow stroma in extramedullary autoimplants and after evacuation of marrow cavity. *Cell and Tissue Research*, *192*(3), 437–450. https://doi.org/10.1007/BF00212324.

Bessis, M. (1958). [Erythroblastic island, functional unity of bone marrow]. *Revue d'hematologie*, *13*(1), 8–11.

Boettcher, S., Gerosa, R. C., Radpour, R., Bauer, J., Ampenberger, F., Heikenwalder, M., Kopf, M. & Manz, M. G. (2014). Endothelial cells translate pathogen signals into G-CSF-driven emergency granulopoiesis. *Blood*, *124*(9), 1393–1403. https://doi.org/10.1182/BLOOD-2014-04-570762.

Branemark, P. I. (1959). Vital microscopy of bone marrow in rabbit *Scandinavian Journal of Clinical and Laboratory Investigation*, *11 Supp 38*, 1–82.

Bruns, I., Lucas, D., Pinho, S., Ahmed, J., Lambert, M. P., Kunisaki, Y., Scheiermann, C., Schiff, L., Poncz, M., Bergman, A. & Frenette, P. S. (2014). Megakaryocytes regulate hematopoietic stem cell quiescence through CXCL4 secretion. *Nature Medicine*, *20*(11), 1315–1320. https://doi.org/10.1038/NM.3707.

Campbell, F. (1967). Fine structure of the bone marrow of the chicken and pigeon. *Journal of Morphology*, *123*(4), 405–439. https://doi.org/10.1002/JMOR.1051230407.

Campbell, F. R. (1972a). Ultrastructural studies of transmural migration of blood cells in the bone marrow of rats, mice and guinea pigs. *American Journal of Anatomy*, *135*(4), 521–535. https://doi.org/10.1002/AJA.1001350406.

Campbell, F. R. (1972b). Ultrastructural studies of transmural migration of blood cells in the bone marrow of rats, mice and guinea pigs. *American Journal of Anatomy*, *135*(4), 521–535. https://doi.org/10.1002/AJA.1001350406.

Chamberlain, J. K. & Lichtman, M. A. (n.d.). Marrow Cell Egress: Specificity of the Site of Penetration Into the Sinus. In *Blood* (Vol. 52, Issue 5). https://ashpublications.org/blood/article-pdf/52/5/959/581435/959.pdf.

Christodoulou, C., Spencer, J. A., Yeh, S. C. A., Turcotte, R., Kokkaliaris, K. D., Panero, R., Ramos, A., Guo, G., Seyedhassantehrani, N., Esipova, T. V., Vinogradov, S. A., Rudzinskas, S., Zhang, Y., Perkins, A. S., Orkin, S. H., Calogero, R. A., Schroeder, T., Lin, C. P. & Camargo, F. D. (2020). Live-animal imaging of native haematopoietic stem and progenitor cells. *Nature*, *578*(7794), 278–283. https://doi.org/10.1038/S41586-020-1971-Z.

Comazzetto, S., Murphy, M. M., Berto, S., Jeffery, E., Zhao, Z. & Morrison, S. J. (2019). Restricted Hematopoietic Progenitors and Erythropoiesis Require SCF from Leptin Receptor+ Niche Cells in the Bone Marrow. *Cell Stem Cell*, *24*(3), 477-486.e6. https://doi.org/10.1016/J.STEM.2018.11.022.

Cordeiro Gomes, A., Hara, T., Lim, V. Y., Herndler-Brandstetter, D., Nevius, E., Sugiyama, T., Tani-ichi, S., Schlenner, S., Richie, E., Rodewald, H. R., Flavell, R. A., Nagasawa, T., Ikuta, K. & Pereira, J. P. (2016). Hematopoietic Stem Cell Niches Produce Lineage-Instructive Signals to Control Multipotent Progenitor Differentiation. *Immunity*, *45*(6), 1219–1231. https://doi.org/10.1016/J.IMMUNI.2016.11.004.

Ding, L. & Morrison, S. J. (2013). Haematopoietic stem cells and early lymphoid progenitors occupy distinct bone marrow niches. *Nature*, *495*(7440), 231–235. https://doi.org/10.1038/NATURE11885.

Gu, Y. C., Kortesmaa, J., Tryggvason, K., Persson, J., Ekblom, P., Jacobsen, S. E. & Ekblom, M. (2003). Laminin isoform-specific promotion of adhesion and migration of human bone marrow progenitor cells. *Blood*, *101*(3), 877–885. https://doi.org/10.1182/blood-2002-03-0796.

Hérault, A., Binnewies, M., Leong, S., Calero-Nieto, F. J., Zhang, S. Y., Kang, Y. A., Wang, X., Pietras, E. M., Chu, S. H., Barry-Holson, K., Armstrong, S., Göttgens, B. & Passegué, E. (2017). Myeloid progenitor cluster formation drives emergency and leukaemic myelopoiesis. *Nature*, *544*(7648), 53–58. https://doi.org/10.1038/NATURE21693.

Histology and Cell Biology An Introduction to Pathology Fourth Edition. (n.d.).

Hoyer, F. F., Zhang, X., Coppin, E., Vasamsetti, S. B., Modugu, G., Schloss, M. J., Rohde, D., McAlpine, C. S., Iwamoto, Y., Libby, P., Naxerova, K., Swirski, F. K., Dutta, P. & Nahrendorf, M. (2020). Bone Marrow Endothelial Cells Regulate Myelopoiesis in Diabetes Mellitus. *Circulation*, *142*(3), 244–258. https://doi.org/10.1161/CIRCULATIONAHA.120.046038.

Inoue, S. & Osmond, D. G. (2001). *Basement Membrane of Mouse Bone Marrow Sinusoids Shows Distinctive Structure and Proteoglycan Composition: A High Resolution Ultrastructural Study*. https://doi.org/10.1002/ar.XXXX.

Kokkaliaris, K. D., Kunz, L., Cabezas-Wallscheid, N., Christodoulou, C., Renders, S., Camargo, F., Trumpp, A., Scadden, D. T. & Schroeder, T. (2020). Adult blood stem cell localization reflects the abundance of reported bone marrow niche cell types and their combinations. *Blood*, *136*(20), 2296–2307. https://doi.org/10.1182/BLOOD.2020006574.

Kolset, S. O. & Gallagher, J. T. (1990). Proteoglycans in haemopoietic cells. *Biochimica et Biophysica Acta*, *1032*(2–3), 191–211. https://doi.org/10.1016/0304-419X(90)90004-K.

Kunisaki, Y., Bruns, I., Scheiermann, C., Ahmed, J., Pinho, S., Zhang, D., Mizoguchi, T., Wei, Q., Lucas, D., Ito, K., Mar, J. C., Bergman, A. & Frenette, P. S. (2013). Arteriolar niches maintain haematopoietic stem cell quiescence. *Nature*, *502*(7473), 637–643. https://doi.org/10.1038/NATURE12612.

Kwon, M., Kim, B. S., Yoon, S., Oh, S. O. & Lee, D. (2024). Hematopoietic Stem Cells and Their Niche in Bone Marrow. *International Journal of Molecular Sciences 2024, Vol. 25, Page 6837*, *25*(13), 6837. https://doi.org/10.3390/IJMS25136837.

Laurie, G. W. (1985). Lack of heparan sulfate proteoglycan in a discontinuous and irregular placental basement membrane. *Developmental Biology*, *108*(2), 299–309. https://doi.org/10.1016/0012-1606(85)90034-X.

Lichtman, M. A., Kaushansky Kenneth, Kipps Thomas J., Prchal Josef T. & Levi Marcel M. (2011). *Williams Manual of Hematology* (M. A. Lichtman, Kaushansky Kenneth, Kipps Thomas J., Prchal Josef T., & Levi Marcel M., Eds.; 8th ed.). McGraw-Hill Education.

Lichtman, M. A. & Kearney, E. (1970). Cellular Deformability during Maturation of the Myeloblast. *New England Journal of Medicine*, *283*(18), 943–948. https://doi.org/10.1056/NEJM197010292831801.

Lo Celso, C., Fleming, H. E., Wu, J. W., Zhao, C. X., Miake-Lye, S., Fujisaki, J., Côté, D., Rowe, D. W., Lin, C. P. & Scadden, D. T. (2009). Live-animal tracking of individual haematopoietic stem/progenitor cells in their niche. *Nature*, *457*(7225), 92–96. https://doi.org/10.1038/NATURE07434.

Lucas, D. (2021). Structural organization of the bone marrow and its role in hematopoiesis. *Current Opinion in Hematology*, *28*(1), 36. https://doi.org/10.1097/MOH.0000000000000621.

Mehdi Tavassoli. (1979). The Marrow-Blood Barrier. *Britishjournal of Haematology*, *41*, 297–302.

Mohandas, N. & Prenant, M. (1978). Three-dimensional model of bone marrow. *Blood*, *51*(4), 633–643.

Nagareddy, P. R., Murphy, A. J., Stirzaker, R. A., Hu, Y., Yu, S., Miller, R. G., Ramkhelawon, B., Distel, E., Westerterp, M., Huang, L. S., Schmidt, A. M., Orchard, T. J., Fisher, E. A., Tall, A. R. & Goldberg, I. J. (2013). Hyperglycemia promotes myelopoiesis and impairs the resolution of atherosclerosis. *Cell Metabolism*, *17*(5), 695–708. https://doi.org/10.1016/J.CMET.2013.04.001.

Neuman, W. F., Neuman, M. W. & Myers, C. R. (1979). Blood:bone disequilibrium. III. Linkage between cell energetics and Ca fluxes. *The American Journal of Physiology*, *236*(5). https://doi.org/10.1152/AJPCELL.1979.236.5.C244.

Neuman, William F., Neuman, M. W., Diamond, A. G., Menanteau, J. & Gibbons, W. S. (1982). Blood:Bone disequilibrium. VI. Studies of the solubility characteristics of brushite: Apatite mixtures and their stabilization by noncollagenous proteins of bone. *Calcified Tissue International*, *34*(1), 149–157. https://doi.org/10.1007/BF02411226/METRICS.

Picker, L. J. & Siegelman, M. H. (1999). *Fundamental Immunology* (W. E. Paul, Ed.; 4th ed.). Lippincott-Raven.

Pinho, S., Marchand, T., Yang, E., Wei, Q., Nerlov, C. & Frenette, P. S. (2018). Lineage-Biased Hematopoietic Stem Cells Are Regulated by Distinct Niches. *Developmental Cell*, *44*(5), 634-641.e4. https://doi.org/10.1016/J.DEVCEL.2018.01.016.

Ross Histology Text and Atlas 6th txtbk (1). (n.d.).

Sato, M., Asada, N., Kawano, Y., Wakahashi, K., Minagawa, K., Kawano, H., Sada, A., Ikeda, K., Matsui, T. & Katayama, Y. (2013). Osteocytes regulate primary lymphoid organs and fat metabolism. *Cell Metabolism*, *18*(5), 749–758. https://doi.org/10.1016/J.CMET.2013.09.014.

Schürch, C. M., Riether, C. & Ochsenbein, A. F. (2014). Cytotoxic CD8+ T cells stimulate hematopoietic progenitors by promoting cytokine release from bone marrow mesenchymal stromal cells. *Cell Stem Cell*, *14*(4), 460–472. https://doi.org/10.1016/J.STEM.2014.01.002.

Shaklai, M. & Tavassoli, M. (1979). Cellular relationship in the rat bone marrow studied by freeze fracture and lanthanum impregnation thin-sectioning electron microscopy. *Journal of Ultrastructure Research*, *69*(3), 343–361. https://doi.org/10.1016/S0022-5320(79)80052-0.

Shi, C., Jia, T., Mendez-Ferrer, S., Hohl, T. M., Serbina, N. V., Lipuma, L., Leiner, I., Li, M. O., Frenette, P. S. & Pamer, E. G. (2011). Bone marrow mesenchymal stem and progenitor cells induce monocyte emigration in response to circulating toll-like receptor ligands. *Immunity*, *34*(4), 590–601. https://doi.org/10.1016/J.IMMUNI.2011.02.016.

Silberstein, L., Goncalves, K. A., Kharchenko, P. V., Turcotte, R., Kfoury, Y., Mercier, F., Baryawno, N., Severe, N., Bachand, J., Spencer, J. A., Papazian, A., Lee, D., Chitteti, B. R., Srour, E. F., Hoggatt, J., Tate, T., Lo Celso, C., Ono, N., Nutt, S., … Scadden, D. T. (2016). Proximity-Based Differential Single-Cell Analysis of the Niche to Identify Stem/Progenitor Cell Regulators. *Cell Stem Cell*, *19*(4), 530–543. https://doi.org/10.1016/J.STEM.2016.07.004.

Siler, U., Seiffert, M., Puch, S., Blood, A. R.-, Journal, T. & 2000, undefined. (n.d.). Characterization and functional analysis of laminin isoforms in human bone marrow. *Ashpublications.OrgU Siler, M Seiffert, S Puch, A Richards, B Torok-Storb, CA Müller, L Sorokin, G KleinBlood, The Journal of the American Society of Hematology, 2000•ashpublications.Org*. Retrieved November 15, 2024, from https://ashpublications.org/blood/article-abstract/96/13/4194/176230.

Sivan, U., De Angelis, J. & Kusumbe, A. P. (2019). Role of angiocrine signals in bone development, homeostasis and disease. *Open Biology*, *9*(10). https://doi.org/10.1098/RSOB.190144.

Spooncer, E., Gallagher, J. T., Krizsa, F. & Dexter, T. M. (1983). Regulation of haemopoiesis in long-term bone marrow cultures. IV. Glycosaminoglycan synthesis and the stimulation of haemopoiesis by beta-D-xylosides. *The Journal of Cell Biology*, *96*(2), 510–514. https://doi.org/10.1083/JCB.96.2.510.

Talmage, R. V., Doppelt, S. H. & Fondren, F. B. (1977). An interpretation of acute changes in plasma45Ca following parathyroid hormone administration to thyroparathyroidectomized rats. *Calcified Tissue Research*, *22*(1), 117–128. https://doi.org/10.1007/BF02010351/METRICS.

Tavassoli, M. (1974). Bone marrow erythroclasia: the function of perisinal macrophages relative to the uptake of erythroid cells. *Journal of the Reticuloendothelial Society*, *15*(2), 163–169.

Tavassoli, M. (1977). Intravascular phagocytosis in the rabbit bone marrow: a possible fate of normal senescent red cells. *British Journal of Haematology*, *36*(3), 323–326. https://doi.org/10.1111/j.1365-2141.1977.tb00655.x.

Tavassoli, Mehdi. (1990). Bone Marrow and Hemopoiesis. *Aplastic Anemia and Other Bone Marrow Failure Syndromes*, 1–24. https://doi.org/10.1007/978-1-4612-3254-4_1.

Tavassoli, Mehdi & Shaklai, M. (1979). *Absence of Tight Junctions in Endotheliurn of Marrow Sinuses: Possible Significance for Marrow Cell Egress* (Vol. 41).

Tavassoli, N. & Friedenstein, A. (1983). Hemopoietic Stromal Microenvironment. In *American Journal of Hematology*.

Travlos, G. S. (2006). Normal Structure, Function, and Histology of the Bone Marrow. *Toxicologic Pathology*, *34*(5), 548–565. https://doi.org/10.1080/019262306 00939856.

Valdez, R., Zutter, M. & Florea, A. D. (2012). *Rubin's Pathology: Clinicopathologic Foundations of Medicine* (6th ed.). Lippincott Williams & Wilkins.

Verfaillie, C., Hurley, R., Bhatia, R. & McCarthy, J. B. (1994). Role of bone marrow matrix in normal and abnormal hematopoiesis. *Critical Reviews in Oncology/Hematology*, *16*(3), 201–224. https://doi.org/10.1016/1040-8428(94)90071-X

Weiss, L. (1965). The structure of bone marrow. Functional interrelationships of vascular and hematopoietic compartments in experimental hemolytic anemia: an electron microscopic study. *Journal of Morphology*, *117*(3), 467–537. https://doi.org/10.1002/JMOR.1051170308.

Weiss, L. (1976). The hematopoietic microenvironment of the bone marrow: An ultrastructural study of the stroma in rats. *The Anatomical Record*, *186*(2), 161–184. https://doi.org/10.1002/AR.1091860204.

Westen, H. & Bainton, D. F. (1979). Association of alkaline-phosphatase-positive reticulum cells in bone marrow with granulocytic precursors. *The Journal of Experimental Medicine*, *150*(4), 919–937. https://doi.org/10.1084/JEM.150.4.919.

Yamada, E. (1975, August 25). Scanning electron microscopy of the bone marrow. *Proceedings of the Tenth International Congress of Anatomists*.

Yu, V. W. C., Saez, B., Cook, C., Lotinun, S., Pardo-Saganta, A., Wang, Y. H., Lymperi, S., Ferraro, F., Raaijmakers, M. H. G. P., Wu, J. Y., Zhou, L., Rajagopal, J., Kronenberg, H. M., Baron, R. & Scadden, D. T. (2015). Specific bone cells produce DLL4 to generate thymus-seeding progenitors from bone marrow. *The Journal of Experimental Medicine*, *212*(5), 759–774. https://doi.org/10.1084/JEM.20141843.

Zhang, J. ;, Huang, Q. ;, Bian, W. ;, Wang, J. ;, Guan, H. ;, Niu, J., Zhang, J., Huang, Q., Bian, W., Wang, J., Guan, H. & Niu, J. (2023). Imaging Techniques and Clinical Application of the Marrow–Blood Barrier in Hematological Malignancies. *Diagnostics 2024, Vol. 14, Page 18*, *14*(1), 18. https://doi.org/10.3390/DIAGNOSTICS14010018.

Zhao, M., Perry, J. M., Marshall, H., Venkatraman, A., Qian, P., He, X. C., Ahamed, J. & Li, L. (2014). Megakaryocytes maintain homeostatic quiescence and promote post-injury regeneration of hematopoietic stem cells. *Nature Medicine*, *20*(11), 1321–1326. https://doi.org/10.1038/NM.3706.

Zhao, M., Tao, F., Venkatraman, A., Li, Z., Smith, S. E., Unruh, J., Chen, S., Ward, C., Qian, P., Perry, J. M., Marshall, H., Wang, J., He, X. C. & Li, L. (2019). N-Cadherin-Expressing Bone and Marrow Stromal Progenitor Cells Maintain Reserve Hematopoietic Stem Cells. *Cell Reports*, *26*(3), 652-669.e6. https://doi.org/10.1016/J.CELREP.2018.12.093.

Zhu, J., Garrett, R., Jung, Y., Zhang, Y., Kim, N., Wang, J., Joe, G. J., Hexner, E., Choi, Y., Taichman, R. S. & Emerson, S. G. (2007). Osteoblasts support B-lymphocyte commitment and differentiation from hematopoietic stem cells. *Blood*, *109*(9), 3706–3712. https://doi.org/10.1182/BLOOD-2006-08-041384.

Chapter 12

The Blood-Air Barrier

Arzu Güneş*, PhD
Department of Histology and Embryology, International School of Medicine, Istanbul Medipol University, İstanbul, Türkiye

Abstract

The blood-air barrier, also called the alveolar-capillary barrier, is crucial for lung function as it allows the exchange of carbon dioxide (CO_2) and oxygen (O_2) between the pulmonary circulation and the alveolar air spaces. The alveolar epithelium, the extracellular matrix, and the pulmonary microvascular endothelium together form this barrier. Structurally, it consists of the cellular extensions of type I alveolar epithelial cells (AEC1s), the cellular extensions of the continuous endothelial cell layer, the common basal lamina of AEC1s and endothelial cells, and the plasma membrane of erythrocytes. The AEC1s cover about 95% of the alveolar surface and are remarkably thin to allow efficient gas exchange. The thickness of the alveolar-capillary barrier ranges from 0.1 to 1.5 μm and allows optimal gas diffusion while maintaining structural integrity. In addition, tight junctions between epithelial cells prevent leakage of fluid into the alveolar space, further supporting efficient gas exchange. Type II alveolar epithelial cells (AEC2s) secrete surfactant, a lipid-protein complex that, although not a structural component of the blood-air barrier, coats the alveolar surface, reduces surface tension, and averts alveolar atelectasis during exhalation. During the development of the respiratory system, the blood-air barrier undergoes significant changes in the shape and structure of the tissue. Although most mammals, including humans, initiate air respiration at birth, the lungs achieve functional maturity before birth. The formation

* Corresponding Author's Email: arzu.gunes@medipol.edu.tr

In: A Histological Approach to Human Body Barriers
Editor: İlknur Keskin
ISBN: 979-8-89530-738-0

of the blood-air barrier is an intricate process involving the differentiation and proliferation of alveolar epithelial cells, the establishment of the capillary network, and the deposition of extracellular matrix components. Proper formation and maintenance of this barrier is critical for normal respiratory function and overall health. Damage to the alveolar-capillary barrier increases lung permeability, disrupts gas exchange and leads to dyspnoea. Such damage can have various causes, including infection, inflammation and mechanical injury.

Keywords: alveolar epithelial cells, blood-air barrier, gas exchange, pneumocytes, respiration, surfactant

Introduction

The blood-air barrier is a crucial interface for gas exchange within the lungs, comprising the alveolar epithelium, an interstitial compartment, and the capillary epithelium (Figure 12.1). In a young adult with an average weight of 70 kg, the area of the alveolar surface is 130 m^2, while the area of the capillary surface is 115 m^2. The blood-air barrier consists of two segments with different thicknesses. Its thin segment, which constitutes about half of the total surface area, is less than 0.5 µm thick and covers an estimated surface area of about 100 m^2. It includes the endothelium, epithelium, and a fused basal membrane that forms the interstitial compartment (Weibel, 2017). In addition to these components, the thick segment comprises the extracellular matrix and various cells, including fibroblasts and immune cells (Mescher, 2021).

The structure-function relationship of the blood-air barrier is an important factor affecting O_2 diffusion and capillary microvascular filtration. O_2 diffusion at rest is approximately 10^{-2} mL/cm^2 per day, while capillary microvascular filtration is 4×10^{-8} mL/cm^2 (Miserocchi, 2009). This indicates that the blood-air barrier efficiently transfers respiratory gases while remaining slightly permeable to water (Miserocchi, 2023).

Understanding the intricacies of the blood-air barrier is essential for comprehending its role in respiratory physiology and its response to various pathological conditions. This chapter sets the stage for a detailed exploration of the functional and structural dynamics of the blood-air barrier, highlighting its significance in maintaining efficient gas exchange and overall pulmonary health.

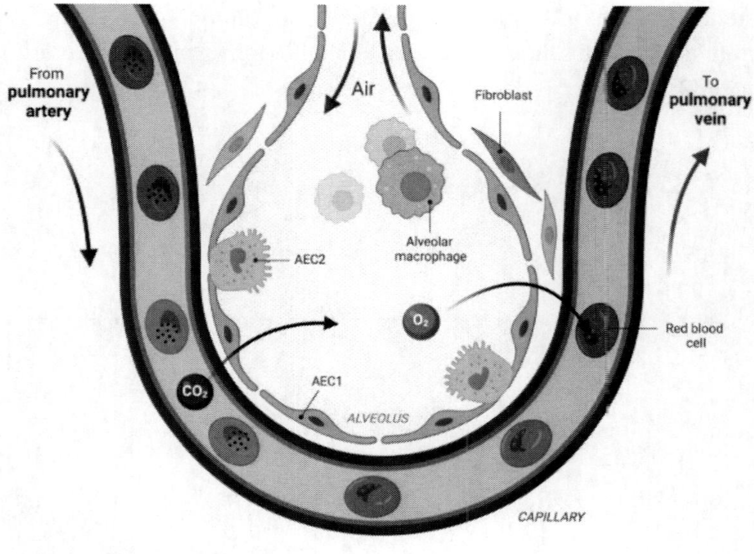

Figure 1. Gas exchange between the alveoli and capillary vasculature. Created with BioRender.com.

Cellular Architecture of Alveoli

Alveoli are sac-like protrusions, each approximately 200 μm in diameter, extending from the respiratory bronchioles, alveolar ducts, and alveolar sacs. Together with the bronchial tree, the alveoli contribute to the spongy architecture of the lungs (Mescher, 2021). An average alveolus, among the 400 million found in the lungs, contains approximately 47 AEC1s and 92 AEC2s, forming a mosaic of around 140 epithelial cells. AEC1s cover about 93% of the alveolar surface, corresponding to roughly 0.22 mm^2 of an average alveolus. Each AEC1 cell spans an extensive area of about 5,098 μm^2 of the alveolar septum, which is substantial compared to AEC2s, typical cuboidal epithelial cells, which cover less than 100 μm^2. In the alveoli, AEC1s are the second most prevalent cell type, with an average volume of 1,763 μm^3, whereas macrophages are the largest, with an average volume of 2,492 μm^3. In contrast, AEC2s cover about 7% of the alveolar surface. Although the average volume of AEC2s is half that of AEC1s, light microscopy can sometimes give the impression that AEC2s are larger. This misconception arises because the thin cytoplasmic extensions of AEC1s, which cover the alveolar surface, do not accurately represent AEC1s' true volume in two-dimensional sections. Despite being larger in volume, AEC1s are highly efficient in maximizing the surface area available for respiration (Figure 12.2) (Crapo, 1982).

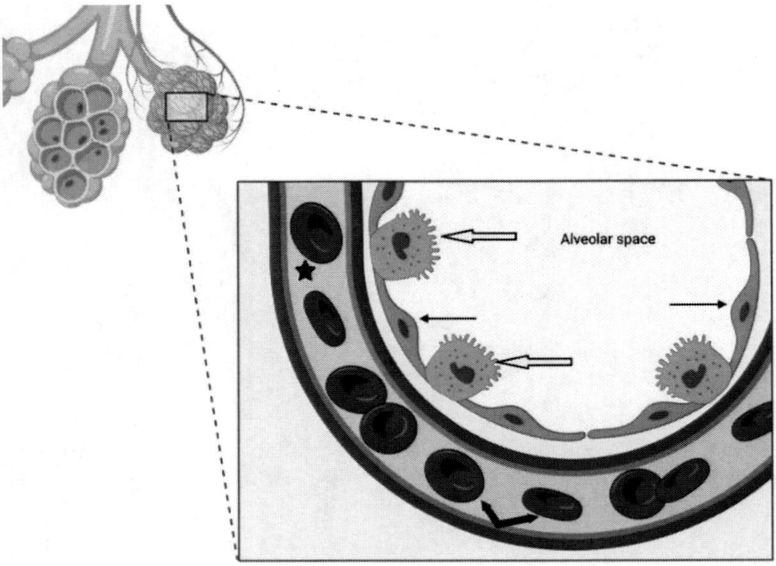

Figure 2. Cellular architecture of alveoli: Black arrows: AEC1s, white arrows: AEC2s, black star: capillary lumen, two-headed arrow: erythrocytes. Created with BioRender.com.

Alveolar Wall

The alveolar wall is located between the alveolar epithelium and the capillary endothelium. This compartment contains the extracellular matrix and various cells, including fibroblasts and immune cells, that provide structural support and facilitate the exchange of substances. The alveolar wall consists of thin interalveolar septa situated between neighbouring alveoli. These septa consist of dispersed fibroblasts and a minimal extracellular matrix (ECM), incorporating elastic and reticular fibres within the connective tissue. The elastic fibres facilitate the expansion of alveoli during inspiration and their passive contraction during expiration. In contrast, the reticular fibres avert both the collapse and overdistension of an alveolus. The interalveolar septa host the body's most extensive capillary networks. The pulmonary capillaries are densely interwoven within the interalveolar septa, reinforced by the alveoli's reticular and elastic fibre meshwork (Mescher, 2021). The capillaries within the alveolar walls are lined with approximately 170 capillary endothelial cells and are associated with around 210 interstitial fibroblasts (Crapo, 1982).

Additionally, macrophages and other leukocytes are present within the septa. Alveolar pores, or pores of Kohn, which range from 10-15 μm in diameter, pierce the interalveolar septa. These pores link adjacent alveoli opening into different bronchioles, aiding in the equalization of air pressure across alveoli and facilitating collateral air circulation if a bronchiole is obstructed (Figure 12.3) (Mescher, 2021). The walls of the alveolar ducts consist of networks that divide the alveolar air space from the capillary compartment. The inter-alveolar septum is structured to offer a thin diffusion barrier and an extensive surface area facilitating efficient exchange of O_2 and CO_2. Additionally, it must ensure stability to prevent collapse of alveoli or over-distension and maintain flexibility to accommodate thoracic movements during the breathing cycle (Knudsen, 2018).

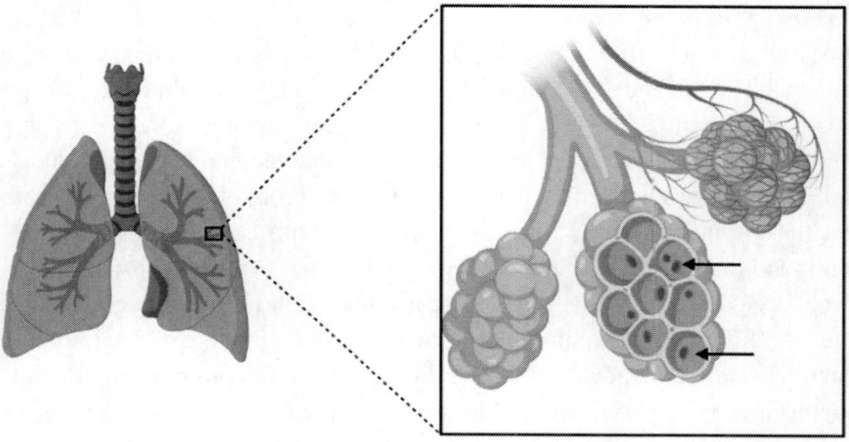

Figure 3. Image of alveoli. Black arrows: Pores of Kohn. Created with BioRender.com.

Components of the Air-Blood Barrier

- AEC1s cover the majority of the alveolar surface and are primarily responsible for gas exchange. Their thin cytoplasmic extensions help minimize the distance gases must diffuse.

- Interstitial space between the alveolar epithelium and capillary epithelium.
- Capillary endothelial cells form the inner lining of the capillaries and are essential in controlling the transfer of gases, nutrients, and waste products between the blood and the alveolar space.
- Plasma membrane of erythrocytes (Mescher, 2019).

AEC1s

AEC1s were historically mischaracterized due to the limitations of early microscopy techniques. The thin cytoplasmic extensions of these cells spread over multiple capillary surfaces, making their nuclei rarely visible in two-dimensional sections. This visibility issue led to a significant misunderstanding, and until the mid-1950s, these cells were incorrectly described as nucleus-free lamellae. Furthermore, the limitations of light microscopy at the time meant that the very thin extensions (approximately 0.1 μm) of AEC1s were not visible. Consequently, the alveolar capillaries appeared devoid of epithelial cells, leading to their characterization as "naked." The advent of electron microscopy brought a revolutionary change in our understanding of AEC1s. It allowed for the detailed visualization of these thin cytoplasmic extensions and revealed that they indeed possess nuclei and complex cellular structures. Electron microscopy studies demonstrated that these thin extensions form tight junctions with each other, providing a continuous and comprehensive cover over the capillary surfaces. This discovery corrected the previous misconceptions and highlighted the critical role of AEC1s in maintaining the integrity and function of the blood-air barrier. In summary, advancements in imaging technologies have significantly enhanced our understanding of AEC1s, rectifying earlier misconceptions and providing a clearer picture of their structure and function within the lungs (Weibel, 1971).

AEC2s

AEC2s are cuboidal-shaped epithelial cells that extend into the alveolar air space, playing crucial roles in alveolar function. These cells display a distinctive morphology, characterized by the presence of microvilli on their apical surface and lamellar bodies within their cytoplasm. Lamellar bodies act as reservoirs for surface active agents, commonly referred to as surfactants. Surfactant is essential for lowering surface tension within the alveoli, aiding in the prevention of collapse of these air sacs during exhalation. As a result, surfactant is essential for maintaining the proper function of the blood-air barrier. Beyond their role in surfactant secretion, AEC2s also have the capacity for self-renewal and can differentiate into AEC1s. This dual functionality enables AEC2s to indirectly support the blood-air barrier not only through surfactant secretion but also by playing a crucial role in the regeneration and upkeep of the alveolar epithelium (Guillot, 2013).

Interstitial Space between AEC1s and Capillary Endothelium

The blood-air barrier, which isolates the air in the alveoli from the blood in the capillaries, consists of two continuous layers of cells: an endothelium that lines the capillary walls and an epithelium that lines the alveolar lumen. Positioned between these two layers is an interstitial space that varies in both thickness and composition. This barrier is characterised by areas of varying thicknesses: the thicker sections are rich in cell nuclei and an extensive network of fibres, which together provide regenerative capabilities and mechanical stability. Conversely, the thinner sections of the barrier feature a shared basal lamina between the capillary endothelium and the alveolar epithelium, which minimizes the thickness of the diffusion barrier and facilitates efficient gas exchange (Leiby, 2020).

The most prevalent cells in the interstitium are fibroblasts, also known as septal cells. These fibroblasts, similar to classical fibroblasts, are responsible for producing and maintaining the extracellular matrix (ECM). Additionally, myofibroblasts, which possess contractile properties, are present. These myofibroblasts possess filaments that link the two epithelial surfaces of the septum and provide support to the interstitial space. They can directly connect the alveolar epithelium and capillary endothelium via pores in the basal lamina. The network of extracellular connective tissue fibers is interlaced with the alveolar capillary network (Kapanci, 1974).

In the thinner segments of the blood-air barrier, the connective tissue is notably absent, leaving behind only the fused basal lamina produced by the AEC1s and endothelial cells. This thin part of the barrier is where gas exchange predominantly occurs. In this region, the alveolar capillaries are in close proximity to the alveolar lumen, a configuration that is relatively unique compared to the lumens found in other organs.

Development of Blood-Air Barrier

During embryonic development, the anterior foregut endoderm forms the lower respiratory system, which includes the larynx, trachea, bronchi, and lungs, as well as the oesophagus, liver, and thyroid. The pulmonary epithelium and the glands of the larynx, trachea, and bronchi arise from the endodermal lining of the laryngotracheal groove. Additionally, the connective tissue, cartilage, and smooth muscle of these structures are derived from the splanchnic mesoderm surrounding the foregut (Moore, 2011).

Lung development progresses through four distinct stages based on histological changes: (i) pseudoglandular, (ii) canalicular, (iii) saccular, and (iv) alveolar. The alveolar stage begins at 24 gestational weeks and continues through microvascular maturation until approximately 8 years of age. This stage may extend up to 18 years. Notably, approximately 50% of the alveolar septa are formed between the ages of 3 and 18 (Leiby, 2020). In the early stages of respiratory system development, the laryngotracheal groove, diverticulum, and lung buds are covered with columnar epithelium. As the pseudoglandular stage progresses, the heights of epithelial cells gradually decrease, with some cells becoming more cuboidal and developing a variety of lamellar bodies, whereas others differentiate into squamous pneumocytes crucial for the formation of the blood-air barrier. This complex process facilitates the proper development of the respiratory tract, which is vital for effective gas exchange and respiratory function (Moore, 2011).

The beginning of the canalicular stage is marked by the appearance of the first portions of the blood-air barrier. The cuboidal cells, rich in lamellar bodies, known as primitive pneumoblasts, later differentiate into AEC1s and AEC2s. Most of these AEC2s differentiate into AEC1s. This conversion involves several processes, including the reduction of intercellular tight junctions, mediated by cytoskeletal proteins and basolateral membranes. Junctions between neighbouring epithelial cells are shifted basally, leading to the protrusion of the apical portion of the cell into the lumen (Herriges, 2014).

The extrusion of lamellar bodies as the airspaces expand, along with cell thinning and the apposition of blood capillaries, resulting in the formation of the thin blood-air barrier. Surfactant, present early in the canalicular stage, plays a vital role in this thinning process by reducing surface tension. This intricate and multifaceted sequence of events is vital for the optimal development and functionality of the respiratory system (Makanya, 2016).

Plasma Membrane of Erythrocytes

In the late 17th century, Dutch biologists Jan Swammerdam and Antonie van Leeuwenhoek made significant early observations of erythrocytes also known as red blood cells (RBCs). Swammerdam first noted erythrocytes in 1668, although his findings were not immediately shared widely. Leeuwenhoek, however, published his detailed observations in 1675 in the Philosophical Transactions of the Royal Society. He described how erythrocytes appeared hard and rigid when a person was ill, but softened and became more pliable as the person recovered. Leeuwenhoek concluded that in a healthy body, erythrocytes must be flexible to pass through the body's capillaries and arteries, changing shape from round to oval and back again as they travel through differently sized vessels. This insight, made over three centuries ago, has proven remarkably accurate, underscoring the necessity of erythrocyte flexibility for efficient circulatory function (Mohandas, 2008).

Building on these early observations, modern research has further elucidated the characteristics of mature erythrocytes. These cells are unique among cells as they lack a nucleus and organelles, yet they are intricately structured to fulfil the vital role of transporting O_2 and removing CO_2 from all other cells in the body. Additionally, they are built to withstand the significant shear stress encountered as they navigate through small vessels and sinusoids. The mammalian RBC has developed into a very specialized cell designed for the efficient delivery of O_2 throughout the circulatory system. Its structure is optimized to ensure survival under continuous shear stress, which is a testament to its advanced differentiation. The cell membrane of the RBC consists of a lipid bilayer that is lined on its cytoplasmic surface by the RBC cytoskeleton. Together, these components form the erythrocyte membrane, a critical feature for maintaining the cell's structural integrity and functionality (Risinger, 2020).

Blood Air Barrier Dysfunction and Homeostasis

In the lungs, the blood-air barrier is a dynamic structure, actively maintained by the capillary epithelium and alveolar endothelium to regulate permeation and remove excess fluid, ensuring that the alveolar surface remains relatively dry. When this delicate balance is disrupted, it can lead to the development of interstitial and alveolar oedema, which may impair gas exchange and, in severe cases, cause alveolar collapse and hypoxia. Pulmonary oedema, which can be classified as hydrostatic or high permeability, may arise from fluid leakage not only from the capillaries but also from the pulmonary arteries and veins. Although this fluid build-up generally spares the gas-exchange surfaces, it can still reduce lung compliance and result in breathlessness. The lungs have protective mechanisms, such as increased lymphatic flow and active fluid clearance (AFC), to limit the extent of oedema. However, when these mechanisms are overwhelmed, fluid first accumulates in the septal interstitium, causing the alveolar walls to thicken, which can significantly hinder the diffusion of O_2 and impair gas exchange. Pulmonary oedema can also occur when the permeability of the alveolar wall is abnormally increased, allowing plasma proteins and fluid to leak through. This type of oedema is usually linked to enhanced capillary endothelial permeability, except in cases of direct damage to the epithelial cells, such as in capillary stress failure. The alveolar epithelium acts as the most selective element of the alveolar wall, effectively regulating the movement of fluids and water-soluble substances. Beyond this regulatory role, the alveolar epithelium is crucial in maintaining the stability of the blood-gas barrier by actively removing fluid and water-soluble substances from the distal airspaces through a process known as AFC. Both AEC1 and AEC2 cells play a role in the active transport of ions, with a particular emphasis on sodium, across the alveolar wall. This ion transport creates an osmotic gradient that drives the removal of water from the alveolar lumen, making AFC the primary mechanism for clearing fluid from the distal airspaces (Leiby, 2020).

The lung's capacity for gas exchange relies on the intricate interplay between the alveolar epithelium and the pulmonary microvascular endothelium. If either of these components of the blood-air barrier is impaired, interstitial and alveolar oedema may occur. Experimental in vitro and in vivo models suggest that blood-air barrier dysfunction is an important factor in the development of acute lung injury (ALI). ALI is marked by non-cardiogenic pulmonary oedema and is linked to elevated morbidity and mortality rates. This condition is frequently associated with clinical issues such as pneumonia, aspiration syndromes, non-pulmonary sepsis, shock, and severe trauma.

Despite numerous clinical trials, no pharmacologic treatment has been found to effectively reduce mortality associated with ALI. The inflammatory responses seen in ALI may be triggered by a primary infectious stimulus, such as pneumonia, or may arise from systemic inflammation that is exacerbated by lung injury. The severity of blood-air barrier damage directly increases the severity of ALI. Endothelial dysfunction also plays an important role in lung injury and repair. Endothelial dysfunction not only contributes to the influx of inflammatory cells and mediators during the exudative phase but also acts as an active source of growth factors and mediators that affect vascular tone, cell proliferation, and angiogenesis. The endothelium is an important site where inflammatory, coagulation and fibrinolysis systems interact and directly influence the outcome of these processes (Cross, 2011).

Conclusion

The blood-air barrier, an essential structure within the lungs, facilitates critical gas exchange between the alveoli and the pulmonary circulation. This barrier, which includes the alveolar epithelium, the surrounding microvascular endothelium and the interstitial matrix, ensures efficient O_2 and CO_2 transfer while maintaining the structural stability necessary for lung function. AEC1 predominantly cover the alveolar surface and optimize it for gas exchange, while AEC2s produce surfactant to maintain alveolar stability and reduce surface tension.

Historical advancements in microscopy have significantly enhanced our understanding of the intricate architecture and functioning of the blood-air barrier. The development of this barrier begins at the embryonic stage and continues postnatally to ensure that the lungs are capable of efficient gas exchange at birth. The delicate balance of this barrier can be disrupted by various factors, resulting in increased lung permeability and impaired gas exchange.

Acute lung injury (ALI) leading to non-cardiogenic pulmonary oedema underscores the critical importance of the blood-air barrier. Conditions such as pneumonia, sepsis, aspiration syndromes and severe trauma can lead to ALI, which is characterized by significant morbidity and mortality. Despite numerous clinical trials, effective pharmacologic interventions for ALI remain limited.

In summary, the intricate structure and function of the blood-air barrier are paramount to respiratory health, and a deeper understanding of this critical interface offers promising avenues for advancing treatments for various pulmonary conditions.

References

Crapo, J. D., Barry, B. E., Gehr, P., Bachofen, M., & Weibel, E. R. (1982). Cell number and cell characteristics of the normal human lung. *American Review of Respiratory Disease, 126*(2), 332–337. https://doi.org/10.1164/arrd.1982.126.2.332.

Cross, L. J., & Matthay, M. A. (2011). Biomarkers in acute lung injury: Insights into the pathogenesis of acute lung injury. *Critical Care Clinics, 27*(2), 355–377. https://doi.org/10.1016/j.ccc.2010.12.005.

Guillot, L., Nathan, N., Tabary, O., Thouvenin, G., Le Rouzic, P., et al. (2013). Alveolar epithelial cells: Master regulators of lung homeostasis. *International Journal of Biochemistry & Cell Biology, 45*(11), 2568–2573. https://doi.org/10.1016/j.biocel.2013.08.009.

Herriges, M., & Morrisey, E. E. (2014). Lung development: Orchestrating the generation and regeneration of a complex organ. *Development, 141*(3), 502–513. https://doi.org/10.1242/dev.098186.

Kapanci, Y., Assimacopoulos, A., Irle, C., Zwahlen, A., & Gabbiani, G. (1974). "Contractile interstitial cells" in pulmonary alveolar septa: A possible regulator of ventilation-perfusion ratio? Ultrastructural, immunofluorescence, and in vitro studies. *Journal of Cell Biology, 60*(2), 375–392. https://doi.org/10.1083/jcb.60.2.375.

Kierszenbaum, A. L., & Tres, L. L. (2015). *Histology and cell biology: An introduction to pathology* (4th ed.). Saunders.

Knudsen, L., & Ochs, M. (2018). The micromechanics of lung alveoli: Structure and function of surfactant and tissue components. *Histochemistry and Cell Biology, 150*(6), 661–676. https://doi.org/10.1007/s00418-018-1747-9.

Leiby, K. L., Raredon, M. S. B., & Niklason, L. E. (2020). Bioengineering the blood-gas barrier. *Comprehensive Physiology, 10*(2), 415–452. https://doi.org/10.1002/cphy.c190026.

Makanya, A. N. (2016). Membrane-mediated development of the vertebrate blood-gas barrier. *Birth Defects Research Part C: Embryo Today, 108*(1), 85–97. https://doi.org/10.1002/bdrc.21120.

Mescher, A. L. (2023). *Junqueira's basic histology: Text & atlas* (17th ed.). McGraw Hill.

Miserocchi, G. (2009). Mechanisms controlling the volume of pleural fluid and extravascular lung water. *European Respiratory Review, 18*(114), 244–252. https://doi.org/10.1183/09059180.00002709.

Miserocchi, G. (2023). The impact of heterogeneity of the air-blood barrier on control of lung extravascular water and alveolar gas exchange. *Frontiers in Network Physiology, 3*, 1142245. https://doi.org/10.3389/fnetp.2023.1142245.

Mohandas, N., & Gallagher, P. G. (2008). Red cell membrane: Past, present, and future. *Blood, 112*(10), 3939–3948. https://doi.org/10.1182/blood-2008-07-161166.

Moore, K. L., Persaud, T. V. N., & Torchia, M. G. (2011). *Before we are born: Essentials of embryology and birth defects* (8th ed.). Elsevier.

Risinger, M., & Kalfa, T. A. (2020). Red cell membrane disorders: Structure meets function. *Blood, 136*(11), 1250–1261. https://doi.org/10.1182/blood.2019000946.

Weibel, E. R. (1971). The mystery of "non-nucleated plates" in the alveolar epithelium of the lung explained. *Acta Anatomica (Basel), 78*(3), 425–443. https://doi.org/10.1159/000143605.

Weibel, E. R. (2017). Lung morphometry: The link between structure and function. *Cell and Tissue Research, 367*, 413–426. https://doi.org/10.1007/s00441-016-2541-4.

Chapter 13

The Blood-Thymus Barrier

Özlem Tuğçe Çilingir-Kaya[1,*], PhD
and Gökhan Cüce[2], MD
[1]Department of Histology and Embryology, Marmara Universtiy School of Medicine, İstanbul, Turkiye
[2]Department of Histology and Embryology, Necmettin Erbakan University School of Medicine, Konya, Turkiye

Abstract

The blood-thymus barrier (BTB) is a specialized structure that is essential for maintaining immune tolerance and supporting T-cell education. These barrier isolates develop thymocytes in the thymic cortex from circulating antigens and inflammatory mediators, ensuring a controlled microenvironment that is critical for T-cell selection. Structurally, the BTB comprises endothelial cells with tight junctions, a basal lamina, pericytes, and squamous Type 1 thymic epithelial cells (TECs) connected by desmosomes. Macrophages in the cortical parenchyma contribute to the protective role of the BTB by phagocytosing macromolecules that penetrate the barrier.

The BTB is intact in most of the thymic cortex but displays structural discontinuity near the corticomedullary junction and the medulla, permitting limited antigen exposure. These features allow for distinct stages of T-cell maturation. The integrity of the barrier can be disrupted by factors, such as sex steroids, stress, and aging, which influence its permeability and functionality. Immunohistochemical studies revealed distinct keratin expression patterns in cortical and medullary TECs, further highlighting the regional variations in BTB characteristics.

---

[*] Corresponding Author's Email: tugce.cilingir@marmara.edu.tr

In: A Histological Approach to Human Body Barriers
Editor: İlknur Keskin
ISBN: 979-8-89530-738-0

The ontogenesis of the BTB begins during embryogenesis, involving interactions between thymic epithelial cells and neural crest-derived cells, and continues postnatally. Age-related changes include thymic involution, increased permeability, compromised immune tolerance, and autoimmune disorders. Experimental models, including genetically modified animals and advanced imaging techniques, have facilitated the understanding of the structure and function of the BTB.
Research into the role of the BTB in thymic function and peripheral tolerance offers insights into autoimmune diseases, infections, and thymic tumors. Future advancements in regenerative medicine and organ-on-chip systems hold promise as therapeutic strategies targeting BTB integrity and immune modulation.

Keywords: blood-thymus barrier, T-cell education, ımmune tolerance, thymic microenvironment, thymic epithelial cells

Introduction

The thymus is a vital organ of the immune system that plays a critical role in T cell maturation. The thymus gland is the site where T cells are produced and is responsible for recognizing foreign antigens and initiating immune responses against them. The thymus enhances the capacity of the immune system to recognize cells and prevent autoimmunity. The functions of the thymus change throughout life, undergoing involution as age increases (Sakaguchi et al., 2008; Thapa & Farber, 2019). In this context, the thymus "trains" immune cells from the blood, ensuring that they can effectively respond to external antigens while preventing damage to the body's tissues (Bruss & Ely, 2019; Ross & Pawlina, 2020).

T lymphocytes are derived from hematopoietic stem cells in the bone marrow and mature in the thymic microenvironment. These cells undergo positive and negative selections during maturation. Positive selection ensures that T cells recognize major histocompatibility complex (MHC) molecules. During this process, only T cells that bind to MHC molecules with low-to-moderate affinity survive and become functional (Hsieh et al., 2012). Negative selection eliminates T cells that bind with a high affinity to self-antigens, thereby reducing the risk of autoimmune diseases (Klein & Petrozziello, 2024). Thymic epithelial and dendritic cells play a critical role in antigen presentation during T cell selection. These cells ensure the functionality of central tolerance mechanisms by suppressing immune responses that may harm the tissues of the body (Sakaguchi et al., 2008).

During the prenatal period, the thymus grows rapidly, forming a repertoire of T-cells that are essential for immune tolerance. Genetic factors and cellular signaling mechanisms play crucial roles in prenatal thymus development (Haniffa et al., 2024). During the postnatal period, the thymus forms the foundation of the adaptive immune system by responding to antigens from the environment (Thapa & Farber, 2019).

Thymus Development

The thymus begins to develop into two separate lobes during the sixth week of gestation. In the eighth week, the lobes began to migrate and fuse within the anterosuperior mediastinum. Hematopoietic cells generated by the fetal liver migrated to the thymus during the 10th week, marking the start of lobule formation. By weeks 14–16, the thymus differentiates into the cortex and medulla (Ross & Pawlina, 2020). The bilateral primordium of the thymus fuses at the midline to form a two-lobe thymus in the superior mediastinum. This bilobed structure persists throughout life. Each lobe has its vasculature, lymphatic drainage, and nerves, which remain separate despite the fusion of the lobes. The epithelium of the third pharyngeal pouch, originating from the endoderm and mesenchyme between epithelial tubules, contributes to thymic development. Epithelial tubes form solid cords, proliferate, and create branches forming the thymic lobules' core. Some epithelial cord cells are arranged around a central axis, forming small cell groups known as thymic corpuscles (Hassall's corpuscles). Other epithelial cord cells form the epithelial reticulum, and lymphocytes appear shortly thereafter. A fine mesenchymal covering, essential for thymic development, envelops the primordium of the thymus. This mesenchyme and some thymic epithelial cells are derived from the neural crest. Isolated cells from this origin can cause thymic developmental defects (Junqueira & Carneiro, 2018).

During the perinatal stage, the thymus is comparatively large and extends from the thorax to the root of the neck. Its size begins to decrease in late childhood until puberty. During adulthood, the cortex becomes indistinct owing to fat infiltration, yet the thymus remains functional and critical for health. It continues to secrete hormones and mature thymocytes.

Histological Structure

The thymus is a small, encapsulated organ with two lobes in the superior mediastinum, above the major vessels of the heart. The organ is surrounded by a dense collagenous capsule that sends trabeculae into the lobes and divides them into lobules. Each lobule comprises a cortex and a lighter-stained medulla (Figure 1).

The cortex is darker because of T lymphocytes (thymocytes) abundance. Immunologically naïve T lymphocytes migrate from the bone marrow to the cortex, proliferate, and acquire immune competence. The cortex also contains macrophages and epithelial reticular cells of ectodermal origin (Gartner & Hiatt, 2013).

Epithelial Reticular Cells in the Cortex

1) *Type 1 Cells:* Located beneath the capsule and trabeculae; they form the blood-thymus barrier (BTB) by enclosing capillaries.
2) *Type 2 Cells:* Found in the middle of the cortex; they possess prominent nuclei and desmosomes between their processes.
3) *Type 3 Cells:* Present at the corticomedullary junction, contributing to a barrier that prevents antigen entry into the cortex.

Epithelial Reticular Cells in the Medulla

- *Type 4 Cells:* Contribution to the corticomedullary boundary.
- *Type 5 Cells:* Form a network for lymphocyte arrangement.
- *Type 6 Cells:* Large, pale cells that form Hassall's corpuscles increase with age and can exhibit keratohyalin granules and calcification.

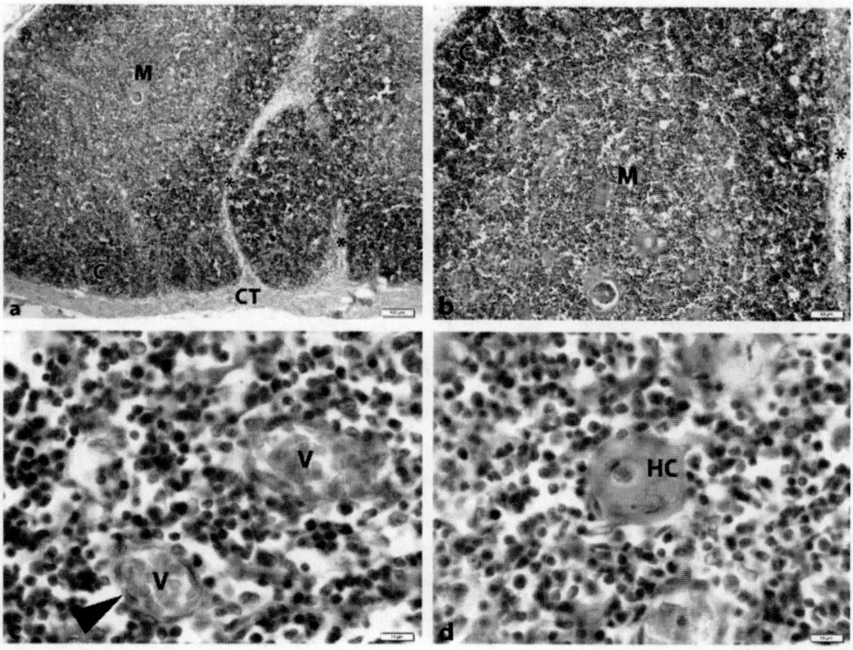

Figure 1. Representative micrographs of the thymus (a-d). C: cortex, M: medulla, CT: connective tissue capsule, *: trabeculae, V: blood vessel/capillary, arrowhead: endothelial cell of the capillary, HC: Hassal's corpuscle. Hematoxylin & Eosin staining.

Vasculature and Lymphatics

Numerous small arteries from the capsule were distributed throughout the organ via the trabeculae. These arteries form capillary beds at the corticomedullary junction, extending into the cortex and medulla (Ross & Pawlina, 2020). The thymus lacks afferent lymphatic vessels, indicating a lack of filtration function. Efferent lymphatics are present (Gartner & Hiatt, 2013). Newly formed, immunologically weak T cells migrate to the corticomedullary junction and cortical periphery, mature, and exit the medulla as immunocompetent cells to colonize thymus-dependent regions of peripheral lymphoid organs (e.g., lymph node paracortical areas, Peyer's patches, and spleen periarteriolar sheaths) (Junqueira & Carneiro, 2018).

Structure of the Blood-Thymus Barrier

The BTB was first discovered after the critical role of the thymus in establishing immune tolerance was understood. Studies conducted by Miller (1961) demonstrated the effects of the thymus on peripheral tolerance mechanisms. This discovery revealed that the thymic microenvironment and the blood-thymus barrier protect against antigens that affect T-cell development (Miller, 2011).

The blood-thymus barrier (BTB) is a specialized, functional, and selective barrier that isolates T lymphocytes from the blood and cortical capillaries. It consists of multiple cellular layers that prevent macromolecules from entering the cortical parenchyma from the vascular compartments. The innermost layer of the BTB is composed of vascular endothelial cells surrounded by pericytes. Above these, squamous Type 1 thymic epithelial cells (TECs), connected by desmosomes and occluding junctions, create an additional layer. TECs exhibit characteristics of both epithelial and reticular cells. Within the cortical parenchyma, macrophages are distributed and play a critical role in phagocytosing macromolecules that penetrate the BTB (Kierszenbaum & Tres, 2020).

The structural components of the BTB are shown (Figure 2).

1) *Capillary endothelial cells:* The capillary structure is composed of nonfenestrated endothelial cells. These cells are interconnected through tight junctions, which limits the entry of circulating antigens into the thymic microenvironment (Pearse, 2006). Tight junction proteins such as zonula occludens-1 and claudin-5 are expressed in endothelial cells and play a regulatory role in barrier permeability (Nagatake et al., 2021).
2) *Basal lamina of the endothelium:* The basal lamina lies between endothelial cells and pericytes, providing mechanical support and facilitating cell-cell interactions. Extracellular matrix proteins, such as laminin and collagen, are the primary components of the basal lamina, ensuring the structural integrity of the barrier (Foster et al., 2008).
3) *Pericytes:* Pericytes located on the outer surface of capillaries are critical for maintaining vascular stability. Additionally, pericytes influence the differentiation of endothelial cells and the regulation of tight junction proteins (Foster et al., 2008). In the thymic microenvironment, pericytes are essential for preserving immune

tolerance and maintaining vascular homeostasis (Nagatake et al., 2021; Foster et al., 2008).

4) *Perivascular connective tissue*
5) *Basal lamina of Type 1 epithelial-reticular cells*
6) *Type 1 epithelial-reticular cells:* Located in the medulla and cortex of the thymus, epithelial-reticular cells are integral cellular components of the BTB. These cells secrete the growth factors and cytokines necessary for the maturation of T cells. Additionally, epithelial-reticular cells form tight junctions to regulate the barrier permeability (Milićević & Milićević, 2004).

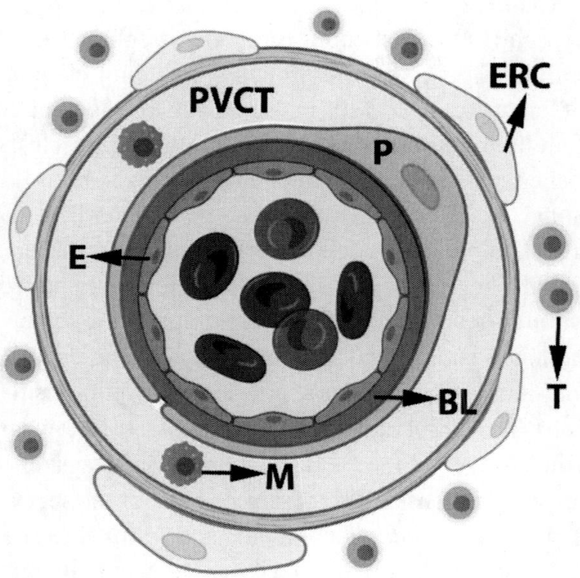

Figure 2. Schematic structure of the blood-thymus barrier. T: T-cell, ERC: epithelial-reticular cell, PVCT: perivascular connective tissue, M: macrophage, P: pericyte, BL: basal lamina, E: endothelium. Created on BioRender.com.

In most of the cortex, the barrier is intact and effectively restricts circulating antigens from accessing developing cortical lymphocytes. These lymphocytes differentiate into various T-cell subpopulations and become peripheral T lymphocytes with distinct markers and immune functions. These peripheral T cells migrate via the bloodstream to specific lymphoid regions (Ross & Pawlina, 2020). T cells exiting the thymus destroy infected cells and reject foreign tissue grafts.

However, the barrier is incomplete in specific regions, such as the juxtamedullary cortex, cortical venules, and the medulla. This allows circulating antigens to enter the thymic parenchyma. In contrast to cortical thymocytes, medullary thymocytes are exposed to circulating macromolecules. Macrophages in the perivascular space phagocytose and retain these molecules, thereby limiting their distribution (Sadler, 2018).

Overall, the BTB plays a critical role in preventing bloodborne antigens from reaching the thymic cortex, where T lymphocytes are formed. This protective mechanism ensures the proper development and maturation of T cells within the thymus.

The histological structure of the blood-thymus barrier (BTB) is analyzed using classical staining techniques such as Hematoxylin and Eosin (H&E) and Periodic Acid-Schiff (PAS) staining. Immunohistochemical staining plays a crucial role in identifying specific proteins, including claudin-5 and zonula occludens-1 (Nagatake et al., 2021). Classical histological features of the thymus include the cortex, medulla, Hassall's corpuscles, and lobules. Immunohistochemical studies using anti-pan-cytokeratin staining have revealed distinct keratin expression patterns in cortical and medullary epithelial cells. The medulla is characterized by a keratin-positive network interspersed with keratin-negative regions. Keratin-negative areas share histological similarities with the connective tissue of the septa.

While the basal lamina remains continuous in the capsule and septa, it exhibits discontinuity at the interface between the keratin-positive and keratin-negative regions. This observation provides the first histological evidence that may explain the absence of the BTB in the medulla. The supporting tissue in the keratin-negative regions closely resembled that of the septa. Blood vessels in the thymic medulla are predominantly located within these keratin-negative regions. As a result, any immunologically competent cells migrating into or through the thymus must traverse this keratin-negative region, designating it as the transitional zone of the thymus (Moore et al., 2020).

Certain factors, such as sex steroids (e.g., estrogen, progesterone) and glucocorticoids, can disrupt the BTB, allowing foreign antigens to infiltrate the thymus. Stress, ACTH, and other factors contributing to thymic involution also affect BTB permeability (Ross & Pawlina, 2020). The BTB is crucial for maintaining a controlled microenvironment within the thymus, facilitating T-cell education, and regulating the interaction of T cells with major histocompatibility complex (MHC) molecules. By preserving this environment, the BTB supports positive and negative selection processes that are essential for T-cell development and immune function (Junqueira & Carneiro, 2018).

The Blood-Thymus Barrier: Its Role in T Cell Education and Interaction with MHC Molecules

The BTB represents a highly specialized structure that is indispensable for the maintenance of T cell education within the thymus. This barrier ensures the creation of a controlled microenvironment, isolating developing thymocytes from circulating antigens and inflammatory mediators, while simultaneously facilitating interactions between T cells and major histocompatibility complex (MHC) molecules. By preserving the thymic environment, the BTB is essential for the precise regulation of both positive and negative selection processes of T cells.

Ontogenesis of the Blood-Thymus Barrier

BTB formation begins during embryogenesis and is complete during the postnatal period. This process is critically important for thymic development and the proper functioning of the immune system. Barrier formation is associated with endothelial cell differentiation, basal membrane organization, and the arrangement of epithelial-reticular cells.

Development of the Barrier during Embryogenesis

During embryonic development, the thymus originates from the third and fourth pharyngeal pouches. Thymic epithelial cells differentiate in interaction with neural crest-derived cells, playing a vital role in the formation of the thymic microenvironment (Foster et al., 2008). As blood vessels develop, endothelial cells become non-fenestrated and form tight junctions, preventing circulating antigens from entering the thymic microenvironment. Additionally, pericytes and basal membrane structures are formed, ensuring vascular stability (Petrie, 2003).

Postnatal Period

After birth, the thymus functions as an organ for peripheral lymphocyte maturation. During this period, the permeability of the BTB decreases, and maturation processes are completed. Tight junctions between endothelial cells strengthen further, while epithelial-reticular cells provide stromal support. These structures are essential for the functionality of central tolerance mechanisms (Boehm, 2008).

Effects of Aging and Thymic Involution on the Barrier

The thymus is an active immune organ in early life but undergoes involution after puberty. During this process, the number of thymic stromal cells and functional epithelial cells decreases, and adipose tissue replaces them. Consequently, the production of new T cells declines, weakening immune responses (Boehm & Swann, 2013). Aging-associated functional decline of the thymus increases susceptibility to infections and age-related diseases such as cancer (Miller, 2011). Structural changes in the BTB during aging include thickening of the basal membrane and increased permeability of endothelial cells, leading to impaired peripheral tolerance and an elevated risk of autoimmune diseases (Cowan et al., 2020; Boehm & Swann, 2013).

Genetic and Molecular Factors

Genetic and molecular signals play a significant role in the formation of the BTB. Molecules such as fibroblast growth factor (FGF) and vascular endothelial growth factor (VEGF) are critically important for vascular development (Petrie, 2003). Additionally, cytokines secreted by epithelial-reticular cells contribute to the regulation of barrier structures.

The ontogenesis of the BTB is a complex process that spans from embryogenesis to the postnatal period. This process is essential for preserving the thymic microenvironment and regulating the central tolerance mechanisms of the immune system. Aging-related changes in this structure can lead to immune dysfunction, highlighting the need for further research on the formation and functionality of BTB.

Pathological Conditions of the Blood-Thymus Barrier

The BTB is a critical structure that supports the healthy functioning of the immune system. However, structural and functional impairments of the barrier in various pathological conditions can result in a wide range of adverse outcomes, including autoimmune diseases, infections, and tumor progression.

Autoimmune Diseases

Disruptions in the BTB may contribute to the development of autoimmune diseases. Barrier permeability facilitates the entry of autoantigens into the thymic microenvironment, thereby compromising immune tolerance. Diseases such as myasthenia gravis and systemic lupus erythematosus are associated with these changes in the BTB (Boehm & Swann, 2013).

- Myasthenia Gravis: Structural changes such as thymic hyperplasia and thymoma are frequently observed in this autoimmune disease. These changes in the thymic microenvironment impair T-cell development and increase autoantibody production (Cowan et al., 2020).
- Systemic Lupus Erythematosus: This systemic autoimmune disease is characterized by the immune system targeting its tissues. Disruptions in the BTB increase autoantigen presentation, contributing to disease progression (Boehm & Swann, 2013).

Infections

Viral and bacterial infections can affect the BTB. During infections, inflammatory cytokines compromise the structural integrity of the barrier and weaken immune tolerance mechanisms. For example, certain viral infections accelerate thymic involution, disrupting T-cell development (Petrie, 2003).

- Viral Infections: Pathogens such as HIV and hepatitis viruses cause structural changes in the thymic microenvironment, resulting in immunodeficiency and weakened responses to infections (Cowan et al., 2020).

- Bacterial Infections: Bacterial endotoxins induce inflammation in the BTB, increasing permeability. This disrupts the regulatory mechanisms of the immune system and contributes to chronic inflammation (Boehm & Swann, 2013).

Tumoral Diseases

The BTB undergoes significant structural and functional changes in thymic tumors. Thymomas, a type of thymic neoplasm, impair barrier function, leading to the loss of immune tolerance and an increase in autoimmune reactions (Cowan et al., 2020).

- Thymoma: This tumor, originating from thymic epithelial cells, causes structural disruptions in the BTB and weakens immune tolerance mechanisms. Myasthenia gravis is the most common autoimmune disease associated with thymoma (Boehm & Swann, 2013).
- Metastatic Cancers: Structural disruptions in the BTB facilitate the access of metastatic cancer cells to the thymic microenvironment, contributing to the transformation of the thymus into an immunosuppressive microenvironment (Cowan et al., 2020).

Experimental Models for Studying the Blood-Thymus Barrier

Disruptions in the BTB during pathological conditions have significant effects on immune system balance. These disruptions can trigger autoimmune diseases, weaken defenses against infections, and accelerate tumor progression. Research on the structural and functional integrity of BTB has contributed to the development of new therapeutic approaches for these pathologies. Thus, the structure and function of the BTB play a crucial role in understanding the fundamental mechanisms of the immune system. Animal models, in vitro systems, and advanced imaging techniques are commonly used to investigate the BTB.

Animal Models

Small mammals, such as mice and rats, are frequently used to study the BTB. These models are ideal for investigating thymic development, barrier permeability, and changes in the immune system.

- Genetically Modified Animals: Genetically modified mouse models are particularly useful for understanding the molecular components of the barrier. For example, mice lacking claudin-5 expression were used to study the effect of tight junctions on barrier permeability (Nagatake et al., 2021).
- Inflammatory and Autoimmune Models: Experimental autoimmune encephalomyelitis (EAE) and lupus mouse models were used to study the effects of inflammatory processes and autoimmune diseases on BTB (Boehm & Swann, 2013).

In Vitro Models

In vitro models have been used to understand the cellular and molecular functions of the BTB.

- Thymic Epithelial Cell Cultures: Culture systems derived from thymic epithelial cells are used to investigate cell-cell interactions, cytokine roles, and permeability mechanisms of the barrier (Milićević & Milićević, 2004).
- Organ-on-Chip Systems: Microfluidic chip technologies have recently been developed to model BTB. These systems enable real-time permeability analysis of the barrier (Foster et al., 2008).

Imaging Techniques

Advanced imaging techniques are used to understand the anatomical and functional features of the BTB.

- Confocal Microscopy: This technique is suitable for examining tight junctions and cellular components of the barrier at high resolution. It is particularly useful in combination with immunohistochemical methods to localize proteins such as claudin-5 and zonula occludens-1 (Nagatake et al., 2021).

- Electron Microscopy: Electron microscopy is ideal for ultrastructural analysis of the barrier, including tight junctions between endothelial cells and detailed structure of the basal membrane (Pearse, 2006).

Pharmacological Experiments

Pharmacological approaches have been used to investigate the effects of molecules and drugs that regulate the barrier permeability. For example, the effects of certain cytokine inhibitors and growth factors on the barrier have been tested in in vitro and in vivo models (Milićević & Milićević, 2004).

The experimental models used to study the BTB are critically important for understanding their structural and functional properties. Animal models, in vitro systems, and advanced imaging techniques are essential tools for elucidating how the barrier operates under both normal and pathological conditions.

Clinical Applications and Future Perspectives

Research on the structure and function of the BTB has provided significant insights into immune system function and has enabled the development of new approaches for clinical applications. Restoring or modifying the thymus and the BTB represents a promising area for the treatment of immunological diseases and the prevention of age-related immune dysfunction.

Thymus Transplantation and Regenerative Medicine

Thymus transplantation has been clinically applied, particularly in cases of immunodeficiency syndromes, such as DiGeorge syndrome. This approach restores immune function, allowing the development of adaptive immune responses. The functionality of the BTB is critical for maintaining the stability of the thymic microenvironment after transplantation (Boehm & Swann, 2013).

In regenerative medicine, efforts to produce thymic organoids in vitro for transplantation into patients are ongoing. These organoids offer a potential solution for reconstructing the BTB (Cowan et al., 2020).

Pharmacological Strategies Targeting the Blood-Thymus Barrier

Pharmacological agents are being developed to regulate the permeability of BTB and to optimize its function. Drugs targeting tight junction proteins may selectively increase or decrease the barrier's permeability.

- Cytokine Modulation: Anti-cytokine therapies used to suppress inflammatory processes may be effective in preserving the functionality of the barrier (Milićević & Milićević, 2004).
- Growth Factors: Molecules such as fibroblast growth factor (FGF) and vascular endothelial growth factor (VEGF) are potential therapeutic options for supporting thymic vascular structures (Petrie, 2003).

Managing Age-Related Thymic Involution

Age-related thymic involution weakens the immune system and increases susceptibility to infections. Structural changes in the BTB during this process also play a significant role. Pharmacological and genetic interventions aimed at preserving the structure and function of the barrier may be important in preventing age-related immunological impairments (Boehm & Swann, 2013).

Future Research Areas

In future studies on the BTB, the following topics are expected to gain prominence:

- Discovery of Molecular Mechanisms: Detailed examination of the molecular regulators of the BTB may enable the identification of new therapeutic targets (Nagatake et al., 2021).

- Organ-on-a-Chip Models: Organ-on-a-chip systems that model the BTB offer an innovative approach to understanding the dynamic processes of the barrier. These technologies can be used in both fundamental research and drug development (Foster et al., 2008).
- Enhancement of Immune Tolerance: Modifying the BTB could establish a new paradigm for the prevention or treatment of autoimmune diseases (Klein & Petrozziello, 2024).

Conclusion

Clinical applications and research on the BTB present promising opportunities for the regulation of the immune system and the treatment of diseases. Thymus transplantation, pharmacological strategies, and regenerative medicine approaches are among the current and future therapeutic methods that target the functionality of this barrier. A better understanding of the fundamental mechanisms of BTB could open new pathways for managing immunological diseases and supporting healthy aging.

References

Anderson, G., Jenkinson, E. J., & Moore, N. C. (2002). Thymic epithelial cells provide unique signals for positive selection of CD4+CD8+ thymocytes in FTOC. *Journal of Immunology.*

Anderson, G., Jenkinson, W. E., & Moore, N. C. (2002). Positive and negative selection in the thymus. *Nature Reviews Immunology.*

Bódi, I., H-Minkó, K., Prodán, Z., Nagy, N., & Oláh, I. (2019). A thymus szerkezete a huszonegyedik század elején [Structure of the thymus at the beginning of the 21st century]. *Orvosi Hetilap, 160*(5), 163–171. https://doi.org/10.1556/650.2019.31224.

Bruss, D. M., & Ely, S. (2019). Anatomy, head and neck, blood-thymus barrier. *StatPearls.*

Bubanovic, I. V. (2003). Failure of blood-thymus barrier as a mechanism of tumor and trophoblast escape. *Medical Hypotheses, 60*(3), 315–320. https://doi org/10.1016/s0306-9877(02)00450-4.

Gartner, L. P., & Hiatt, J. L. (2013). *Color textbook of histology* (4th ed.). Elsevier.

Junqueira, L. C., & Carneiro, J. (2018). *Basic histology: Text & atlas* (15th ed.). McGraw Hill Education.

Keilholz, W. U., Weber, G., & Schuetz, G. (2010). Barrier mechanisms in the thymus and implications for immune tolerance. *Trends in Immunology.*

Kierszenbaum, A. L., & Tres, L. L. (2020). *Histology and cell biology: An introduction to pathology* (5th ed.). Elsevier.

Kyewski, B., & Klein, L. (2006). A central role for central tolerance. *Annual Review of Immunology.*

Miller, J. F. A. P. (2020). The function of the thymus and its impact on modern medicine. *Science, 369*(6503), eaba2429. https://doi.org/10.1126/science.aba2429.

Moore, K. L., Persaud, T. V. N., & Torchia, M. G. (2020). *The developing human: Clinically oriented embryology* (11th ed.). Elsevier.

Murphy, K., & Weaver, C. (2016). *Janeway's immunobiology* (9th ed.). Garland Science.

Ribatti, D. (2015). The discovery of the blood–thymus barrier. *Immunology Letters, 168*, 325–328.

Ritter, M. A., & Boyd, R. L. (1993). Development in the thymus: it takes two to tango. *Immunology Today.*

Ross, M. H., & Pawlina, W. (2020). *Histology: A text and atlas with correlated cell and molecular biology* (8th ed.). Wolters Kluwer Health/Lippincott Williams & Wilkins.

Sadler, T. W. (2018). *Langman's medical embryology* (14th ed.). Wolters Kluwer.

Starr, T. K., Jameson, S. C., & Hogquist, K. A. (2003). Positive and negative selection of T cells. *Annual Review of Immunology.*

Wekerle, H. (2005). Immune protection by the blood–brain and the blood–thymus barriers. *Nature Reviews Immunology.*

Zikherman, J., Parameswaran, R., & Weiss, A. (2012). Endogenous antigen tunes the responsiveness of naive B cells but not T cells. *Nature Immunology.*

Chapter 14

The Blood-Brain-Tumor Barrier

Begum Sahin*, MSc
Talat Yasin Acar, MSc
and Aysenur Kurt, BSc
Department of Histology and Embryology, The School of Medicine,
Istanbul Medipol University, Istanbul, Türkiye

Abstract

The Blood-Brain-Tumor Barrier (BBTB) is a modified version of the blood-brain barrier (BBB) that forms in the presence of brain tumors. This barrier plays a critical role in the progression and treatment of primary and metastatic brain tumors. While it supports tumor growth by supplying nutrients and enabling metastasis, it also impedes the delivery of therapeutic drugs. Tumors originating from organs like the lungs, breast, and kidneys alter the BBB, leading to the development of the BBTB, which exhibits structural differences like increased permeability and reduced functionality. These changes make drug delivery to brain tumors challenging, often requiring higher drug doses that result in toxicity with limited treatment effectiveness. The BBTB is structurally complex, involving various cellular components such as endothelial cells, astrocytes, and pericytes, which interact to either protect or promote tumor growth. Several methods, such as nanoparticles and focused ultrasound, are being explored to bypass the BBTB and enhance drug delivery. Diagnostic methods like MRI and PET imaging are useful in assessing BBTB disruption, but treatment remains complex due to the heterogeneous nature of this barrier.Efforts are ongoing to better understand the molecular and cellular mechanisms behind the formation

---

* Corresponding Author's Email: beggumsahin@gmail.com

In: A Histological Approach to Human Body Barriers
Editor: İlknur Keskin
ISBN: 979-8-89530-738-0

of the BBTB and develop more effective treatment strategies. These include chemical modifications to increase drug permeability and using innovative delivery methods to overcome the BBTB's resistance to chemotherapy.In conclusion, while the BBTB presents a significant challenge to cancer treatment, advancements in medical technology and understanding of the BBTB's structure offer potential solutions to improve drug delivery and patient outcomes.

Keywords: blood-tumor barrier, tumor, permability, drug resistant, blood barrier

Introduction

BBTB is a modified version of BBB, a semi-permeable membrane that maintains homeostasis in the brain (Upton, Ung et al. 2022). BBTB occurs due to differentiation of the BBB structure due to tumors occurring in the brain. Metastatic brain tumors predominantly originate from lung (~50%), breast (~15%), melanoma (~10%), and kidney cancers (~5%). Brain metastasis occurs when a primary systemic tumor (breast, melanoma, kidney) detaches from the tumor mass, lodges in the brain's microvascular capillary network, extravasates into the perivascular space, survives, proliferates, and forms a new lesion (Sprowls, Arsiwala et al. 2019).

The progression of primary or metastatic intracranial tumors within the BBB leads to tumor cell colonization (Steeg 2021). The tumor vasculature becomes increasingly heterogeneous, compromising the structural integrity of the BBB (Sarkaria, Hu et al. 2017, Arvanitis, Ferraro et al. 2020). This transformation results in the BBB evolving into the BBTB. The newly formed BBTB exhibits distinct characteristics in terms of pharmacokinetics and therapeutic efficacy compared to the BBB (Sprowls, Arsiwala et al. 2019).

The BBTB, which forms from the capillaries within brain tumors, exhibits uneven permeability and actively removes molecules, setting it apart from the BBB. The BBTB includes both existing and newly formed blood vessels that supply the tumor with nutrients and oxygen and help tumor cells spread to other parts of the brain. It tends to be more permeable than the BBB. The structural integrity of the BBB and BBTB can differ depending on the type of tumor and the nature of metastatic lesions, leading to varied permeability. This variability can cause water and metabolic waste to accumulate in the brain tissue, raising interstitial and intracranial pressure due to the leaky and partially functional vessels (Upton, Ung et al. 2022).

BBTB Structure

The BBB is composed of non-fenestrated endothelial cells in contact with pericytes and astrocytes. These cells are connected by adherens junctions, gap junctions, and tight junctions (e.g., occludin and claudin-5), which protect the brain from pathogens and toxins. Additionally, this barrier limits drug penetration to lipophilic, low molecular weight molecules (Narsinh, Perez et al. 2024).

The BBTB consists of three different microvascular populations: continuous capillaries, fenestrated capillaries, and sinusoids. The cellular and molecular characteristics of the BBTB are influenced by astrocytes, pericytes, and microglia. Astrocytes protect neuronal cells from damage by secreting various inflammatory cytokines like TNFα and IL-6. These cytokines promote tumor cell proliferation. Additionally, astrocytes secrete exosomes containing miRNA-19a, which induces PTEN loss and further promotes tumor cell growth in the brain. Microglia surrounding brain tumors are known to secrete growth factors and cytokines, and various metalloproteinases. These molecules promote tumor cell proliferation, invasion, and angiogenesis (Sprowls, Arsiwala et al. 2019).

The abnormal distribution of pericytes, loss of astrocytic end-feet, and neuronal connections are characteristic features of the BBTB (Figure 1). Tumor cells can displace astrocytic end-feet, compromising the integrity of the BBB. BBTB endothelial cells reduce junctional proteins (Upton, Ung et al. 2022). Compared to the BBB, the BBTB also contains pinocytic vesicles and large vacuoles (Rathi, Griffith et al. 2022). Studies have shown that zonula occludens-1 (ZO-1), occludin, and claudin-5 proteins increase BBTB permeability (Wang, Cai et al. 2016). TNF receptors 1 and 2 are present in the BBTB formed as a result of brain metastasis, regulating the expression of adherens junction proteins, while these receptors are absent in the BBB (Steeg 2021). In a glioma mouse model, tight junctions were disrupted, and the distance between the endothelial surface and astrocytic end-feet increased. Similarly, in human glioblastoma, the expression of claudin-1 and claudin-5 was reduced. These findings indicate that the BBB structure is compromised in tumors (Patel, Yang et al. 2020). Inconsistencies in the expression of junctional proteins can allow passive permeability of cytotoxic therapies into tumor tissue. The major facilitator superfamily domain 2a (Mfsd2a), which plays a role in the growth of mammalian tissues and organs and lipid metabolism, has been shown to downregulate the BBTB and promote metastatic brain growth due to the lack of astrocytes, thus contributing to BBB leakage in brain tumors (Sprowls, Arsiwala et al. 2019). Astrocytic end-feet surround the growing lesion, triggering a neuroinflammatory response, and play a role in brain metastasis. An in vitro model study showed that astrocytes reduce the expression of sphingosine-1-phosphate receptor 3 (S1P3), decreasing the permeability of both the BBB and BBTB. Additionally, reductions in the levels of secreted chemokines, growth factors, and interleukins were observed (Allen and Limoli 2022).

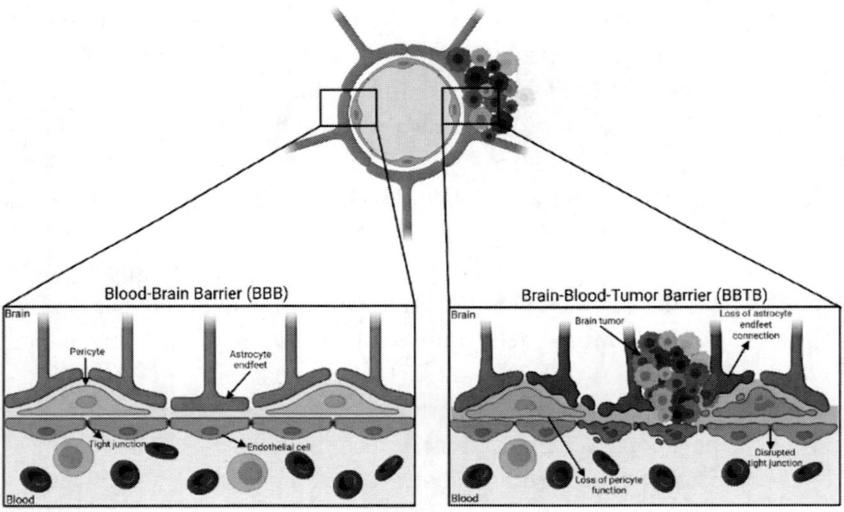

Figure 1. BBB and BBTB structure (Created with Biorender.com).

Several hypotheses have been evaluated to clarify the mechanisms leading to the formation of the BBTB. One hypothesis suggests that structural disruptions occur due to the loss of the tight junction protein claudin-3, increasing intercellular and perivascular spaces. Another hypothesis links the formation of the BBTB with an increase in desmin+ pericyte populations and a decrease in the astrocytic basal membrane component laminin α2, observed in breast cancer brain metastasis models with increased BBTB permeability (Rathi, Griffith et al. 2022).

The BBTB supports tumor growth by serving as a niche for cancer cell migration, proliferation, and invasion (Steeg 2021). The progression of glioblastoma leads to increased vascularization, affecting BBB permeability. Newly formed vessels exhibit abnormal morphology and function, with varying diameters and permeability, and irregular basal lamina in histological samples. A major factor contributing to this is the high levels of vascular endothelial growth factor (VEGF) in the tumor mass. VEGF mediates communication between tumor cells and endothelial cells. Similar to VEGF's effects on the BBB, aquaporins also play a role in tumor progression. Aquaporins are channel proteins from the integral membrane transport protein family involved in water transport between cells. AQP1, AQP8, and AQP9 within this family are associated with tumor development. Aquaporins also have regulatory effects on the structural integrity of the BBB. Increased expression of AQP4 is thought to act as a protective mechanism in gliomas by reversing the loss of astrocytic end-feet in the BBB and increasing perivascular space. As tumor formation progresses, significant disruptions in the BBB structure begin. The vascular structure deteriorates, endothelial cells detach from the vessel structure, and new angiogenic regions associated with the developing tumor form. These morphological changes and formations in blood vessels lead to the disruption of tight junctions and the formation of fenestrations. Consequently, the thickness of the basal lamina changes, and the number of pericytes associated with vessels and the perivascular space increases (Dubois, Campanati et al. 2014). Additionally, invasive tumor cells settle in the perivascular space, while glioma stem-like cells or pericytes differentiating into endothelial cells support the BBTB to contribute to tumor growth.

The development of the BBTB through the differentiation of tumor cells into endothelial cells increases resistance to chemotherapy. Increasing the dose of chemotherapy drugs causes toxicity, but the dose increase provides limited benefit (Chen, Momin et al. 2023). Due to its impact on drug passage and therapeutic efficacy, medulloblastoma shows heterogeneity in its four histological/molecular subtypes (Mo, Pellerino et al. 2021). Medulloblastoma is among childhood brain tumors. A treatable subtype, wingless (WNT)-medulloblastoma, exhibits paracrine signals mediated by β-catenin, allowing the intracellular accumulation of chemotherapeutics in fenestrated endothelial cells (Patel, Yang et al. 2020). Additionally, by downregulating the Notch3 pathway, it affects the development of the CNS vascular structure through the WNT pathway, leading to vascular branching. Sonic hedgehog (SHH) activation likely plays a role in maintaining the development and integrity of the CNS vascular structure (Mo, Pellerino et al. 2021). Therefore, another resistant subtype, SHH-medulloblastoma, has a BBTB that is less permeable compared to other types. This results in resistance to chemotherapy and reduced treatment efficacy due to limited drug delivery to the target tissue (Patel, Yang et al. 2020). The decreased permeability of the BBB observed in SHH-medulloblastoma, compared to the WNT subtype, shows lower sensitivity and response to chemotherapy with vincristine. In cases of brain metastasis originating from breast cancer, the BBB is often disrupted in triple-negative or basal-like subtypes, while it remains intact in HER2-positive breast cancer. Additionally, the expression of ATP-binding cassette (ABC) proteins on the surface of cells varies across different histological subtypes of brain metastases. Specifically, HER2-positive breast cancer generally exhibits higher levels of GLUT1 and breast cancer resistance protein (BCRP) compared to other subtypes (Mo, Pellerino et al. 2021).

BBTB Diagnosis Method

The failure of drugs to distribute into brain tumor tissues has caused advancements in techniques aimed at disrupting the BBB (Sprowls, Arsiwala et al. 2019). Deterioration of the BBB is indicated by higher drug accumulation and the detection of circulating brain tumor markers compared to unaffected brain tissue. Imaging techniques like magnetic resonance imaging (MRI) and positron emission tomography (Chen, Momin et al.) are used to confirm BBTB disruption (Arvanitis, Ferraro et al. 2020). However, correlating diagnostic imaging with drug distribution and treatment efficacy is not straightforward. Contrast-enhanced MRI is commonly used in the diagnosis of brain tumors. The BBTB may be permeable to contrast agents, resulting in high-intensity regions on T1-weighted MRI in certain brain areas, aiding in identification. However, due to the heterogeneous nature of the BBTB, accumulation in brain tumors is not uniform (Rathi, Griffith et al. 2022). PET is another method used to identify brain tumors and assess BBB disruption. The most used PET tracers that can penetrate the BBB are 18F-fluorodeoxyglucose (FDG), 18F-3’-deoxy-3’-fluorothymidine (18F-FLT) (Patel, Yang et al. 2020).

BBB/BBTB Treatment Methods

In recent years, numerous studies have been conducted to enhance drug delivery to brain tumors (van Tellingen, Yetkin-Arik et al. 2015). The BBB poses a barrier to drug transport and targeting. While the BBB protects the brain from various harmful substances, it also restricts the transport and targeting of therapeutic agents, complicating the treatment of brain tumors (Yang, Barth et al. 2000). In brain tumors, the BBB structure can be disrupted, resulting in the formation of the BBTB, which is more permeable than the BBB. However, due to its irregular permeability, it leads to non-uniform drug distribution within the tumor (Rathi, Griffith et al. 2022). Major treatment methods include intratumoral, intranasal, intrathecal, or intravenous drug administration, physical and osmotic disruption of the BBB, chemical modification of molecules, and targeting BBB transporters/receptors to enhance transcytosis (Haumann, Videira et al. 2020, Mo, Pellerino et al. 2021, Mitusova, Peltek et al. 2022). Researchers are developing new strategies to more effectively bypass the BBB and BBTB using nanoparticles and other drug delivery systems, aiming to deliver higher concentrations of therapeutics to the tumor region (Belykh, Shaffer et al. 2020). Additionally, focused ultrasound and convection-enhanced delivery techniques are being investigated to temporarily disrupt the BBB/BBTB structure, allowing more effective drug delivery to the tumor (Virtanen, Ortiz et al. 2024).

Intratumoral, Intranasal, Intrathecal, or Intravenous Drug Administration

Intratumoral Injection

This method involves the local implementation of drugs to increase drug concentration in the tumor region and reduce systemic toxicity. Polymer structures composed of liposomal DOX have been clinically approved for intracranial treatment of glioblastoma. Direct infusion of fluid into the tumor has been clinically investigated, demonstrating local drug effects and prolonged retention in the tumor region. However, the complex application procedure, risk of infection, local toxicity of drugs, and rapid clearance from brain parenchyma are disadvantages of this method (Mitusova, Peltek et al. 2022).

Intranasal Administration

This alternative method bypasses the BBB, allowing access to the brain parenchyma without interfering with the BBB. Drugs are delivered to the CNS through paracellular, transcellular, and neural transport pathways from the nasal cavity's neuroepithelium. However, this method is not suitable for all drugs due to specific physicochemical properties and formulations. Lipophilic drugs with low molecular weight show better bioavailability after nasal administration compared to charged hydrophilic drugs. While nasal drug administration offers the advantage of avoiding first-pass metabolism, the small volume that can be administered intranasally is a disadvantage (Haumann, Videira et al. 2020).

Intrathecal implementation involves the direct injection of therapeutic drugs into the cerebrospinal fluid (CSF) (Mo, Pellerino et al. 2021). Direct application of antineoplastic drugs into the CSF allows the drug to pass through the BBB's selective permeable filter, reducing the likelihood of systemic toxicity. Intrathecal drug delivery is performed via the lumbar thecal sac or through a subcutaneous reservoir and ventricular catheter known as the Ommaya reservoir, allowing intraventricular injection into the lateral ventricles. The Ommaya reservoir is a subcutaneous device that provides direct access to cerebrospinal fluid (CSF) via a catheter inserted into one of the brain's lateral ventricles. After cleansing the CSF with 2-4 ml of a 0.9% sodium chloride solution, medications are injected into the ventricular reservoir using a syringe. Ommaya reservoirs are advantageous because they allow for more uniform drug distribution and higher concentrations of medication in the subarachnoid space. However, their use can lead to catheter blockage, bleeding, and infections.

Intralumbar injection, another method for delivering drugs directly into the subarachnoid space, can also cause complications like post-puncture headaches, back pain, or bleeding. Additionally, there is a risk that the drug may inadvertently enter or leak into the subdural or epidural space (Triarico, Maurizi et al. 2019).

Intra-arterial drug delivery involves administering drugs directly into an artery near the tumor. After cannulating the target area, the drug is delivered into the blood vessel. In addition to chemotherapeutic drugs, hyperosmolar agents like mannitol can be used to locally open the BBB. However, toxicity and low drug efficacy are disadvantages of intra-arterial drug applications in primary brain tumors (Haumann, Videira et al. 2020).

Intravenous administration offers the advantage of simply injecting the required dose of therapeutic drug into the bloodstream and adjusting the dosage. The application can be stopped if unwanted side effects occur. However, it can lead to non-specific accumulation of drugs in the liver, kidneys, and spleen, and cause complications like aphasia, hemiparesis, or intracranial herniation (Mitusova, Peltek et al. 2022).

Physical and Osmotic Disruption of the BBB

Hyperosmotic agents and focused ultrasound (FUS) are physical methods that increase permeability by applying pressure on endothelial cells and tight junction proteins (Allen and Limoli 2022). MRI-guided focused ultrasound is a new technique for disrupting the BBB/BBTB structure. At higher energies, focused ultrasound (high-intensity focused ultrasound, HIFU) can destroy the tumor mass in the brain. In contrast, at lower energies (low-intensity focused ultrasound, LIFU) in the presence of microbubbles (MB), focused ultrasound can open the BBB (Blethen, Arsiwala et al. 2021).

The osmotic disruption method involves temporarily disrupting the BBTB by injecting a hyperosmotic solution (a concentrated mannitol solution) into the carotid or vertebral artery immediately before drug administration. This application causes the connections between endothelial cells to open by drawing water from the endothelial cells that form the BBTB structure, allowing more drugs to be transported across the BBTB. Osmotic disruption is temporary and reversible. A local regional application protocol is needed to avoid systemic effects. However, due to the invasive nature of the procedure, it has disadvantages like neurological deficits, strokes, seizures, and new tumor formation, often due to temporary edema caused by increased bulk fluid flow (Allen and Limoli 2022).

One of the most promising and less invasive methods for mechanical BBB disruption involves the combined use of circulating MB and FUS (Allen and Limoli 2022). Without the use of MBs, structural disruption of the BBB/BBTB does not occur (Mungur, Zheng et al. 2022). MBs consist of a core and shell, each with different physicochemical properties (Kim, Lee et al. 2023). MBs are used as contrast agents in ultrasound to evaluate blood flow for diagnostic and therapeutic purposes. The concentration of MBs used increases the rate of BBB/BBTB disruption (Mungur, Zheng et al. 2022). To enhance the stability and efficiency of MBs, the structural components of the core and shell are made from various materials. In brain cancer treatment, the MB core uses components with higher molecular weight and lower blood solubility than atmospheric air, such as sulfur hexafluoride (SF6) or perfluorocarbons. Commercially, SonoVue® (SF6), Definity® (perfluoropropane [C3F8]), and Optison® (C3F8) are used. Additionally, various studies use perfluorochemicals like perfluorobutane (C4F10) and perfluoropentane (C5F12) as core components. C5F12 is in liquid form during production and transitions to gas at body temperature after injection, forming MBs. The shell structure, made of proteins, surfactants, polymers, or phospholipids, prevents gas leakage, MB fragmentation, and coalescence. The shell structure affects MB stability by reducing surface tension. MBs create hydrogen bonds between water and gas molecules at the gas-water interface, resulting in a contraction force on the MB surface. This creates inward surface tension, increasing pressure. High pressure increases gas dissolution rates, reducing MB stability, while the shell structure covering the core surface prevents hydrogen bond formation, reducing internal pressure and increasing MB stability. In brain cancer treatment, phospholipids and phospholipid-derived materials are used as shell components. The hydrophobicity of phospholipids increases the drug-loading capacity and stability of MBs. Recent studies have enabled the innovative design of MBs to be encapsulated or conjugated with drugs, improving circulation times and targeting specific ligands more effectively. In addition to traditional small MBs, studies with smaller nanoscale bubbles (nanobubbles, nanodroplets, and nanocomposites) are also being conducted. These nanoscale bubbles have stronger penetration power and enhanced permeability and retention effects.

Microbubble-assisted FUS is one of the most invasive methods targeting small brain structures with low toxicity to surrounding normal brain cells. Numerous studies have shown that FUS can open the BBB. However, this method varies depending on various parameters, including dose, duration, timing, and cycles.

High-Intensity Focused Ultrasound (HIFU) is a method used to deliver high-intensity energy (100-10,000 W/cm^2) through the skull. This method raises the temperature to approximately 500°C, providing ablation in the target tumor area. Cell death is induced by accumulated thermal energy, frictional vibration between cells, or non-thermal changes in peak rarefaction pressure amplitude. HIFU has been approved by the FDA for creating thalamic ablation to regulate tremors in essential tremor and dominant tremor Parkinson's disease. The currently used HIFU system is limited in terms of brain tissue volume for tumor ablation. Interstitial HIFU can be used as an alternative with cooling elements and single or multi-element catheters generating high acoustic energy (Arsiwala, Sprowls et al. 2021).

Low-Intensity Focused Ultrasound (LIFU) can be directed to different regions of the brain in various ways, hence referred to as FUS. FUS allows the destruction of targeted cell clusters through thermocoagulation while preserving surrounding cells and tissues (Allen and Limoli 2022). The LIFU technique involves the intravenous injection of MBs (1-10 μm in diameter) (Marcucci, Corti et al. 2021). Under FUS exposure, MBs oscillate within the vascular system, affecting the endothelial cell membrane. The pressure applied by MBs in the gaps between endothelial cells temporarily increases the aqueous diffusion of drugs into the brain (Blethen, Arsiwala et al. 2021). In the selected brain region, MBs oscillate in response to FUS waves, temporarily (4-6 hours) disrupting the barrier and increasing permeability (Marcucci, Corti et al. 2021). Following LIFU application, there is an increase in the release of heat shock protein 70 (Hsp70), IL-8, TNF-α, and damage-associated molecules in the parenchyma (Blethen, Arsiwala et al. 2021).

Although treatment with FUS in targeted regions has been observed to cause ischemia or adverse behavioral effects, it is defined as an excessive immune response and brain hemorrhage caused by the mechanical shear force generated by MBs. Therefore, FUS parameters must be appropriately controlled to prevent significant erythrocyte extravasation (Mo, Pellerino et al. 2021).

Laser-Induced Thermal Therapy (LITT) is a technique used to selectively and locally open BBB (Mo et al., 2021). When lasers are applied to the skull, the energy from the photons can have various effects depending on how the laser is used. LITT is particularly valued in neuro-oncology for its ability to effectively destroy tumor cells. The photons from the laser are absorbed by chromophores in the tumor cells, which generating thermal energy and heating the surrounding tissue. For tumor cells to die, the temperature must be maintained at a certain level for a specific period. While the exact heat requirements can vary based on cell type and target organ, a specific thermal dose can induce cellular necrosis and tissue coagulation. Research using a mouse model found that laser ablation temporarily increased the permeability of the BBB and BBTB, with the greatest permeability observed one week after treatment and lasting up to 30 days. This increased permeability is likely due to heightened transcytosis or the disruption of tight junctions (Patel, Yang et al. 2020).

Small Molecules

In the treatment of both primary and metastatic brain tumors in peripheral tumors, drug selection is generally based on the tissue from which the cancer originates. Temozolomide (TMZ), an orally administered alkylating agent, is the most commonly used chemotherapeutic in the treatment of glioblastoma multiforme (GBM). Nitro-urea compounds; lomustine (CCNU) are used alone or in combination with drugs like procarbazine and vincristine, carmustine (BCNU), and fotemustine as a treatment method for high-grade gliomas.

Chemotherapy options are limited for secondary brain tumors and are preferred as salvage therapy in patients who do not respond to surgery or radiotherapy (Rathi, Griffith et al. 2022).

Epidermal growth factor receptor (EGFR) inhibitors (gefitinib, erlotinib, and lapatinib) are therapeutic drugs showing promising results, but these results have not been clinically replicated. Secondary and tertiary generation inhibitors (afatinib, dacomitinib, and osimertinib) have been developed. Afatinib and osimertinib have shown survival benefits in mutant EGFR-positive tumors, while dacomitinib has shown limited activity in preclinical mouse models of GBM tumors. Other multikinase inhibitors like imatinib, dasatinib, sunitinib, tandutinib, and regorafenib have not shown significant clinical benefits in clinical trials (Rathi, Griffith et al. 2022).

Lapatinib and neratinib, inhibitors of human epidermal growth factor receptor 2 (HER2), show limited activity alone but demonstrate improved response when used in combination with capecitabine. Mitogen-activated protein/extracellular signal-regulated kinase (MEK) has been identified as a target in melanoma. The MEK inhibitor E6201 is used as a potential inhibitory drug in MEK-induced brain metastasis (Rathi, Griffith et al. 2022).

Chemical Modification

Various methods have been developed for the biochemical modulation of the BBB. Studies have shown that minoxidil sulfate, a selective activator of ATP-sensitive potassium channels (KATP), increases BBB permeability in glioma via the transcellular route (Mo, Pellerino et al. 2021). While KATP channels are lowly expressed in normal brain endothelial cells, they are overexpressed in vascular endothelial cells in brain tumors. This leads to increased selective permeability in the brain tumor area. The mechanism of increased tumor BBB permeability may involve pinocytosis, as pinocytic vesicles have been confirmed in vivo in brain tumor endothelium and brain tumors (Luo and Shusta 2020). Additionally, both in vivo and in vitro studies have shown decreased expression of caveolin-1 and tight junction proteins occludin and claudin-5 (Mo, Pellerino et al. 2021).

Similarly, it has been shown that NS1619, an antagonist of calcium-activated potassium channels (KCa), increases BBB permeability by regulating endocytic and transcellular pathways when injected intravenously (Mo, Pellerino et al. 2021). Researchers have demonstrated that KCa channels are expressed at lower levels, or almost not at all in some tissues, in the BBTB tumor and tumor vasculature area compared to normal brain tissue. When examining mRNA levels and protein analyses, it has been shown that the KCa channel subunit alpha-1 (KCNMA1) is more highly expressed in advanced glioma tissues and the glioma cell line U-87 compared to normal brain tissues. In this case, KCa channels become an effective target for BBTB permeability and can enhance the delivery of chemotherapeutics to the tumor region (Luo and Shusta 2020).

It has been shown that the phosphodiesterase 5 inhibitor (PDE5) increases the permeability of brain capillaries by inhibiting degradation and leading to the accumulation of cyclic guanosine monophosphate (cGMP) within the cell (Mo, Pellerino et al. 2021). PDE5 is known to be highly expressed in glioblastoma cells. It has been demonstrated that the use of PDE5 inhibitors in patients can modulate the BBTB. The uptake of the chemotherapeutic drug adriamycin by the tumor was significantly increased compared to normal brain tissue after the administration of the PDE5 inhibitor vardenafil (Levitra) in rats bearing 9L gliosarcoma tumors. The inhibitor has been shown to increase the survival rate in rats compared to the control. The increased vesicular transport in blood vessels surrounding the tumor, which causes an increase in BBTB permeability compared to the BBB, can be attenuated by iberiotoxin, a selective inhibitor of KCa channels that is also effective in cGMP signaling (Luo and Shusta 2020).

In rats with RG2 gliomas, administering low doses of bradykinin (BK) at 10 micrograms/kg/min, which activates bradykinin type 2 (B2) receptors, significantly enhanced permeability in tumor capillaries for six different tracers with varying molecular weights. This resulted in a notable increase in the BBTB permeability. Specifically, the permeability of RG2 gliomas to high molecular weight dextran (70,000) surged 12-fold following bradykinin treatment. However, bradykinin administration did not affect the vascularity or permeability of normal brain tissue (Inamura and Black 1994). The B2 receptor peptide agonist RMP-7, used in clinical trials, can selectively increase BBTB permeability, enhancing the delivery of administered drugs to tumor tissue. To overcome the limitations of bradykinin degradation in clinical applications, an analog called retro-inverso bradykinin (RI-BK), which is more resistant to proteolysis and has 40 times higher binding affinity to the B2 receptor, has been developed. In a study conducted in mice, RI-BK showed an anti-glioma effect by increasing coumarin-6 levels in glioma compared to normal brain tissue. The BBTB permeability induced by bradykinin and RI-BK is temporary and lasts approximately 20 minutes (Luo and Shusta 2020).

Caveolae-1 and caveolae-2-mediated transcellular pathways are effective in increasing BBTB permeability induced by bradykinin. After the induction of BBTB with bradykinin, the expression of ZO-1, claudin-5, and occludin decreases, and the cytoskeleton is reorganized. Additionally, the increase in BBTB permeability is associated with the depolymerization of F-actin. Bradykinin leads to an increase in intracellular Ca2+ levels by facilitating the release of Ca2+ within the cell or increasing Ca2+ entry. The increase in intracellular Ca2+ activates nitric oxide synthase (NOS), thereby increasing NO production (Luo and Shusta 2020).

Adenosine is an endogenous ligand for the A2A receptor (A2AR), which belongs to the G protein-coupled receptor family. The expression level of A2AR in human glioma tissue is higher compared to normal brain areas. Activation of A2AR increases BBTB permeability by reducing the expression of VE-cadherin and claudin-5 junction proteins and reorganizing cytoskeletal actin associated with cAMP/RhoA. Although Lexiscan, an FDA-approved A2AR agonist, increases BBTB permeability in mice, its clinical success is limited. Studies have shown that Lexiscan (0.4 mg/kg) does not have a significant effect in humans (Luo and Shusta 2020).

Another molecule effective on BBTB permeability is papaverine, a natural opioid. In the C6 glioma rat model, it has been shown that papaverine can temporarily increase BBTB permeability through the modulation of protein kinase A (PKA) and heat shock protein 70 (HSP70). The combination of papaverine with the chemotherapeutic bis-chloronitrosourea enhances its effect on patients with malignant glioma. Additionally, it has been shown that papaverine can reduce the expression of claudin-5, occludin, and F-actin in tumor tissue compared to normal brain tissue, thereby suggesting that BBTB permeability may result from TJ dysfunction (Luo and Shusta 2020).

MicroRNAs (miRNAs) are a new class of non-coding RNAs and are important regulators of cellular processes (Bartel 2004). Recently, miRNAs have also been shown to have regulatory effects on vascular permeability. It has been found that the expression levels of miR-132-3p in glioma endothelial cells are higher compared to normal brain tissue and that it increases BBTB permeability, thus suggesting that miRNAs could be a new target for BBTB modulation in brain tumors (Bartel 2004, Luo and Shusta 2020).

Nanoparticles in BBB/BBTB

Nanoparticles are classified as liposomes, polymersomes, dendrimers, carbon nanotubes, solid lipid nanoparticles, quantum dots, gold nanoparticles, and magnetic nanoparticles. Using these methods, small molecule drugs such as siRNA, DOX, and TMZ, as well as products like iron oxide, antibodies, antibody-drug conjugates, and plasmids, can be delivered to the brain via oral, ocular, intralymphatic, intrathecal, intracerebral, intraventricular, intranasal, and intravenous routes (Rathi, Griffith et al. 2022).

Even when the structure of the BBB/BBTB remains intact, there is often an overexpression of various receptors and transporters. These molecules play a crucial role in regulating the movement of specific ligands and substances across the barrier. Furthermore, the membrane of the BBB/BBTB is negatively charged, which increases its affinity for positively charged particles. This triggers cells to uptake these contents. Such ligands can regulate the penetration of nanoparticles into the BBB/BBTB (Table 1) (Gao 2016).

Table 1. Transporter types of the BBB (Gao 2016)

Receptor-Mediated Transport	Active Efflux-Mediated Transport	Transporter-Mediated Transport
Transferrin receptor	Adenosin triphospate-binding cassette (ABC) transporter, subfamily B, member 1 (P-glycoprotein)	Glucose transporter member 1
Insulin receptor	ABC transporter, subfamily C	Large neutral amino acid
Low-density lipoprotein receptor related protein	ABC transporter, subfamily G, member 2	Cationic amino acid transporter, member 1
Nicotinic acetylcholine receptor	Organic anion transporter	Monocarboxylic acid transporter, member 1
Insulin-like growth factor receptor	Organic anion-transporting polypeptide	Concentrative nucleoside transporter
Diphtheria toxin receptor	Glutamic acid, amino acid transporter	Concentrative nucleoside transporter
Scavenger receptor class B type	Taurine transporter	Nucleobase transporter
Leptin receptor		
Neonatal Fc receptor		

The transferrin (Tf) receptor, a transmembrane glycoprotein, is the most extensively studied protein in receptor-mediated transport and is overexpressed in brain endothelial cells. The specific protein of the receptor that regulates iron transport to the brain, Tf, can be functionalized onto various nanoparticles to enhance the brain delivery process (Qian, Li et al. 2002, Pang, Gao et al. 2011, Pang, Gao et al. 2011). tudies have shown that Tf-modified NPs exhibit better affinity for brain capillary endothelial cells and carry more cargo to the brain compared to unmodified NPs. For example, in a study conducted on rats, the group with doxorubicin-loaded Tf-NPs showed better anti-tumor effects and a 70% longer survival time compared to the doxorubicin-treated group (Kumar, Wu et al. 2007, Pang, Lu et al. 2008, Gao 2016). Although the use of endogenous ligands allows for enhanced brain targeting, endogenous ligands can bind to receptors, reducing the binding efficiency of ligand-modified NPs. To overcome this, antibodies have been designed for these receptors. By designing the binding regions of antibodies differently from ligands, ligand competition can be prevented. For example, in a study in which the OX26 antibody was conjugated onto NPs and NC1900 was administered intravenously to rats, the concentration in the brain tissue of the OX26-NPs group was found to be 2.62 times higher than that of the unmodified nanoparticle group 2 hours after injection (Pang, Lu et al. 2008, Gao 2016).

The glutathione transporter, one of the most studied proteins in transporter-mediated transport, is overexpressed in the BBB. Researchers have conjugated it onto liposomes to deliver various drugs to the brain (Gaillard, Visser et al. 2012). Using a fluorescent probe, it was observed that when glutathione-modified liposomes were administered intravenously, there was a fourfold increase in brain accumulation compared to unmodified liposomes (Rip, Chen et al. 2014).

Adsorptive-mediated brain targeting is based on the interaction of positively charged drug delivery systems with the negatively charged brain. Cationized bovine serum albumin (CBSA) can be used for adsorptive-mediated brain-targeted delivery (Gao 2016). When CBSA was transferred onto nanoparticles, the cellular uptake rate increased twofold compared to unmodified nanoparticle groups (Lu, Zhang et al. 2005). In studies using an in vitro BBB model, BBB permeability increased between 2.7 and 9.0 times when CBSA-NPs were used (Lu, Wan et al. 2007). In in vivo studies, brain accumulation increased 1.6 times compared to unmodified NPs when CBSA-NPs were used (Lu, Wan et al. 2007). In a study in which aclarubicin was encapsulated in CBSA-NPs, the concentration of aclarubicin in brain tumors was 2.6 times higher in the CBSA-NPs group compared to the unmodified group (Lu, Wan et al. 2007). Cationized immunoglobulins and cationized monoclonal antibodies and histones have brain-targeting properties through similar mechanisms. However, due to the negative charge of most biological membranes, they are rarely used in systemic applications (Guo, Ren et al. 2012).

Cell-penetrating peptides (CPPs) were discovered in 1988 and have been noted for their ability to facilitate cargo transport across cell membranes (Bechara and Sagan 2013). The negatively charged BBB membrane also shows affinity for CPPs. Various research groups have used CPPs for BBB penetration. A study demonstrated that conjugating liposomes with transactivating-transduction (TAT) (TAT-liposomes) resulted in 2.54 times greater brain accumulation compared to the unmodified liposome group (Qin, Chen et al. 2011). Another study showed that TAT-conjugated chitosan nanoparticles increased gene transfer to the brain (Malhotra, Tomaro-Duchesneau et al. 2013). Although it has been suggested that the passage of CPP molecules through the cell membrane may be mediated by fatty acids, this pathway does not provide cell selectivity for CPP molecules and carries the risk of accumulation in the liver and spleen. Therefore, CPP-modified nanoparticles are rarely used for brain targeting (Koren and Torchilin 2012, Malhotra, Tomaro-Duchesneau et al. 2013, Herce, Garcia et al. 2014). To overcome this, a bi-ligand method was developed. CPPs were conjugated with a specific targeting ligand, thereby gaining cell selectivity (Kibria, Hatakeyama et al. 2011). In one study, Tf poly-L-arginine conjugation was performed to obtain Tf-PR-liposomes. In vivo, Tf-PR-liposomes showed twice as much brain targeting compared to Tf-liposomes. As a result, gene-loaded Tf-PR-liposomes caused 1.66 times more gene expression in the brains of mice compared to gene-loaded Tf-liposomes (Sharma, Modgil et al. 2012, Sharma, Modgil et al. 2013).

Conclusion

BBTB constitutes a significant obstacle to cancer treatment. Although studies have provided enlightening information on the morphology, function and function of the BBTB structure, the structure has not yet been fully explained. Studies have shown that BBB permeability changes in primary or metastatic brain tumors, and the barrier structure and function are impaired. The molecular and cellular pathways by which this change occurs are still a matter of research. BBTB exhibits structural heterogeneity in different cancer subtypes. Therefore, revealing the molecular and cellular pathways of BBTB and knowing the characteristics that change specific to the cancer type are important for stopping tumor progression and treating the tumor (Arvanitis,

Ferraro et al. 2020). Considering the studies conducted in recent years, new treatment approaches continue to be developed for the possible effects of the changing permeability of BBTB on drug transport to the tumor site.

References

Allen, B. D., & Limoli, C. L. (2022). Breaking barriers: Neurodegenerative repercussions of radiotherapy-induced damage on the blood-brain and blood-tumor barrier. *Free Radical Biology and Medicine, 178*, 189–201. https://doi.org/10.1016/j.freeradbiomed.2021.12.028.

Arsiwala, T. A., Sprowls, S. A., Blethen, K. E., Adkins, C. E., Saralkar, P. A., Fladeland, R. A., Pentz, W., Gabriele, A., Kielkowski, B. N., Mehta, R. I., Wang, P., Carpenter, J. S., Ranjan, M., Najib, U., Rezai, A. R., & Lockman, P. R. (2021). Ultrasound-mediated disruption of the blood-tumor barrier for improved therapeutic delivery. *Neoplasia, 23*(7), 676–691. https://doi.org/10.1016/j.neo.2021.06.001.

Arvanitis, C. D., Ferraro, G. B., & Jain, R. K. (2020). The blood–brain barrier and blood–tumor barrier in brain tumors and metastases. *Nature Reviews Cancer, 20*(1), 26–41. https://doi.org/10.1038/s41568-019-0205-x.

Bartel, D. P. (2004). MicroRNAs: Genomics, biogenesis, mechanism, and function. *Cell, 116*(2), 281–297. https://doi.org/10.1016/S0092-8674(04)00045-5.

Bechara, C., & Sagan, S. (2013). Cell-penetrating peptides: 20 years later, where do we stand? *FEBS Letters, 587*(12), 1693–1702. https://doi.org/10.1016/j.febslet.2013.04.031.

Belykh, E., Shaffer, K. V., Lin, C., Byvaltsev, V. A., Preul, M. C., & Chen, L. (2020). Blood-brain barrier, blood-brain tumor barrier, and fluorescence-guided neurosurgical oncology: Delivering optical labels to brain tumors. *Frontiers in Oncology, 10*, 739. https://doi.org/10.3389/fonc.2020.00739.

Blethen, K. E., Arsiwala, T. A., Fladeland, R. A., Sprowls, S. A., Panchal, D. M., Adkins, C. E., Kielkowski, B. N., Earp, L. E., Glass, M. J., Pritt, T. A., Cabuyao, Y. M., Aulakh, S., & Lockman, P. R. (2021). Modulation of the blood-tumor barrier to enhance drug delivery and efficacy for brain metastases. *Neuro-Oncology Advances, 3*(Suppl 5), v133–v143. https://doi.org/10.1093/noajnl/vdab172.

Chen, X., Momin, A., Wanggou, S., Wang, X., Min, H. K., Dou, W., Gong, Z., Chan, J., Dong, W., Fan, J. J., Xiong, Y., Talipova, K., Zhao, H., Chen, Y. X., Veerasammy, K., Fekete, A., Kumar, S. A., Liu, H., Yang, Q., ... Huang, X. (2023). Mechanosensitive brain tumor cells construct blood-tumor barrier to mask chemosensitivity. *Neuron, 111*(1), 30–48.e14. https://doi.org/10.1016/j.neuron.2022.10.020.

Dubois, L. G., Campanati, L., Righy, C., D'Andrea-Meira, I., Spohr, T. C., Porto-Carreiro, I., Pereira, C. M., Balça-Silva, J., Kahn, S. A., Dos Santos, M. F., Oliveira, A., Ximenes-da-Silva, A., Lopes, M. C., Faveret, E., Gasparetto, E. L., & Moura-Neto, V. (2014). Gliomas and the vascular fragility of the blood-brain barrier. *Frontiers in Cellular Neuroscience, 8*, 418. https://doi.org/10.3389/fncel.2014.00418.

Gaillard, P. J., Visser, C. C., Appeldoorn, C. C. M., & Rip, J. (2012). Enhanced brain drug delivery: Safely crossing the blood–brain barrier. *Drug Discovery Today: Technologies, 9*(2), e155–e160. https://doi.org/10.1016/j.ddtec.2012.04.002.

Gao, H. (2016). Progress and perspectives on targeting nanoparticles for brain drug delivery. *Acta Pharmaceutica Sinica B, 6*(4), 268–286. https://doi.org/10.1016/j.apsb.2016.05.001.

Guo, L., Ren, J., & Jiang, X. (2012). Perspectives on brain-targeting drug delivery systems. *Current Pharmaceutical Biotechnology, 13*(12), 2310–2318. https://doi.org/10.2174/138920112803341885.

Haumann, R., Videira, J. C., Kaspers, G. J. L., van Vuurden, D. G., & Hulleman, E. (2020). Overview of current drug delivery methods across the blood–brain barrier for the treatment of primary brain tumors. *CNS Drugs, 34*(11), 1121–1131. https://doi.org/10.1007/s40263-020-00757-7.

Herce, H. D., Garcia, A. E., & Cardoso, M. C. (2014). Fundamental molecular mechanism for the cellular uptake of guanidinium-rich molecules. *Journal of the American Chemical Society, 136*(50), 17459–17467. https://doi.org/10.1021/ja507790z.

Inamura, T., & Black, K. L. (1994). Bradykinin selectively opens blood-tumor barrier in experimental brain tumors. *Journal of Cerebral Blood Flow & Metabolism, 14*(5), 862–870. https://doi.org/10.1038/jcbfm.1994.114.

Kibria, G., Hatakeyama, H., Ohga, N., Hida, K., & Harashima, H. (2011). Dual-ligand modification of PEGylated liposomes shows better cell selectivity and efficient gene delivery. *Journal of Controlled Release, 153*(2), 141–148. https://doi.org/10.1016/j.jconrel.2011.04.009.

Kim, K., Lee, J., & Park, M. H. (2023). Microbubble delivery platform for ultrasound-mediated therapy in brain cancers. *Pharmaceutics, 15*(2), 290. https://doi.org/10.3390/pharmaceutics15020290.

Koren, E., & Torchilin, V. P. (2012). Cell-penetrating peptides: Breaking through to the other side. *Trends in Molecular Medicine, 18*(7), 385–393. https://doi.org/10.1016/j.molmed.2012.04.012.

Kumar, P., Wu, H., McBride, J. L., Jung, K. E., Kim, M. H., Davidson, B. L., Lee, S. K., Shankar, P., & Manjunath, N. (2007). Transvascular delivery of small interfering RNA to the central nervous system. *Nature, 448*(7149), 39–43. https://doi.org/10.1038/nature05906.

Lu, W., Wan, J., She, Z., & Jiang, X. (2007). Brain delivery property and accelerated blood clearance of cationic albumin conjugated pegylated nanoparticle. *Journal of Controlled Release, 118*(1), 38–53. https://doi.org/10.1016/j.jconrel.2006.12.017.

Lu, W., Wan, J., Zhang, Q., She, Z., & Jiang, X. (2007). Aclarubicin-loaded cationic albumin-conjugated pegylated nanoparticle for glioma chemotherapy in rats. *International Journal of Cancer, 120*(2), 420–431. https://doi.org/10.1002/ijc.22297.

Lu, W., Zhang, Y., Tan, Y. Z., Hu, K. L., Jiang, X. G., & Fu, S. K. (2005). Cationic albumin-conjugated pegylated nanoparticles as novel drug carrier for brain delivery. *Journal of Controlled Release, 107*(3), 428–448. https://doi.org/10.1016/j.jconrel.2005.07.023.

Luo, H., & Shusta, E. V. (2020). Blood-brain barrier modulation to improve glioma drug delivery. *Pharmaceutics, 12*(11), 1085. https://doi.org/10.3390/pharmaceutics 12111085.

Malhotra, M., Tomaro-Duchesneau, C., & Prakash, S. (2013). Synthesis of TAT peptide-tagged PEGylated chitosan nanoparticles for siRNA delivery targeting neurodegenerative diseases. *Biomaterials, 34*(4), 1270–1280. https://doi.org/10.1016/ j.biomaterials.2012.10.074.

Marcucci, F., Corti, A., & Ferreri, A. J. M. (2021). Breaching the blood-brain tumor barrier for tumor therapy. *Cancers, 13*(10), 2391. https://doi.org/10.3390/cancers13102391.

Mitusova, K., Peltek, O. O., Karpov, T. E., Muslimov, A. R., Zyuzin, M. V., & Timin, A. S. (2022). Overcoming the blood–brain barrier for the therapy of malignant brain tumor: Current status and prospects of drug delivery approaches. *Journal of Nanobiotechnology, 20*(1), 412. https://doi.org/10.1186/s12951-022-01590-8.

Mo, F., Pellerino, A., Soffietti, R., & Rudà, R. (2021). Blood-brain barrier in brain tumors: Biology and clinical relevance. *International Journal of Molecular Sciences, 22*(23), 12654. https://doi.org/10.3390/ijms222312654.

Mungur, R., Zheng, J., Wang, B., Chen, X., Zhan, R., & Tong, Y. (2022). Low-intensity focused ultrasound technique in glioblastoma multiforme treatment. *Frontiers in Oncology, 12*, 903059. https://doi.org/10.3389/fonc.2022.903059.

Narsinh, K. H., Perez, E., Haddad, A. F., Young, J. S., Savastano, L., Villanueva-Meyer, J. E., Winkler, E., & de Groot, J. (2024). Strategies to improve drug delivery across the blood-brain barrier for glioblastoma. *Current Neurology and Neuroscience Reports, 24*(5), 123–139. https://doi.org/10.1007/s11910-024-01219-5.

Pang, Z., Gao, H., Yu, Y., Chen, J., Guo, L., Ren, J., Wen, Z., Su, J., & Jiang, X. (2011). Brain delivery and cellular internalization mechanisms for transferrin conjugated biodegradable polymersomes. *International Journal of Pharmaceutics, 415*(1–2), 284–292. https://doi.org/10.1016/j.ijpharm.2011.05.060.

Pang, Z., Gao, H., Yu, Y., Guo, L., Chen, J., Pan, S., Ren, J., Wen, Z., & Jiang, X. (2011). Enhanced intracellular delivery and chemotherapy for glioma rats by transferrin-conjugated biodegradable polymersomes loaded with doxorubicin. *Bioconjugate Chemistry, 22*(6), 1171–1180. https://doi.org/10.1021/bc2000564.

Pang, Z., Lu, W., Gao, H., Hu, K., Chen, J., Zhang, C., Gao, X., Jiang, X., & Zhu, C. (2008). Preparation and brain delivery property of biodegradable polymersomes conjugated with OX26. *Journal of Controlled Release, 128*(2), 120–127. https://doi.org/10.1016/j.jconrel.2008.02.008.

Patel, B., Yang, P. H., & Kim, A. H. (2020). The effect of thermal therapy on the blood-brain barrier and blood-tumor barrier. *International Journal of Hyperthermia, 37*(2), 35–43. https://doi.org/10.1080/02656736.2020.1733141.

Qian, Z. M., Li, H., Sun, H., & Ho, K. (2002). Targeted drug delivery via the transferrin receptor-mediated endocytosis pathway. *Pharmacological Reviews, 54*(4), 561–587. https://doi.org/10.1124/pr.54.4.561.

Qin, Y., Chen, H., Yuan, W., Kuai, R., Zhang, Q., Xie, F., Zhang, L., Zhang, Z., Liu, J., & He, Q. (2011). Liposome formulated with TAT-modified cholesterol for enhancing the brain delivery. *International Journal of Pharmaceutics, 419*(1–2), 85–95. https://doi.org/10.1016/j.ijpharm.2011.07.015.

Rathi, S., Griffith, J. I., Zhang, W., Zhang, W., Oh, J. H., Talele, S., Sarkaria, J. N., & Elmquist, W. F. (2022). The influence of the blood-brain barrier in the treatment of brain tumours. *Journal of Internal Medicine, 292*(1), 3–30. https://doi.org/10.1111/joim.13474.

Rip, J., Chen, L., Hartman, R., van den Heuvel, A., Reijerkerk, A., van Kregten, J., van der Boom, B., Appeldoorn, C., de Boer, M., Maussang, D., de Lange, E. C., & Gaillard, P. J. (2014). Glutathione PEGylated liposomes: Pharmacokinetics and delivery of cargo across the blood-brain barrier in rats. *Journal of Drug Targeting, 22*(5), 460–467. https://doi.org/10.3109/1061186X.2014.920897.

Sarkaria, J. N., Hu, L. S., Parney, I. F., Pafundi, D. H., Brinkmann, D. H., Laack, N. N., Giannini, C., Burns, T. C., Kizilbash, S. H., Laramy, J. K., Swanson, K. R., Kaufmann, T. J., Brown, P. D., Agar, N. Y. R., Galanis, E., Buckner, J. C., & Elmquist, W. F. (2017). Is the blood–brain barrier really disrupted in all glioblastomas? A critical assessment of existing clinical data. *Neuro-Oncology, 20*(2), 184–191. https://doi.org/10.1093/neuonc/nox175.

Sharma, G., Modgil, A., Layek, B., Arora, K., Sun, C., Law, B., & Singh, J. (2013). Cell penetrating peptide tethered bi-ligand liposomes for delivery to brain in vivo: Biodistribution and transfection. *Journal of Controlled Release, 167*(1), 1–10. https://doi.org/10.1016/j.jconrel.2013.02.001.

Sharma, G., Modgil, A., Sun, C., & Singh, J. (2012). Grafting of cell-penetrating peptide to receptor-targeted liposomes improves their transfection efficiency and transport across blood-brain barrier model. *Journal of Pharmaceutical Sciences, 101*(7), 2468–2478. https://doi.org/10.1002/jps.23126.

Sprowls, S. A., Arsiwala, T. A., Bumgarner, J. R., Shah, N., Lateef, S. S., Kielkowski, B. N., & Lockman, P. R. (2019). Improving CNS delivery to brain metastases by blood-tumor barrier disruption. *Trends in Cancer, 5*(8), 495–505. https://doi.org/10.1016/j.trecan.2019.06.005.

Steeg, P. S. (2021). The blood–tumour barrier in cancer biology and therapy. *Nature Reviews Clinical Oncology, 18*(11), 696–714. https://doi.org/10.1038/s41571-021-00551-9.

Triarico, S., Maurizi, P., Mastrangelo, S., Attinà, G., Capozza, M. A., & Ruggiero, A. (2019). Improving the brain delivery of chemotherapeutic drugs in childhood brain tumors. *Cancers, 11*(6), 824. https://doi.org/10.3390/cancers11060824.

Upton, D. H., Ung, C., George, S. M., Tsoli, M., Kavallaris, M., & Ziegler, D. S. (2022). Challenges and opportunities to penetrate the blood-brain barrier for brain cancer therapy. *Theranostics, 12*(10), 4734–4752. https://doi.org/10.7150/thno.73274.

van Tellingen, O., Yetkin-Arik, B., de Gooijer, M. C., Wesseling, P., Wurdinger, T., & de Vries, H. E. (2015). Overcoming the blood–brain tumor barrier for effective glioblastoma treatment. *Drug Resistance Updates, 19*, 1–12. https://doi.org/10.1016/j.drup.2015.02.002.

Virtanen, P. S., Ortiz, K. J., Patel, A., Blocher, W. A. III, & Richardson, A. M. (2024). Blood-brain barrier disruption for the treatment of primary brain tumors: Advances in the past half-decade. *Current Oncology Reports, 26*(3), 236–249. https://doi.org/10.1007/s11912-024-01391-1.

Wang, Z., Cai, X. J., Qin, J., Xie, F. J., Han, N., & Lu, H. Y. (2016). The role of histamine in opening blood-tumor barrier. *Oncotarget, 7*(21), 31299–31310. https://doi.org/10.18632/oncotarget.8816.

Yang, W., Barth, R. F., Rotaru, J. H., Boesel, C. P., Wilkie, D. A., Bresnahan, J. C., Hadjiconstantinou, M., Goettl, V. M., Joel, D. D., & Nawrocky, M. M. (2000). Boron neutron capture therapy of brain tumors: Functional and neuropathologic effects of blood-brain barrier disruption and intracarotid injection of sodium borocaptate and boronophenylalanine. *Journal of Neuro-Oncology, 48*(3), 179–190. https://doi.org/10.1023/A:1006485606895.

Index

A

B

N

O

P

R

S